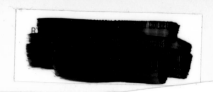

DATE DUE

A History of Nursing

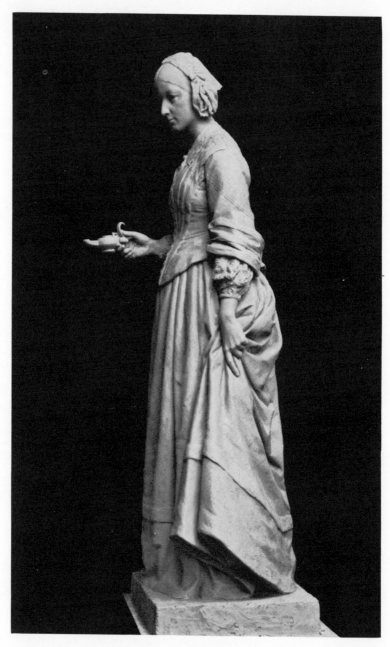

Florence Nightingale. From the Crimean Memorial that stands on the Thames embankment at Waterloo Place, London, England.

A History of Nursing

FROM ANCIENT TO MODERN TIMES

A WORLD VIEW (Fifth Edition)

19039

By Isabel M. Stewart

PROFESSOR EMERITUS, TEACHERS COLLEGE,
COLUMBIA UNIVERSITY

and Anne L. Austin

FORMERLY PROFESSOR OF NURSING,
WESTERN RESERVE UNIVERSITY

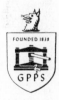

G. P. Putnam's Sons   New York

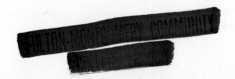

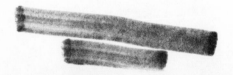

Dedication

THIS edition of *A History of Nursing* is dedicated to the memory of M. Adelaide Nutting and Lavinia L. Dock, to whom the whole nursing world is indebted for their pioneer explorations in nursing history and their scholarly four-volume *History of Nursing* published more than half a century ago. They also did much to stimulate the teaching and study of nursing history in both basic and advanced programs for nurses and sponsored the first textbook on this subject, which in this Fifth Edition still incorporates much of Miss Dock's original writing. As voluntary secretary for twenty years of the International Council of Nurses and in charge of the Foreign Department of the *American Journal of Nursing* from 1900 to 1923, she was one of the foremost leaders in the organization and growth of the ICN and in the worldwide spread of current information about nursing. Adelaide Nutting's influence as a distinguished educator, historian, writer, and international leader was also far reaching. Her philosophy is briefly expressed in this extract from a tribute to Florence Nightingale: "We who are nurses are inheritors of a great tradition. It is ours to guard, to strengthen, to enlarge where needed and to equip ourselves worthily for so doing."

Preface to First Edition

THIS little volume has been prepared especially for the use of student nurses. Most of the material has been condensed from the four volumes of the larger *History of Nursing,* and those who wish a more detailed and complete account of nursing history will find it necessary to refer constantly to this earlier and fuller edition. Certain of the more recent developments will, however, be found only in this volume.

It is generally believed that the best place in the nursing curriculum for the History of Nursing is in the early part of the first year, when the student is just beginning to form her conception of nursing and is being initiated into its practices. It is hoped that this story of her very ancient and honorable vocation will serve to fire her zeal and to strengthen her purpose and that the examples of many distinguished nursing leaders of the past will help her to understand and carry on the splendid traditions they have established.

It is suggested that the detailed study of the modern period and the discussion of modern professional problems might better be postponed till the final year of training, when the student will be able to appreciate more fully the issues involved and when she will be preparing more definitely for her professional responsibilities as a graduate nurse. The final chapter is intended to introduce the young nurse to some of the fundamental principles of nursing ethics and to show how these principles have grown up out of the history of nursing and are linked to it.

The references will suggest something of the rich body of historical material that is available for those who are interested in following up special topics or who wish to enjoy a rather fuller acquaintance with the characters and the incidents that are necessarily so briefly discussed in this short book. Although Miss Nutting's name does not appear on this volume, it was at her suggestion that the work was undertaken, and we are greatly indebted to her not only for helpful criticism but for her share in the original *History of Nursing* from which much of this has been drawn.

L. L. D.

I. M. S.

Preface to the Fifth Edition

IN planning the revision of *The Short History of Nursing,* we have considered a number of questions concerned with its original purpose as a text for student nurses and its close relationship to the parent four-volume *History of Nursing.* To these books has now been added the *History of Nursing Source Book,* all three issued by the same publisher and supplementing each other in several ways. A close relation, though belonging to another series,[1] is the *Education of Nurses—Historical Foundations and Modern Trends,* written primarily for nurses preparing as administrators and teachers in schools of nursing. There are now available many other publications deal-

---

[1] The Macmillan Nursing Education Monographs.

ing with nursing history, several of which focus on more recent developments in one particular country. A notable example is Mary M. Roberts' *American Nursing: History and Interpretation,* which covers the period 1900 to 1950 in the United States. Another widely used American text, *Professional Nursing—Trends, Responsibilities and Relationships,* by Eugenia K. Spalding, also contains extensive references to modern nursing, especially in the United States. These and similar publications fill a definite need, but we believe that there is still an important place in nursing school programs for the longer and broader view of nursing history herein presented.

Because of the critical situation in the world today, the growing emphasis on the international health movement, and the increasing demand for nurses who are qualified to participate in such programs, graduate nurses as well as students in basic courses are recognizing the need to broaden their views of nursing by study and travel far beyond their own national boundaries.

These and other considerations have led to the rather extensive changes in this edition which have been discussed with many colleagues in nursing and have been generally approved by them. One of these changes is the division of the book into two parts, the first giving a long view of nursing history from earliest times to the beginning of modern nursing, the second covering the period from 1860 to the present and tracing the spread of the new movement over large sections of the globe. Special attention is given to the countries that took an active part in developing nursing as a self-governing profession and in organizing nurses on a national and international basis. Included in this new plan are broad revisions of the early chapters and the complete rewriting of the remainder of the book, beginning with Chapter 7.

With reference to the use of this text in schools of nursing, it is suggested that Chapter 1 be placed early in the course, when students are being introduced to their new profession, and that the remainder of Part I be studied during the first year. Part II would fit best into the last-year program, when students are considering their opportunities and obligations as graduate nurses and the problems they are likely to meet. Though it is assumed that special attention will be given to the history of nursing in their own country, this takes on added significance when it is compared with the nursing systems and conditions in at least a few other countries. We believe also that all nurses today should have a world view of the nursing situation, including the general stage of nursing development in different countries and the more important national and international organizations and agencies that are playing a significant part in the spread of the modern nursing movement.

As to the teaching of nursing history, we have provided illustrations, maps, and charts which we hope will help to identify important events, leaders, and movements and to provide guideposts for students in their study of this subject. We believe it is unnecessary to require much memorization of dates and other purely factual material, also that if students can be encouraged to do a little searching for themselves, they are more likely to enjoy their study of the subject and to continue it long after their student days. Many have developed a life-long interest which has led them to make a valuable contribution to the search for important source materials and to the writing and teaching of nursing history.

The reading lists are intended as an aid to teachers and various groups of basic and graduate nurse students and other readers. Teachers are expected to guide the basic students in their choice of readings by using the selected bibliographies at the ends of the chapters. The assignments will, of course, depend upon time, interest, and the availability of materials. It is hoped that graduate nurses who need clues to further sources relating to special areas of nursing and those who are teachers of nursing history will find the additional suggestions given at the end of the text of value. General readers who wish to acquire further information about the evolution of the profession of nursing will also find helpful references in the bibliography. It is not expected that the members of any of the groups mentioned will read all the references given.

In conclusion we would like to acknowledge our debt to our own teachers and colleagues and to our students who have been an inspiration in this and other studies of nursing history. We are greatly indebted also to a large number of nurses from many lands who have helped with suggestions and criticisms and often with source materials. It would be quite impossible to mention all of their names, but the following list includes most of those who have read and criticized sections, supplied important information, charts, or similar material, and otherwise contributed substantially to the preparation of this volume: Grace Alt, Virginia Arnold, Olive Baggallay, Bettina Bennett, Elizabeth Brackett, Daisy Bridges, Ellen Broe, Gwen Buttery, Shulamith Cantor, G. B. Carter, Agnes Chagas, Mai Yu Chow, Lyle Creelman, Maja Foget, Hazel Goff, Celia Guzman, Yvonne Hentsch, Grace Seki Hora, Ruth Ingram, Ethel Johns, Mary Lambie, Elizabeth Lind, Margaret McElfactrick, R. Louise McManus, Athena Messalora, Mary Mills, Helen Mussallem, Killiki Pohjala, Grace Reid, Mary Roberts, Lucy Seymer, Gladys Sharpe, Venny Snellman, Eugenia Spalding, M. Elizabeth Tennant, Mildred Tuttle, Florence Udell, Louisa White and Asiye Yuccsan.

Librarians have been relied on for assistance at every turn and have willingly responded to the many general and specific demands made on them. The staffs of Butler and Teachers College Libraries of Columbia University and the New York Public Library have been most helpful, especially in the early stages of the work. In particular, we wish to express our great appreciation to Lois Miller, Librarian at the Sophia F. Palmer Library, for her generous response to our requests at every stage of this revision.

And, finally, our thanks are gladly given to Mr. Asa B. Elliott and Mr. Richard H. Miller of G. P. Putnam's Sons for their understanding, help, and patience in the preparation of this volume. This includes those who supplied the maps and the many secretaries who have helped in the preparation of the manuscript.

Isabel M. Stewart
Anne L. Austin

CONTENTS

Part I

Part II

DIAGRAMS, CHARTS
and ILLUSTRATIONS

Part I

As stated in the preface, the first part of this History of Nursing *is intended primarily for beginning students of nursing. Chapter 1 introduces them to the origin of nursing and to its history and in some measure to their new vocation. It discusses the meaning and nature of nursing, the roots from which it springs, and the cultural and other influences which have determined its rate of growth and its gradual evolution as a modern vocation or profession. The next chapters follow a chronological order, beginning with primitive man and noting the main stages through which nursing has passed, up to and including the launching of the Nightingale system in Great Britain and North America about a century ago. Each stage is seen in its historical and cultural setting. Since nursing has been influenced greatly by the Greek-Hebrew-Christian cultural stream, special attention is given to that part of the earlier history and to the humanitarian, scientific, and liberal movements of later centuries which had their origin in these ancient cultures. It is hoped that this discussion will throw some light not only on the profession of nursing as it now exists in the world (as presented in Part II) but on the various studies that are a part of its curriculum: the biological, physical, and social sciences as well as various courses dealing with the principles and practice of nursing, including its ethical ideals and standards.*

CHAPTER 1

Orientation to Nursing History

No occupation can be understood or intelligently followed if it is not, to some extent at least, illumined by the light of history. The origin of its various activities, the spirit that animated its founders, the long struggle to realize its ideals and potentialities—these vivify and ennoble the most prosaic labors and inspire workers with the consciousness of being part of a mighty drama to which the uninformed may be quite blind. Without such a view, students of nursing are not only deprived of a rich source of interest and inspiration but may be working partly in the dark, unable to understand many of the traditions or viewpoints they will find in this field of work or to appreciate fully the contributions made by their predecessors who laid the foundations on which they build.

Those who enter nursing today or who observe nurses in action in many modern countries will find an organized profession recognized and accepted by the public; a service that reaches out into hospitals, homes, industries, schools, and communities; a well-established system of education with a wide variety of programs for individuals in all stages and branches of

this work; state laws that regulate nursing preparation and
practice; organizations whose members reach into the hundreds
and thousands. Naturally one wonders how all this came into
being. From what sources did it spring? When did it begin? Who
built it up?

Analogies and speculations based on the study of newer vocations are likely to be misleading. Nursing, which has been called
the oldest of the arts and the youngest of the professions, has
gone through many stages and has been an integral part of many
different movements. Terms such as "nursing," "vocation," and
"profession," have also changed through the ages. Some of these
points are discussed and a few guide posts suggested in this introductory chapter.

ORIGIN, NATURE, AND ROOTS OF NURSING

The word "nursing," which is derived from the Latin *nutrio*
(to nourish), had its origin in the mother-care of helpless infants.
Gradually it came to be used also for the care of sick, injured, or
infirm persons of all ages. "Nurture," which stems from the same
root, has been associated more closely with education, especially
the rearing, training, and general upbringing of the young.
This accounts for the two kinds of helpers who appeared quite
early in some households—child-nurses and sick-nurses. Sick-
nurses became more closely associated with the healing arts and
child-nurses with the teaching and training of children. Often,
the two functions were combined.

The words "health" and "healing" come from an old Anglo-
Saxon word meaning hale or whole—sound in body, mind, and
spirit. Healers who helped to restore health originally included
priests as well as those who used physical remedies for the care of
"dis-eased," injured, or mentally disturbed individuals. Nurses
also applied remedies of various kinds but were somewhat restricted after the early medicine men appeared and began to
organize their healing cults. There was always a demand, however, for the nurse who kept watch at the bedside, provided food
and other physical requirements, gave comfort and support,

and otherwise helped to sustain the strength and courage of their patients and to minister to their needs.

As to the roots of the nursing impulse and their relative strength in different individuals, it was long believed that women, because of their maternal functions, were "born nurses." This is now questioned by social scientists, who hold that the nursing impulse has two roots. The first is found in such conditions as the helplessness of infancy and old age, the threat to human life from disease and injury, and the depletion of group strength by wars, epidemics, and other calamities. The other root is the natural tendency of normal human beings of both sexes to respond to such needs. Because of their role in the family, women had more experience in such activities, but many men have shared in nursing services and in both sexes there are wide differences in native nursing aptitudes and abilities.

HOW THE CULTURE INFLUENCES NURSING

At all times and in all parts of the world nursing has been a part of an existing culture, has been shaped by it, and in turn has helped to develop it. The term "culture" is used here in the modern sense of the total man-made or social environment at any given time or place. For example, it includes not only language and literature, science and art, and tools and methods of work but such matters as marriage customs, child care, economic conditions, and the whole way of life. Since culture is the product of group life, it varies greatly in different racial and national groups and at different periods in history. Biologically, human beings are much the same wherever we find them and have probably been so for many thousands of years. The differences in their customs are the result of conditions in environment and upbringing—that is, of the culture into which they are born which forms the normal setting for their lives. Where life is cheap, where there is little or no regard for the individual, where fatalistic philosophies or superstitious taboos hold sway so that sickness is held inevitable or is intensely feared, the natural nursing impulses, found in all races, have much less outlet or encouragement than in cultures in which the dignity and welfare of the individual are held high and in which there is a strong tradition of mutual aid and of cooperative effort to assist the weak and helpless.

Although cultures differ greatly, all peoples have some tendencies based on common human needs for food, shelter, security, sociability, and the propagation and protection of offspring. These needs lead to some form of organized group life centered first in a common language and related through common ancestors. In the course of time such groups develop customs governing their ordinary relationships and activities. As these customs become regulated, they crystallize into institutions such as the family, the various occupational and social classes, and specialized political, economic, and religious systems. Groups also develop certain ideas, beliefs, and taboos which become standardized as folkways and govern the relations of young and old, men and women, rulers and ruled, and all the common aspects of group living.

Even in more highly developed and complex societies, some primitive institutions, beliefs, and, in a sense, taboos and folkways still dominate the culture. Modern civilizations, though more flexible than the ancient cultures, nevertheless stamp the human beings who live in them with their own imprint. Because civilized people today have developed educational and scientific methods for modifying their cultures and have multiplied their contacts with people of other cultures, changes are much more rapid than in older days. That changes are not always constructive and progressive we know from the serious tension, instability, and unrest of our own times.

HOW CULTURES ARE TRANSMITTED AND CHANGED

Cultural heritage passed from one generation to another by the training of the young in folkways—what we nowadays call education. Training was at first chiefly informal, acquired by living in the family and the tribe and absorbing their ways of thinking and behaving. Later it became more organized, and various institutions, particularly schools, were set up to promote such learning. Most of the older cultures like those of China and Egypt were relatively static over long periods of time and few changes took place in them. As peoples settled down, their institutions became more coordinated and therefore more rigid and difficult to alter. Then, too, human beings in general have tended to resist change and to believe that traditional ways are good and safe, whereas new and strange ways are bad and dangerous.

Nevertheless, many influences for change have been at work, especially where people of different cultures have come into direct contact in migration, war, trade, and intermarriage or have been indirectly affected by writings, pictures, and other modes of communication. Times of crisis which compel unprecedented action often lead to rapid changes as do marked variations in economic conditions, new inventions and discoveries, religious and social movements, and the like. In such periods there often arise creative and dynamic leaders who help to modify traditional modes of thinking and to assist other members of the group to adjust to new conditions and needs. The following chapters give many illustrations of such influences in the field of nursing.

EVOLUTION OF NURSING AS A VOCATION OR PROFESSION

Though nursing had its start as a branch of mother-craft and continued to be one of many domestic arts carried on by members of the household, it also emerged at a fairly early stage as a distinct occupation. The word "care," which is closely associated with nursing, carries with it a wide assortment of meanings, including concern, solicitude, and affection, as well as responsibility for observation, oversight, and ministration. Nurse care-takers soon acquired a number of specific duties to add to certain traditional attitudes, skills and bits of knowledge passed down from one generation to another.

The early stages of nursing and medicine are so closely interwoven that it is impossible to distinguish one from the other.

Historically, the mother-nurse must have come before the priest-magician or medicine man. The two types of service were probably united at first in the wise old crone who learned to gather and use the healing and nourishing roots, leaves, and grasses of the forest. As time went on two branches of the healing art appeared, represented by the medicine-giver and the care-taker. Their relationship was close but not always harmonious, as will be seen in later chapters.

The terms "vocation" and "profession" came into general use with the Christian era. The first meant, originally, a divine call or summons to some form of religious or charitable service. The second meant that the individual had openly professed faith in the new religion and as a rule had made a vow dedicating his or her life sometimes to meditation and study but more often to active works of charity. Gradually the meaning of both vocation and profession was broadened to include a wide variety of secular occupations, the latter usually restricted to those requiring advanced study and higher ethical standards. They have also retained some of their earlier meaning, implying a higher motive than that of simply making a living.

These terms obviously exclude many volunteer workers and "amateurs" who have served as nurses. As the root of amateur (lover) indicates, such persons were expected to serve for love, not gain, and they were also distinguished from professionals as having little or no systematic preparation. Though there have been some conflicts between these two groups, especially in modern times, it will be seen that a good many of the early nursing leaders were voluntary workers of this type who did much to bring about needed reforms.

Some kinds of organization and training will be found in the nursing field in past centuries, but it was not until quite recent times that nursing functions were clearly distinguished from domestic, charitable, religious, medical, or other activities, and nursing became a recognized secular vocation or profession in its own right. This was largely the work of the founder of modern nursing, Florence Nightingale, whose little book, *Notes on Nursing—What It Is and What It Is Not*, clearly placed nursing in the group of healing arts and health services and led to the elimination of many extraneous functions. The Founder also expanded the nurse's field of service to include the care of patients of all ages, classes and kinds and health-nursing as well as sick-nursing. She set up for the first time a definite plan for the training of nurses and for their continued growth in service. She also succeeded in freeing this new-old vocation from the control of various groups that tended to dominate it. As a result of her distinguished example, leadership, and wide popularity, the modern nursing movement was successfully launched and soon spread into many parts of the world.

SOME ESSENTIAL ELEMENTS IN THE NURSE'S EQUIPMENT AND SERVICE

The diagram (p. 10) represents a concept of nursing that has been evolving through the ages and is still in process of development. It suggests not only the personal qualifications required for nursing practice and the three-sided preparation needed for this particular branch of work but the widening spheres of nursing service and the major functions of modern nurses. These include the newer function of rehabilitation, which is now receiving more attention in nursing, as it is in medicine.

It is suggested that these points be kept in mind in following the evolution of nursing as a vocation or profession. One can recognize most of them in embryo even at the primitive stage of nursing, but it took many centuries to develop the fine art of nursing out of a simple handicraft, to accumulate a sound body of tested scientific knowledge in place of the early superstitions and to strengthen the animating spirit or soul of nursing which grew out of love and concern for family and tribe and later extended to neighbors and strangers. Nurses also developed a strong vocational or professional purpose that included a loyalty to co-workers as well as to patients and public and a sense of responsibility for continuously strengthening and extending the usefulness of their service.

Needless to say, nursing has not yet reached its full growth. It can never rise higher than the human instruments by which it is administered and the resources they are able to draw upon in the culture of their age and their group. This culture includes not only the knowledge, techniques, and ideals handed down from the past but the whole political, religious, educational, social, and economic framework within which nurses and other

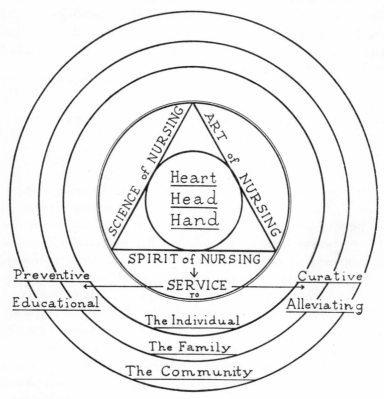

Diagram showing professional equipment of the modern nurse and the scope of her responsibilities

workers function in the practice of their vocations. In all ages such influences have made their chief impact through creative individuals of great social insight, courage, initiative, and spirituality, who broke through the "crust of custom" and led the group to higher levels of achievement. Some were regarded as saints and miracle workers, but even they could not get very far until technical and scientific knowledge had advanced suffi-

ciently to give them a safe and sound foundation for their work
and until proper educational facilities suited to nurses' needs
were made available.

SELECTED BIBLIOGRAPHY

Fuerst, Elinor V., and Lu Verne Wolff. *Fundamentals of Nursing.* Philadelphia:
Lippincott, 1956. Esp. Unit One, Part 1.

Goodrich, Annie W. *The Social and Ethical Significance of Nursing.* New York:
Macmillan, 1932.

Harmer, Bertha, and Virginia Henderson. *Textbook of the Principles and Practice
of Nursing.* New York: Macmillan, 1955. Esp. Part I, Ch. 1.

Linton, Ralph. *The Tree of Culture.* New York: Knopf, 1955.

Montag, Mildred L., and Margaret Filson. *Nursing Arts.* Philadelphia: Saunders,
2nd ed., 1953.

Mumford, Lewis. *The Conditions of Man.* New York: Harcourt, Brace, 1944.

Price, Alice L. *The Art, the Science, and Spirit of Nursing.* Philadelphia: Saunders, 1954. Esp. Ch. I, III.

Selected Papers of Joseph W. Mountin, M. D. Joseph W. Mountin Memorial
Committee, 1956.

Stewart, Isabel M. "The Spirit of Nursing in the Light of History," *ICN,* July
1926, 161-168.

Wolf, Lulu K. *Nursing.* New York: D. Appleton-Century, 1947. Esp. Ch. I-III.

CHAPTER 2

Care of the Sick in the Ancient World

DIFFERENCES BETWEEN PRIMITIVE AND CIVILIZED PEOPLES

The term "ancient world," as used here, includes primitive societies—what modern anthropologists call preliterate or arrested states of civilization. Many such societies exist today and can be studied in the writings of individuals who have lived among them and observed them closely. Some of these individuals are trained anthropologists and sociologists; others are missionaries or travelers who write of their experiences and observations. A notable pioneer and scholar in this field was Sir James Frazer, who in *The Golden Bough* collected examples of primitive customs from a wide variety of sources. From such records a great deal is now known about the customs, beliefs, and behavior of our primitive ancestors and of similar contemporary peoples, and many of our old ideas about them and their ways of thinking and behaving have been revised. Some striking examples of the wide diversity of primitive cultures and behavior patterns are found in Ruth Benedict's *Patterns of Culture,* in which she describes and contrasts two

Indian societies in New Mexico and Vancouver Island, respectively, and another primitive group in Melanesia. Such studies are not only intensely interesting from the human standpoint, but they show us how hazardous it is to generalize about primitive peoples. Civilized countries have richer and more varied cultures than have those at a preliterate stage. Obviously, a written language, the discovery of paper, and other means of preserving and passing on the experience of the race brought greater possibilities of intellectual and moral growth for human beings. The accumulation of such literature in temples or other safe places and the development of a literate class that could read, write, and interpret such records were remarkable steps forward. Such advances, together with the development of agriculture, the domestication of animals, the discovery of weaving, pottery, metal working, and similar arts and the stabilization of governmental and other institutions are marks of the stages of human development. Historians place the beginnings of such a transition about 8000 years ago. By 4000 B.C., a few of the ancient civilizations had begun to establish themselves in the fertile valleys of the Tigris, the Euphrates, and the Nile and in other parts of the ancient world.

THE CARE OF THE SICK IN PRIMITIVE SOCIETIES

As stated earlier, the care of the sick and other aspects of the life of primitive peoples can best be understood as part of the total cultural pattern of the group. Disease is, of course, a universal phenomenon and every society has to find some way of dealing with it, but the methods used will depend on the general attitudes, beliefs, and customs of the people, their social organization, and the resources they have at their command. A fundamental principle in all such societies is that the survival of the group comes before the welfare of the individual. It would be a mistake to conclude, however, that because the weaker and more helpless members of the tribe—babies, old folks, invalids, and others—may be left to die in periods of famine or other crises all primitive peoples are cruel and unfeeling. Kindliness is common among them, and children as a rule receive affection and care, even when infanticide is practiced as an economic policy. Mutual aid is seen even in animal societies, and such cooperation, especially in life saving, seems to be characteristic of all human groups. The old and sick of the tribe are fed and tended, except in severe stress, and even strangers may be cared for and kindly treated. Pre-eminent among the primitive virtues is hospitality, the entertaining of strangers from which come our words, hospital, hospice, and hotel. Hospitality is probably the most ancient expression of man's altruism, and the obligation to provide food, clothing, shelter, and protection to strangers is recognized as sacred and binding by early societies in all parts of the world. It came to be endowed with religious significance and embodied in religious codes, which gave special claims to the sick, infirm, and helpless.

PRIMITIVE MAN'S CONCEPT OF DISEASE

Human beings began quite early to speculate about the inexplicable phenomena of nature and the mysteries connected with birth, life, disease, and death. This led to what seems to be a common belief among primitive peoples which goes by the name of animism. Observing the ceaseless motion in nature, primitive man assumed that everything was alive and that all human beings, animals, and even inanimate objects had in them a spirit or double endowed with powers that might bring evil or good to him and his group. The waters, trees, winds, storms, and lightning were personalities, potential enemies, and the air around him was peopled with invisible spirits that filled his life with fear and dread. Disease might be due to the anger of the offended gods, devils, demons, or malevolent spirits, the supernatural powers of a human enemy, or the displeasure of the dead. So arose the infinite variety of superstitions concerning sickness that have persisted with an extraordinary strength and universality down to the present day.

The treatment of disease was perfectly logical in that it took its cue from the supposed cause; the evil spirit must be driven out, the offended gods placated, the human enemy punished, and the dead appeased. Some of the methods used were material and manual, others were magical. The magical were supposed to require a higher type of ability and more influence with the supernatural than the strictly manipulative. They included in-cantations, exorcisms, elaborate ceremonials, magical rites,

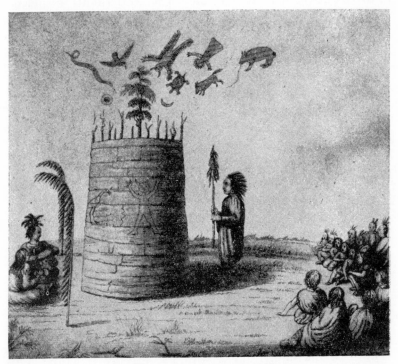

Medicine Lodge of American Indians

and songs and dances with ugly masks and weird noises. Often the medicine man went into a trance or convulsion, and such abnormal conditions as epilepsy were considered an evidence of supernatural powers. Primitive healers also used a wide variety of fetishes, amulets, and other objects believed to have healing power or to be capable of warding off evil spirits with their magical properties.

Manual and material forms of treatment were supposedly **less** potent, but they had a similar purpose. The genealogy of many reputable therapeutic methods used today can be traced back to animistic theories. Thus the practice of massage arose from pummeling and pounding the patient's body to drive out the evil spirit. In trephining the malign spirit was supposed to escape through the hole in the skull. Therapeutic baths began by plunging the patient into hot or cold water or sweating him to drive out the demon of sickness. Counterirritants, blistering appliances, and fire were used to burn out the evil spirits. Purgatives and emetics were given to expel them through the orifices of the body, deodorants to drive them away by strong odors, and horrible medicines to nauseate or kill them. This superstition even dominated the materia medica of certain periods in the Middle Ages, when the most loathsome drugs, composed of insects, excrement, and other unpleasant things, were administered to the sick. Undoubtedly it lingers today in the popular superstition that to be efficacious medicine must be strong and bad-tasting. The cruel methods used down to very recent times in the treatment of the insane who were believed to be possessed by devils are another indication of the persistence of such superstitions.

BEGINNINGS OF SPECIALIZATION IN MEDICAL WORK

From the differentiation between magical and practical modes of treatment used by the primitive medicine man arose the concept of higher and lower ranks among healers and the association of the higher ranks with the priestly function. This distinction is clearly marked at the dawn of history. We shall meet the two forms, theurgic and practical, in Egypt and Greece. In Persia there were three, the knife doctor, the herb doctor, and the word doctor, of which the last, the shaman or magician, was considered the highest. Sometimes the practical doctors served as assistants to the priest-physicians and sometimes they practiced independently.

The surgeon is easily recognized by his skill in the use of the knife and his manipulation of broken bones and dislocations.

All primitive tribes had some kind of wound treatment. Herbs or roots, many having astringent or disinfectant properties, were applied in the form of poultices, powders, or infusions. Various materials were used as sutures; the North American Indians employed sinews; some African tribes used thorns; and among the Somali and the Brazilian Indians, the heads of termites were used for this purpose. Cauterization has been widely used to control bleeding. The treatment of fractures and dislocations with splints was universal among primitives, massage of the broken bone being started early in some tribes. Bleeding and the incision of boils and abscesses were common practice, and cupping was a substitute for the actual sucking out by the medicine man of material believed to cause sickness. Even such dangerous operations as trephining and amputations were performed in some early societies.

The herb doctor probably learned much of his art from the women who usually were responsible for the cultivation and gathering of roots, seeds, and berries, while the men supplied the flesh food for the tribal larder. According to some authorities (for example, Otis Tufton Mason in *Women's Share in Primitive Culture*[1]), women were the chief discoverers of medical herbs and the first empirical physicians who learned to brew and prepare the different potions and to use them as home remedies in the treatment of their families and neighbors. It is believed also that primitive peoples learned a good deal about such matters by observing the habits of animals and that they are better guided than civilized people by instincts which prompt them to use the correct natural remedy and to avoid injurious plants or places where disease lurks. In any case, whether by accident or instinct or acute observation, they acquired many valuable methods of prevention and cure which they explained in their own way. For example, they learned not to eat certain berries or rotten fish containing spirits that kill man; not to touch the leaves of certain vines that harbored demons which crept under the skin, causing uncomfortable rashes; to avoid marshes inhabited by other enemies which caused chills and fever; and to

[1] (New York: Appleton, 1894.)

isolate or destroy individuals or animals believed to be the source of especially malignant disease-producing agents.

So developed the beginnings of hygiene, sanitation, and public health as well as medicine, surgery, psychiatry, midwifery, and all other branches of the healing and health arts. Nursing was inextricably bound up with all of these practices and was associated especially with the feeding and care of infants, the tending of invalid and aged relatives, and the administration of practical household remedies, such as herbs, fomentations, poultices, blisters, baths, and other applications of heat, cold, and counterirritation.

THE RELATIONS OF LEGITIMATE AND OTHER HEALERS

Much of the store of medical knowledge and skill referred to above was originally the possession of the common people, and even after a special group of experts developed, the practice of domestic or "folk" medicine persisted as it does today in civilized communities. To protect themselves from competition, and to exclude unqualified practitioners, medicine men in some groups formed castes or guilds, often requiring for membership painful and exacting initiatory rites. In other tribes admission to such a group was a hereditary privilege. There were some tribes that selected medicine men because they were great dreamers or diviners or were definitely psychopathic or otherwise abnormal. Twins in some cultures were believed to have supernatural powers and so to have special favors from the gods. In a few primitive societies women as well as men were admitted to this select group if they showed convincing evidence of magical powers.

In time there came to be a distinction between white magic, which was occult power or supernatural knowledge used benignly, and black magic, its malign application for evil and destructive purposes. As this distinction grew, the conception of what we now call quackery, an illegitimate encroachment on the province of the physician, began to appear and the difficulty of drawing the line between "folk" medicine, including home nursing, and the officially recognized practice of medicine must have led to serious conflicts. No doubt practical attendants and nurses were often accused of being rivals of the priest-physician or may have been mistrusted by him from jealous motives. The "wise women" who, in ancient countries and among primitive tribes, were often revered as healers and caretakers of the sick would be in special danger, and it is not unreasonable to assume that the witch idea may have grown out of such conflicts. Cases are known in which accusations of witchcraft (black magic) were used to eliminate the competition of women who had long shown a special aptitude for the healing arts. In all the old records witches were credited with uncanny powers of causing illness and wasting disease, and this superstition must have arisen in a remote period. It lingers today in modified form in some isolated communities, always based on some knowledge of herbs and medicinal or magic powers.

In this connection, it is interesting to note that in early Celtic society the druids were recognized as the official medical and religious class. The dark oak groves were their temples and certain plants were used for magical and medical purposes. Chief of these were the mistletoe, called the "all healer," the oak, the rowan (ash), and the yew. In their shade the druids performed their mystic rites. There is some evidence that in Ireland at an early date women had been especially successful as magic wielders but had been ousted by the druids. When this order was suppressed by Christianity, these "wise women" took the name of druidesses, healed diseases, and had charge of the holy wells. Many of the superstitions that exist in Ireland today had their origin in the early practitioners of magic.

MEDICINE AND NURSING IN ANCIENT CIVILIZATIONS

There was no sharp break between preliterate and literate stages of human development or between the ways of thinking of primitive and more civilized peoples. Gradually knowledge accumulated, man's world broadened, new ideas were spread through trade, war, and other contacts, and in some of the ancient civilizations, notably Greece, the human mind began to release itself from the stranglehold of custom and tradition and to explore more freely the secrets of the universe. It was a long time, however, before superstitious ideas and practices concerned with health and sickness changed much. To be sure, the deities took different forms as man's imagination and knowledge developed. Nature gods of complex attributes are to be found in different civilizations and their legends and myths are included in religious and legal codes. From sacred books and other sources we learn most of what we know about health and nursing practices in the pre-Christian world.

It is not easy to affix time periods to the ancient civilizations, since antiquarian research is constantly revealing new remains that carry recorded history further back. In the light of present knowledge, the nations of Africa and Asia show the greatest antiquity, but they do not give equal clues to medical progress in the sphere of nursing. China, for instance, with her strange and antique medical lore, leaves us completely in the dark about the work of men or women in the nursing care of the sick, whereas her neighbors, India and Ceylon have venerable records showing a relatively high state of development in these arts.

EGYPT AND HER MEDICAL CODES

Though some claims have been made for Babylonia, the oldest medical records thus far discovered and deciphered by scholars appear to be Egyptian. Among the medical papyri, the Ebers Papyrus (medical) and the Smith Papyrus (surgical) are perhaps the most celebrated. The Ebers Papyrus has been described as an encyclopedia of medicine as it was practiced by the Egyptians in the sixteenth century before the Christian era. Many diseases and surgical operations known today are described and classified, and more than seven hundred drugs of the vegetable, mineral, and animal kingdom are enumerated. The description of the preparation of these drugs shows that the Egyptian pharmacists made decoctions, infusions, solutions for injection, pills, tablets, troches, capsules, powders, inhalations, lotions, ointments, plasters, and other forms in use today. They knew a great deal about the therapeutic action of drugs, and laid the foundations of chemistry.

The Egyptians also developed the art of embalming in which they employed aromatics, resins, and probably other preservatives now unknown. They attained a rare skill in bandaging, as shown on their mummies, often winding one thousand yards of bandage about one body. Many of their methods are now a lost art. They became skilled in dentistry and filled teeth with gold. Their priest-physicians understood hypnotism and practiced it, using their occult powers to treat the sick and interpret dreams. Egypt had learned astronomers, and this study led to the development of astrology and the belief that disease, as well as the general destiny, was influenced by the stars.

The medical books go back to mythological days when the god Horus, the Sun, learned medicine from his mother Isis, the Earth. There is nothing to be found in these records about nurses and their work, which seems a little strange, since medicine, pharmacy, and sanitation were so well developed. Nor is there any description of hospitals as such. There were temples to which the sick may have resorted, but what their facilities were is not clear. The position of women in ancient Egypt is supposed to have been extremely good in comparison with others of the older days. Women of good family, at least, enjoyed considerable freedom and dignity, but we learn nothing of any professional career, though social and family conditions then are often compared with those of modern times.

The religion of Egypt inculcated kindliness, justice, and charity, and these precepts were observed in some, if not all, circles of Egyptian life. Hospitality was emphasized in the laws, and women especially were enjoined to feed the hungry, clothe the naked, and care for the sick. Their public services were probably limited to the alleviation of suffering. The Egyptian religion forbade the dissection of the human body, and thus surgery and anatomy were crippled. Because of this restriction and the growth of extreme formalism, the medical laws of Egypt gradually became extremely rigid and crystallized into a set of fixed codes. With this tendency, research died away and medicine as a progressive science became extinct.

BABYLONIA, ASSYRIA, AND CHALDEA

The literature of these ancient civilizations has little to tell us of our special subject of nursing. The royal correspondence of the Assyrian empire and other cuneiform writings, however, refer frequently to practices which, though performed by royal physicians, would be done by nurses today. These civilizations were the homes of so many beliefs that have descended to modern times as rank yet widespread health superstitions that their scanty records are of great interest. Assyria and Babylonia gave the securest asylum to the theory of demonology, or possession of the sick person's body by evil spirits. In elaborating this belief, the Assyrians created whole armies of good and bad spirits, leaving man helpless before them except as he could invoke the aid of one against another. The idea, too, of sin as a cause of disease seems to have been emphasized if not originated by these peoples. It led to the adoption of ceremonials, such as purification by fire and water to atone for and cleanse from sin, and of sacrifices, often of a very cruel character, requiring the offering of human life. These characteristics were reflected in many of the beliefs and medical practices of the warlike Assyrians. The legend of sin as the cause of illness lasted long, for we remember the question put to Christ by His disciples, "Did this man sin, or his parents?" We may, indeed, trace it down to our own day, for when chloroform was discovered, and was first used in lessening the pains of childbirth, numerous sermons were preached to show that the curse laid upon Eve made these pains a punishment for sin and it was therefore an impiety to interfere by mitigating them.

Others of the Assyrian, Chaldean, and Babylonian beliefs were based on nature study. Such were their ideas as to the potency of numbers, based on observations of the heavenly bodies and the movements of the stars and planets. They were fond of the number seven, which has always held and still holds a high place in mystic lore, and they tied it in knots on cords. Other occult regulations arose from agricultural experience and fixed the times and seasons for gathering roots and herbs. So persistent have these traditions been that many country people still plant by the moon. Still other remedies were symbolic and doubtless had for ancient people a poetic quality lost to modern minds. They may well have included the use of charms and amulets, the custom of sprinkling with holy water, and the ceremonial of passing certain objects through fire. The latter at least had a practical value as a method of sterilization.

The legal aspect of Assyrian lore is given in the Code of Hammurabi, King of Babylonia about 2000 B.C., which shows an organization of medical treatment and of surgery, with fixed fees and with definite penalties for failure to effect cures. The Babylonian story of the creation and other Babylonian literature refer to wet nurses and children's nurses. Nothing has been found, however, on nursing as it is understood today.

THE HEALTH RELIGION OF INDIA

Centuries before the Christian era, we are told, India had attained to an advanced and enlightened civilization in which women held an enviable position. The Vedas, the sacred books of India, tell of these ancient things. With respect to health matters, it was believed that originally there had been no sin or disease in the world but that man, gradually falling away from his original purity, had brought these sorrows upon himself, whereupon Brahma in pity had given him the Ayur-Veda, the books treating of the cure and prevention of disease.

There were in the ancient mythology, twin brothers, children of the life-giving Sun, one of whom practiced medicine and the other surgery, and two famous mortals, Charaka and Sushruta, about whose human talents myths may have clustered. The dates assigned to these Indian physicians differ, some writers placing Charaka as early as 800 to 600 B.C., and others as late as the first century of our era. Sushruta is usually stated to have lived in the second century, after Charaka. Charaka was believed to have inherited all the wisdom of the serpent-god of the thousand heads, who was the repository of all the sciences, especially that of medicine. Sushruta represented the surgical aspect of Indian medicine. By this time the sciences had attained a rare eminence in India, and in the writings of both physicians definite reference is made to the qualifications and functions of nurses.

The long period of India's Golden Age was that in which the religion of Buddha prevailed. It was a religion of mercy, compassion, and justice which enjoined humane treatment for animals as well as man. King Asoka, who lived in the third century before Christ, was the great apostle of Buddhism, and it was during his reign that the greatest advances were made in charitable and sanitary work.

The records dwell at length on the prevention of disease and show that medicine, surgery, hygiene, and sanitation must have been, for that period, highly developed. The importance of prenatal influence and the principles of care needed before and after childbirth were well understood. Hospital construction had reached a high standard, and in hospital procedures the records would seem to indicate some practice of asepsis. As might be expected, therefore, the annals of India give more complete details of nursing principles and practice than are to be found in any other ancient writings. Indeed, so clear, intelligent, and scientific are many of them that they might fit into any modern textbook. The nurses, to whom frequent reference is made, seem to have been young men; only in special cases are elderly women mentioned. The position of women during this high curve of Indian civilization was socially a favored one, though their liberty was restricted and their activities were limited to the home.

HEALTH OFFICERS AND COMMUNAL HOSPITALS

The ancient communes of India had their health officers and public hospitals. There were also hospitals for animals, supported at public expense. Hygienic procedures were enforced by making them a part of religious observance, and early morning devotions were health measures, quaintly described in poetic phrases.

In the writings of Charaka and Sushruta an estimate is given of the desirable qualifications of "the Physician, the Drugs, the Nurse, and the Patient." The nurse must know how to compound drugs, must be clever, devoted to the patient, and pure in mind and body. Again, in the description of a model hospital, the nurse's qualities are dwelt on in more detail: "Skilled in every kind of service that a patient may require, endowed with general cleverness, competent to cook food, skilled in bathing or washing the patient, well conversant with rubbing or massaging the limbs, lifting the patient or assisting him to walk about, well skilled in making or cleaning beds, ready, patient, and skilful in waiting upon one who is ailing, never unwilling to do anything that may be ordered." In those hospitals of India there were employed, also, professional musicians and storytellers who cheered and diverted the patients by singing and by reciting poetry to them.

It appears that the young men nurses described in these medical writings belonged to subcastes of the Brahmins, or priestly orders. Thus the organization of the nursing profession as a semipriestly caste is of high antiquity, and India lent its pattern to the religious orders of the Christian era, whose "lay brothers" in hospital work corresponded to the subcastes of the older system.

The brilliant period of Hindu medicine began to fade a century or two before Christ. With the fall of Buddhism, hospitals were abandoned. The religion of Brahma in its later manifestations intensified caste and created numerous taboos, so that intelligent medical and nursing care gradually became impossible. This situation prevailed until quite recent times when modern concepts of nursing and health work were introduced and began to make headway in many parts of India.

CHINA, JAPAN, AND KOREA

Very little is known concerning nursing in these countries, but it is possible to trace the influence of Buddhism, which was carried by Indian missionaries, first to China in the first century A.D., and from there in the sixth century to Korea and Japan. Different sects of Buddhists developed and their beliefs and practices varied. Works of charity, including the art of healing, were generally fostered, the motive being philanthropic rather than scientific. The Buddhists built hospitals which they called "Houses of Benevolence or Compassion" and "Halls of Healing."

Most beloved and popular of all the incarnations of Buddha was Kwan-Yin (or Kwannon), sometimes represented as a man but most frequently as a beautiful woman of benign expression, often holding a child in her arms. She was known as the Goddess of Mercy and was regarded as a bodily healer as well as savior from many ills. There are many different manifestations of Kwan-Yin, some with a thousand arms, others with as many eyes, indicating her watchful care and her boundless benefactions. Seven causes of distress in which her help was considered especially effective were the sword, fetters, fire, water, demons, goblins, and enemies. She is still worshipped by millions of people in the Orient, chiefly by women who importune her for easy childbirth and for sons. We are probably justified in looking upon Kwan-Yin as a symbol of nursing and perhaps also of medicine. It is significant that she is represented as returning to earth in repeated reincarnations, refusing to accept release from the wheel of life until her rescue work is done.

Chinese medicine developed a vast pharmacopoeia of remedies, mainly animal and vegetable, rich in symbolism and often of practical value. The Chinese made a specialty of acupuncture and also used cupping, massage, and baths. Korea and Japan took most of their early medical ideas from China, but much superstition was mixed up with all their practices and few leaders of medical science were developed until modern times.

THE CONTRIBUTIONS OF THE JEWS

In the time before Christ the Jews formed a striking contrast to the nations around them, for they discarded the many deities and myths of Egypt, Assyria, and Babylonia and, under the leadership of Moses, declared their adherence to one God. However, the myth of the serpent, symbol of wisdom and knowledge, always closely associated with medicine, was apparently accepted, according to the Biblical account of the healing miracle in the wilderness. Moses' command not to allow a witch to live shows that even he was not entirely free from superstition. Who were the witches of Moses' day? Were they the same old women whose inherited knowledge of herbs and potions brought them into competition with men then engaged in formulating a more complex and probably more scientific health cult? We do not know. But it is known that Jewish women have had in remote times a remarkable skill in medicine, and they must have become experienced in the care of the sick, though this care was exercised perhaps only within the home.

Moses developed remarkable codes of sanitation and hygiene both for family and community life. He is supposed to have learned these sciences from the Egyptians, but he surpassed all the ancients in the clearness of his teachings about diet and sanitary precautions. He stands out in history as one of the great sanitarians of the world.

The Jewish religion emphasized human brotherhood and social justice. The duties of hospitality to the stranger and relief for the widow, the fatherless, and the oppressed were constantly urged as righteous. The Jews showed a strong sense of personal and social responsibility which led them to form benevolent associations to relieve the sick and to provide them with medicine and other things needful. In ancient times they also supported free public inns or hostels for travelers, to which houses for the sick were sometimes attached. It is not supposed, however, that these were organized hospitals such as the Hindus maintained but were rather for temporary care in emergency cases. References to nurses in the Talmud and the Old Testament do not suggest nurses as care-takers of the sick but rather as wet nurses or children's nurses. The Jews have continued down to present times to show the marked interest in medicine and public health and many distinguished nurses have come from this group.

GREECE: THE SOURCE OF MODERN MEDICAL SCIENCE

There is historical abundance in the medical records of ancient and classic Greece. Beginning like other nations in ages of myth and legend, Greek culture brings us in time to the great Hippocrates, the father of modern medicine, whose teaching was based definitely on the natural sciences.

In the mythical ages it was Apollo the sun god who was the deity of health and medicine. His son Asklepios, (in Rome, called Aesculapius) a marvelous physician, in turn became deified and worshiped. The Asklepios myth was doubtless woven about a mortal of fame and skill, for it is traced to a fairly definite date, about thirteen centuries before Christ, and the two sons of Asklepios were surgeons with the Greek army in the Trojan wars. The whole family of Asklepios has significance for the medical and nursing arts, for, if its members were only symbolic, they must have been meant to depict those arts as they existed at that time, and if they were actual persons they combined in their careers all the main lines of specialism that we consider modern.

Of the two sons, Machaon was a surgeon, with "skilled hands to draw out darts and heal sores," and Podalirius, representing internal medicine, "was given cunning to find out things impossible and cure that which healed not." The women of the family typify skill in nursing and in health conservation. The wife, Epigone, was "the soothing one." Among the six daughters, there were Hygeia, the goddess of health, Panacea, the restorer of health, represented as presiding over the administration of medicines, Aegle, whose name is translated as "light of the sun," and Meditrina, the preserver of health. From her title we may suppose her to have been the most ancient known forerunner of the modern public health nurse. Iaso, another daughter, personified recovery from illness. Asklepios is usually represented with a staff, derived from Mercury's staff of office, which indicated that he traveled from place to place, and with a serpent, the emblem of wisdom and of rejuvenescence or immortality (from casting its skin). This symbol of staff and serpent, which is still used by practitioners of the healing arts, is called the caduceus. It has been found in many forms from ancient to modern times. Grateful patients offered as a sacrifice to the gods either a cock or a goat; hence the use of these symbols in some of the pictures of Asklepios.

The Asklepios myth became highly involved and developed a dream-cure, based upon the worship of the serpent as its leading characteristic. As time went on, the priests of Asklepios specialized in two branches, one purely medical, the other occult. From the medical branch there developed a recognized class of physicians, known as the Asclepiades, who founded centers for the teaching of medicine where, in time, important medical schools with hospitals and related institutions grew up.

A GREEK HEALTH RESORT

Among the most famous of these centers was Epidauros, and, since its remains may still be seen, it is easy to get an idea of the Greek medical world in that day. The temple and all the buildings were of white marble, built in the classic style and on an ample scale. There were hospital wards and corridors, baths, gymnasia, libraries, rooms for visitors and attendants, houses for the priests and physicians, and a beautiful outdoor theater, the whole set in a location of ideal beauty among pine-covered hills. The patients on arriving at the hospital were given beds on a long open portico, where, in their sleep, the dream gods were supposed to appear to them and prescribe their treatment. There were two of these sleeping porches, one for men and one for women, so that there may also have been women nurses or attendants. After the patients had received their prescriptions, they were distributed among the small wards. Epidauros accommodated about 500 patients. It had a chief administrator whose position was like that of our hospital superintendent, and various grades of attendants, among them two sets of priestesses, one that assisted in the holy mysteries and the other as "basket-bearers." These priestesses, as head nurses, may have had supervisory charge of the patients, for under them were bath at-

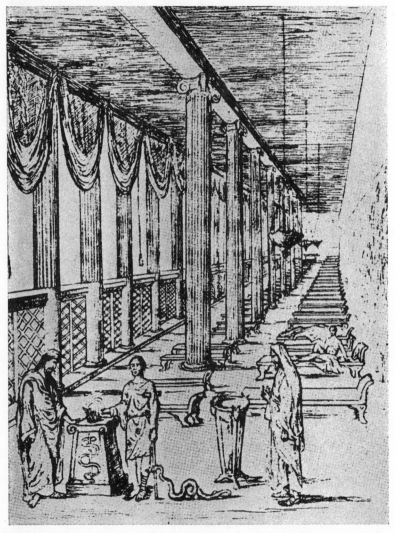

Restoration of the interior of the Abaton at Epidauros. Patient sacrificing and having injured leg licked by the sacred serpent. From *The Temple and Ritual of Asklepios* by permission of Richard Caton, M.D.

tendants and helpers who waited on the sick and carried those
who were unable to walk.

HIPPOCRATES, FATHER OF MODERN MEDICINE

Medical schools maintained by the Asclepiades are traced back
as far as 770 B.C., and under their influence a public system of
free medical relief for the poor grew up which lasted down to
the Christian era. An especially famous school was at Cos, and
there Hippocrates was born in 460 B.C. He is believed to have
been a direct descendant of Asklepios. Hippocrates' time was
the age of Pericles, the Golden Age of Greece, and his genius
ranks him with the other brilliant intellects of that day. In
his medical teachings he openly rejected all myths and superstitions and declared that disease was caused by disobedience to
natural laws. He called Nature "The Just," banished mystery
and reticence from the discussion of natural truths and medical
subjects, and expounded scientific facts in so simple a way that
his style might be called "popular." His medical writings cover
the entire medical field and are still regarded as classics.

Hippocrates[2] left no mention of nurses by name, but in his
medical writings and in those of his followers the technique of
what we now call nursing is taught in minute detail and with
perfect understanding. In all probability the medical students
then carried on these more skilled parts of the nursing service. Hippocrates emphasized the necessity of observation and
experiment in the pursuit of medical knowledge. He was
essentially practical and made the patient the object of his study.
His high ethics, and the generally fine standards of medicine
under his influence, were embodied in the Hippocratic Oath,
the classic statement of medical ethics. This well-known pledge
has had a marked influence on both medicine and nursing.

The followers and disciples of Hippocrates practiced dissection and observed his precepts for a long time, but as their
era passed Greek physicians abandoned clinical medicine for

[2] It is now believed that several authors contributed to these writings and that
there may have been more than one physician named Hippocrates. To avoid confusion, however, the singular term is used here.

philosophical dissertations. Practical work came to be despised, and a bookish and theoretical learning brought on the slow decay of real science in Greece which lasted for many centuries.

Greek culture did not give women of virtuous character much liberty, nor did these women share in men's intellectual, social, or political life. Wives and mothers were restricted to domestic duties, which, if the home were a large estate, included management of the household and care of the health of the servants. It is true that legends tell of high accomplishment in medicine by Greek women, but that was in the heroic, not the classic age. The Greek intellect was clear and rational. It rejected superstition and hampering traditions and developed an ethical philosophy which elevated reason, temperance, justice, and civic integrity to the highest plane. The Greeks worshiped beauty and physical perfection and showed little interest in the sickness or misery of the unfortunate. Their religion did not especially enjoin duty or charity, though hospitality was considered a virtue. In organizing the functions of the state, however, they paid some attention to the problems of poverty. There was state relief for orphans, vagrants, and defectives at public cost, and the poor were attended in sickness by state physicians. Brotherhoods of hospitality provided inns and resting places for travelers, and mutual help associations were fairly common. The literature of the Greeks contains many references to nurses, but these were children's nurses and wet nurses and should not be regarded as the archetype of the modern professional nurse. In Greece, as in other early civilizations, the family servant shared in home nursing.

ROME'S EMINENCE IN SANITATION

The early history of Rome began when Greece was at the height of her civilization and was dotted with health resorts and medical schools. The older Etruscan civilization is dim with mystery, and the simple medical art of the old peasants of the Abruzzi, which they took with them to Rome, preceded the worship of the goddesses of fever, of drains, of the evil eye, and of microbes. It is supposed that Rome applied to Greece for advanced medical teaching. In the third century B.C., during a severe plague, the Sibylline books were consulted, and the Oracle counseled the Romans to import the god Asklepios (Aesculapius) from Greece. A mission was sent, and a staff of physicians and attendants came and settled in the little island in the Tiber. One of the sacred serpents was said to have chosen the spot by jumping out of the galley onto the island. This has been a hospital site ever since.

No doubt Rome had other medical teachers. Among her thousands of Greek and Asiatic slaves were men of high education and attainment, many of whom understood medical treatment and procedure. Of nursing there is no record, apart from the work of military orderlies in the army, an occasional old woman, and children's nurses. It is probable that in the homes of the rich all nursing was done by slaves.

Though the Romans were never distinguished for compassion or pity, they did make a remarkable cult of health preservation. The remains of their public baths, aqueducts, and other engineering and sanitary works found in Rome, Nîmes, Bath, and other parts of Europe amaze modern tourists and testify to the advanced stage of the Romans in these technical arts and in their provisions for public health. In the earlier days in Rome medicine was given a dignified place in civic life, in which public health service with free dispensaries was developed and professors of medicine and sanitation were honored. Later, the practice of medicine fell into the hands of quacks and slaves.

The best and perhaps the only genuine hospitals of ancient Rome were for the army. Sick and wounded soldiers in earlier times had been billeted in private families for their care, but the military hospitals developed later, as shown by excavations in Pompeii, were well built and equipped. The nursing of the orderlies or "nosocomi" was probably of the same kind that every army nurse has seen wherever orderlies have charge. The great talents and ability of the Roman ladies, to whom we shall come presently, had no field in nursing in the old regime but found one under the new order of the Christian era.

PRE-CHRISTIAN NURSING IN IRELAND

A definite organization of such service appeared in Ireland before Christianity arrived there. The *Catholic Encyclopedia* states that the Brehon Laws, an ancient code regulating domestic and social relations, made provisions for a hospital in every military camp and for women to be trained to care for the sick and wounded. There were also district hospitals for each territory. The Brehon Laws state "that the hospital shall be free from debt, shall have four doors and a stream of water running through the middle of the floor. Dogs, fools and female scolds must be kept away from the patient lest he be worried. Whoever inflicted bodily injury on another had to pay for his maintenance either in a hospital or a private house." The laws provided also that the sick should have a physician, food, proper bed, furniture, and a proper house. They distinguished between "lawful" and "unlawful" physicians, and stated the amount of their fees. A "nurse-tender" was also mentioned, that is, "the man who is employed to lift him [the patient] up and lay him down." Dr. James Walsh, in his *History of Nursing*, points out that the homes of physicians were also used to accommodate the sick and came under regulations laid down by the Brehon Laws. The women of the physician's family were supposed to have special knowledge of the healing virtues of plants and to be qualified to assist in the care of the sick.

In looking back from this point, having regard to the slenderness of our sources, it may be conceded that the care of the sick in ancient days compares favorably with that of some more recent periods. It is not only historically incorrect to assume that all neighborly kindness and charity began with the Christian era, it is also a temperamental error that narrows the mind by shutting out the view of the essential humaneness of the human race. The older religions had their merciful aspects, as shown in the charitable works of the Hindus and the Jews. The pagan Greeks and Romans had, in the cult of Orpheus, a softening spiritual influence, which, so far as it reached, inculcated kindness and a horror of suffering. Perhaps the chief deficiency in our eyes in the ancient nursing systems is the small part played by women; yet on the whole we know little about it. There may have been more than has been told. Allusions to the eminence of women among the Norsemen, Teutons, and Celts and to their superior skill in medicine and surgery suggest a larger field for women in the western world than in the Orient. In the medical and surgical arts there were epochs in ancient times that were clearly more brilliant and distinguished than certain centuries of the era that we are about to discuss. And it should not be forgotten that at least three ancient civilizations, India, Greece, and Rome, were comparatively free of the superstition that demons were the cause of illness.

SELECTED BIBLIOGRAPHY

Adams, Francis. (Tr.) *The Genuine Works of Hippocrates*. Baltimore: Williams and Wilkins, 1946.

Austin, Anne L. *History of Nursing Source Book*. New York: Putnam's, 1957. Ch. I.

Benedict, Ruth. *Patterns of Culture*. Boston: Houghton Mifflin, 1934.

Bick, Edgar M. "The Cult of Asklepios: A Critical Study," *Ann. Med. Hist.*, December 1927, 327-331.

Charr, Robert. "Ancient Chinese Medicine," *Ann. Med. Hist.*, May 1936, 242-248.

Chiera, Edward. *They Wrote on Clay: The Babylonian Tablets Speak Today*. Chicago: University of Chicago Press, 1938.

Elsberg, Charles A. "The Edwin Smith Papyrus," *Ann. Med. Hist.*, May 1931, 271-279.

Healy, E. Nellie. "Some Glimpses of Life in Ancient Ireland," *Int. Nurs. Rev.*, May 1931, 233-238.

Hume, Edward H. "Medicine in China: Old and New," *Ann. Med. Hist.*, May 1930, 272-280.

Leake, Chauncey D. "Roman Architectural Hygiene," *Ann. Med. Hist.*, March 1930, 135-163.

Maddox, John L. *The Medicine Man*. New York: Macmillan, 1923.

Major, Ralph H. "The Papyrus Ebers," *Ann. Med. Hist.*, September 1930, 547-555.

Nutting, M. Adelaide, and Lavinia L. Dock, *A History of Nursing*. New York: Putnam's, 1907-1912. 4 vols. Vol. I, Part I, Ch. I-IX.

The Old Testament.

Rivers, W. H. R. *Medicine, Magic, and Religion.* New York: Harcourt, Brace, 1924.

Robinson, Victor, "The Nurse of Greece," *Bull. Inst. Hist. Med.,* November 1938, 1001-1009.

Sarma, P. J. "Hindu Medicine and Its Antiquity," *Ann. Med. Hist.,* May 1931, 318-324.

CHAPTER 3

Influence of the Early Church

THE ROMAN EMPIRE AT THE DAWN
OF CHRISTIANITY

At the opening of the Christian era the Roman Empire extended over the greater part of Europe, a part of Britain, and vast tracts of Asia Minor and Northern Africa. Pre-eminent as a conquering military force, it was equally distinguished for its elaborate political, legal, and administrative organization. The Roman genius was extremely practical and businesslike, and Roman officials allowed the freemen of conquered populations freedom of action and thought on all but two topics—economics and politics. As in Russia under the Czars, subjects who never forgot these taboos might live in peace. The political economy of Rome was based on slavery, the institution that finally undermined the empire. The age was a callous, even a cruel one, yet there were tendencies alive that prepared a welcome for better things.

Women belonging to the patrician families had been strengthening their position in the 200 years of the Republic, and in addition to a notable dignity in home life they had gained a social liberty which allowed them to go freely about in public, to dine out, and receive their husbands' guests at home, in marked contrast to the seclusion in which Greek women lived. It will be remembered that Roman matrons once formed a deputation to the Forum to protest against sumptuary legislation. Such women had also quite exceptional advantages in educational matters.

An alternative to the old pagan religious ceremony of marriage had been evolved in the free marriage contract. This gave the wife entire control over her own property and made her the social equal of her husband, whereas the old law had made her his chattel, with her fortune, her children, and her own life and death at his disposal. The independent and dignified position thus held by women in Roman society was to prove of great importance to the development of nursing, for Roman matrons were presently to turn their abilities and their money toward its organization.

THE TEACHING OF CHRIST

Christ's teachings of love and brotherhood coming into the midst of a hard materialistic society transformed the face of the earth for His disciples, and set free a boundless current of spiritual joy and hope. The disciples' love for their great Teacher took the form of service to those who needed it, especially to the sick, neglected, and destitute. Christ's own parables and miracles had dealt much with disease and death, and He had told His followers that in ministering to the poor and sick they were ministering to Him. We recall the quaint phraseology of the account of all those who were brought to Him to be healed, "sick people that were taken with divers diseases and torments, and those which were possessed with devils, and those which were lunatic, and those that had the palsy; and He healed them." The practical test of the new faith was "not to be ministered unto, but to minister." In later years the Golden Rule was often carved on the seats of hospitals.

THE ALTERED POSITION OF WOMEN

The most striking feature of the new religion was the active strenuous work it brought to women, especially to the single ones. The flat statement sometimes made that women, hopelessly degraded under paganism, were forever exalted by Christianity cannot indeed be accepted unconditionally. The more we learn of ancient society the more evidence we find, in certain periods at least, of respect and consideration for women and often of a just legal status for them; whereas during the long Middle Ages canon law subjugated women in family life and gave them an inferior status by ranking marriage below celibacy. If it is said that Christ's precepts placed women and men on an equal footing, this must be unconditionally agreed to. His answer to Martha, when Mary left the kitchen to hear His words, signified His recognition of women's intellectual aspirations and of their right to share in practical work.

While His influence remained paramount in the early church, men and women worked together on an equal basis, and unmarried women had opportunities for social service on a varied scale never before known. In the older societies there had been no career open to single women, save in special castes with restricted duties, such as the temple women or priestesses and the vestal virgins. But now women, both married and single, threw themselves with the utmost devotion into all the works of the community, chief among which was the care of the sick.

Deaconesses, Virgins, and Widows of the Early Church

It was in all probability Phoebe, the friend of St. Paul, who organized on a wide scale the nursing of the poor. It is known that she was a church deacon (*diakonos*, "one who serves"), that she made journeys to Rome, evidently in connection with her work, and that "she succored many," St. Paul among the number. In spite of this evident approval of Phoebe and other women of good works, St. Paul unfortunately held some prejudices on the subject of women, and the doctrine of inferiority and subordination he laid down in some of his letters was used as a potent argument for the subjection of women up to the modern era.

The literature referring to various women workers of the early Christian church is confusing and contradictory in its allusions to the status, qualifications, and functions of the deaconesses, virgins, and widows. It outlines in some detail, however, their duties and responsibilities, and is helpful toward an understanding of these women and their ministration to the sick. The early Church, at one stage of its development, made men and women deacons with equal rank. Their duties included the performance of certain parts of the church service, teaching and mission work, spreading the gospel, and carrying out all the relief work and charitable undertakings of the church. The care of the sick, including visiting nursing, became their special work (more often that of the women), and the spirit of community service was intensified by the conditions under which the Christian brotherhood lived.

For the first two centuries of the early church the deaconess, whether single, married, or widowed, was chosen or accepted by the higher clergy and ordained by the bishop. She might wear her ordinary garb, live in her own home, and retain her own property. Such favorable conditions gave able women ample scope to realize their plans for nursing and friendly aid. Many distinguished women of that time, widows and daughters of Roman officials, of gentle breeding, culture, and wealth, entered the deaconess sisterhood in order to direct the work. Such women organized groups of deaconesses and sent them far and wide to the parishes of the Eastern Church and west as far as Gaul and Ireland. The highest point of the movement was shown in Constantinople under the bishopric of St. John Chrysostom, about A.D. 398 to A.D. 407. A staff of some forty deaconesses—who had adopted the community life—lived there under the direction of Olympia, a woman who combined great spiritual gifts with worldly prestige.

The order of deaconesses remained organized in the Eastern Church until the eighth century, but its importance began to diminish in the fifth and sixth, after church decrees had deprived its members of their clerical duties and rank. This order did not itself emerge into monasticism, but as it died away its place was taken by groups of monastic women whose origin may be found in the early orders of virgins and widows. The deaconess order had brief periods of renascence in the Middle Ages, generally in connection with religious movements, then regarded as heretical, which attempted a return to the simple life of the apostolic church. It became active again in the nineteenth century when it was revived by Lutheran and some other Protestant churches.

The virgins and widows were also classed among the clergy of the early Church, though their rank at first was somewhat less than that of the deaconesses. The ecclesiastical widows had a claim upon the Church for support and served in various ways, presiding over meetings, teaching the gospel, and forming a bench of "elders." Their position became so dignified and important that many widows of independent means dedicated themselves to church work, donned a special widow's dress, and from their own homes pursued their charitable labors. These widows were not church clergy. Their order became especially important in Rome, and Roman matrons, not necessarily widowed, joined it on their conversion to Christianity. In the third century the ecclesiastical widow, like the deaconess, became the object of some jealous disapproval on the part of men, and her sphere of public work was gradually curtailed.

The virgins were a consecrated order and for several centuries lived in their homes with no special restrictions, devoting themselves freely to the work of their choice, visiting or nursing the sick or pursuing missionary labors, and going about in public without restraint. They are regarded by many as the forerunners of latter-day nuns.

THE ROMAN MATRONS

The first converts to Christianity among the highborn women of Rome have been described in the letters of St. Jerome. Among them were Marcella, the leader, who turned her palace on the

Aventine into the first Roman monastery for women and who was so learned that the clergy often consulted with her on Scriptural passages; Fabiola, who founded in her home the first free public hospital under Christian auspices (about A.D. 390) and worked in it as a nurse, carrying the patients into it and bathing their wounds and sores; and Paula, who knew classic languages and assisted St. Jerome in translating the prophets and who with her daughter devoted immense wealth to the building and maintenance of hospitals and inns for travelers on the routes to Jerusalem.

Probably no group of women ever associated with hospital and nursing organization has surpassed these in intellectual powers and commanding force of character. The period of their activity was after the early persecutions of Christians, for Constantine had made Christianity the state religion in 330. But they lived to see the Goths and barbarians penetrate the empire, and, during the sack of Rome by Alaric, Marcella was killed. The gradual disintegration of Roman power and the general disorganization of society following upon repeated invasions brought the Church prominently to the front as the one uniting and subduing influence, and the Roman matrons bent their energies to the founding of monasteries in which women might find, not only refuge and security, but the opportunity to conserve and upbuild civilization under Christian auspices.

MONASTICISM

From the Roman pattern created in Marcella's home, monastic groups were formed in Marseilles, then in Arles, and so throughout western Europe. In no other way could women have led occupational careers of their own choosing in that time of political and social chaos. In the monastery directed by an abbess, and sheltered by a constitution or "rule" granted by the Church, they were free and safe to pursue intellectual studies or practical interests. There they could establish hospitals and nursing staffs, cultivate and prepare medicinal drugs, receive and attend the sick and afflicted, perfect the household arts, make gardens, study music and languages, illuminate and copy precious manuscripts, and read and write poetry and drama.

This kind of well-balanced useful life was common in communities under the Benedictine rule founded in the sixth century at Monte Cassino, Italy, by Benedict of Nursia. Such monasteries became centers of great activity, which because of their form of internal government have been compared to small republics. The scheme of life as planned by St. Benedict included seven or eight hours a day to be spent in useful and productive labor. The "rule" was introduced as a means of regulating the austerities and self-inflicted tortures which were then practiced by many who sought to follow the religious life.

ASCETICISM

A marked feature of the religious life of that early period was asceticism. In this cult of Oriental origin there were all degrees of self-mortification, but in the monasteries organized for active work asceticism seems not to have been carried beyond a very strict discipline. Some groups that inculcated neglect of body, dress, and physical surroundings and cultivated an intense and mystical spiritual life were extremely popular in the Eastern Church, and St. John Chrysostom tried to persuade the deaconesses under Olympia to go unwashed. In fastidious Rome asceticism was at first disliked, but St. Jerome in his letters lauded Paula, Fabiola, and other Roman matrons for their neglect of personal appearance, comfort, and health and the austerity of their lives, which had formerly been of great luxury. However, we are told that they bathed and cleansed their patients, clothed the naked, dressed their sores, and carried out the other works of charity stressed especially by the Christian church.

St. Augustine, who evidently knew something of Greek medicine, did not despise the body and considered the welfare of both soul and body essential. What benefited the body he called medicine and included in it food, drink, clothing, shelter, and every means of covering and protection to guard it against injuries and mishaps from without as well as from within. What benefited the soul he called discipline. This included teaching. There were other doctrines, however, which held that the body was a product of demons, as against the soul, which was the work of God. The inference of extreme asceticism is that the body is vile, or at least negligible, and that the severest repressions and bodily sufferings are necessary to subdue the flesh and save the soul. In its pure and symbolic essence, on the other hand, asceticism meant training in self-discipline for the attainment of unselfishness, or, in the words of a modern teacher, "the complete conquest of the spirit over the world and the senses." That such training is essential for service to humanity is self-evident. The point of difference came in methods—practical ascetics lived with people and led useful lives instead of withdrawing to solitary cells to meditate.

Monastic Women

The early monasteries required neither "enclosure" nor a regulation dress, at least outside the walls. The period of greatest freedom in monastic life for women seems to have been between the fourth and the twelfth centuries. A remarkable development of that period was the double monastery under a woman's rule, in which an abbess directed two related houses, one of monks, the other of nuns. Such institutions often divided the hospital nursing, the monks taking the men's, the nuns, the women's wards. Famous heads of double monasteries were Queen Radegunde at Poitiers, Hilda of Whitby, and Hersende of Fontevrault. The last named monastery had 3000 members. The social position of the medieval abbess was most respected and dignified. As the feudal system arose, she was politically the equal of men who held fiefs, and there are instances in which abbesses ranked as peers and cast their votes in religious and political meetings.

Among the earlier monastic women was Saint Brigid of Kildare, daughter of an Ulster prince and disciple of St. Patrick. She is said to have introduced female monasteries into Ireland as early as the fifth century and was known as "the patroness of healing." There are references to her miracles, her healing of lepers, and her attendance on the sick with her nuns.

There were many other commanding figures in the monastic life of the early Middle Ages. Among them were Hrotswitha,

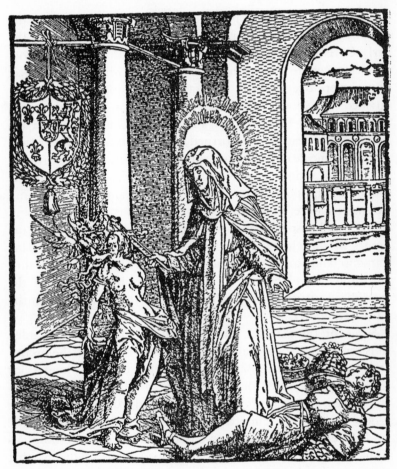

St. Radegunde performing a healing miracle

who knew the Latin classics and wrote dramas, Lisba, Walburga, and Berthgythe who went from Ireland and England to help evangelize Germany, and Hildegarde, "Sybil of the Rhine," whose medical knowledge and political insight were alike remarkable. Such leaders as these trained the women who, amidst other duties, carried on hospital nursing and much medical work over a period of eight centuries.

CHARITABLE WORK UNDER THE CHURCH

The age-old custom of hospitality, which had prevailed in the nations of antiquity, was practiced with religious fervor by the early Christians. Their aim was to hold all things in common. The rich were to give or share all they had with the poor. Their houses were opened wide to every afflicted applicant, and, not satisfied with receiving the needy, the deacons, men and women alike, went out to search for and bring them in. The private homes of the deacons were turned into hospitals called *diakonia*, and the name deacon became synonymous with that of a director of hospital relief. As the bishops' dwellings were especially sought by the poor and sick, they soon became too small, and extensions were added to them. In this way clusters of inns, refuges, and hospital wards grew up about the cathedrals and the homes of the clergy, and these communities in time became immense and varied institutions. The Christian home was thus an ampler development of primitive hospitality, and all the specialized institutions of a later day had their inception in the Christian family.

Some of these larger clusters, called *xenodochia*, included inns for strangers and travelers, hospitals for the sick, the insane, and lepers, asylums for foundlings and orphans, homes for the aged, almshouses for the destitute, dwellings for physicians and nurses, and offices for consultation and administration. This group system was adopted by monasteries until about the twelfth century when it became customary to separate hospitals from other branches of relief and build them singly. At that time towns and cities began to found hospitals as a civic obligation.

SOME EARLY CHRISTIAN HOSPITALS

One of the most famous of the early hospitals was the Basilias, founded and directed by Basil, Bishop of Cesarea, about A.D. 370.

It was like a small city. St. Basil had formed a rule that was adopted by many of the eastern monasteries just as St. Benedict's rule, which was formed nearly two centuries later, became the law for most of the western ones. Both put emphasis on service to one's fellow man, but especially on the care of the sick and homeless.

Still earlier, about A.D. 350, at the time of a severe plague, a notable example of an emergency hospital was created by St. Ephrem at Edessa in Asia Minor. Fabiola's hospital in Rome has been mentioned. It seems to have been strictly a hospital, without almshouse features, for it is called in early writings a *nosocomium* or place for the sick. It is often referred to as the "first hospital," but since Rome had had military hospitals in pagan days it would be more accurate to call it the first Christian hospital in Rome.

Charity in the Eastern Church was developed earlier than in Rome, and there may have been hospitals there, now forgotten. One of the earliest in the West of which mention is made was founded in Spain by Bishop Masona. It is not in existence now, but three of the most ancient hospitals are still in full activity; namely, the Hôtel Dieu in Lyons (A.D. 542), the Hôtel Dieu in Paris (c. A.D. 651), and the Santo Spirito in Rome (thirteenth century). Provisions were also made at a very early date for the sick at the inns and refuges for travelers on the high mountain passes of the Alps and Pyrenees. Every monastery had an infirmary for its own aged or ailing members, as well as a guest house or hospital, varying from a small lodge for emergency cases to a large and well-organized group of wards or buildings.

STATUS OF MEDICINE UNDER MONASTICISM

In the earlier Christian period the medical profession retained to some extent the light of Hippocratic science. Basil, Bishop of Cesarea, was educated at Athens, and in addition to classic subjects he had there gained a thorough knowledge of medicine taught by the Hippocratic school. After the Roman conquest of Greece, Alexandria became the center of Hippocratic medical learning, and medical men practiced dissection. Museums and libraries were opened as scholars of many countries and specialties gathered there, but the passion for metaphysical speculation gradually transformed medicine to mysticism. The last of the great medical men of the ancient world was Galen, who collected all the writings of the past. Though he himself contributed little that was new, he became the medical authority of the world for a thousand years. Dioscorides, author of the first materia medica, should also be mentioned. These two belonged to the first and second centuries A.D.

The early Benedictine monks were advised by Cassiodorus to read the works of Hippocrates, if possible in the original, but other Fathers of the Church retained the old ideas of demonology connected with disease and there was a long struggle between science and superstition, between the spirit of free enquiry and experimentation and the tendency to explain everything in terms of the supernatural and miraculous. The rapid expansion of monastic life had the effect of limiting medical practice to the religious orders for many centuries, and had it not been that the ruling religious thought of that time was out of sympathy with natural science this might have been a great advantage to medical research and progress, for the sick were then gathered together in monasteries, with men and women, the flower of their day, to tend them.

The Benedictine monasteries were especially noted as centers of learning up to the time when universities began to develop (twelfth century), and medical study continued in some degree under their roofs. Hildegarde, in the eleventh century, must have dissected at least the bodies of animals, and possibly the human body, but her records show only that she had to conceal her work under the veil of mystery and protect herself by a claim of supernatural revelation. Her books, remarkable as they are now known to be, were not included in the list of those approved by the Church. The widespread opposition to dissection was, of course, a basic hindrance to the progress of medical knowledge, but from the viewpoint of religious thought at the time dissection seemed a blasphemy, as the body was, in a very special sense, regarded as the temple of the Holy Spirit.

The firm belief in the doctrine of bodily resurrection also inspired popular aversion to the idea of dissection. Then too, rational medicine seemed destructive of the miracle and so of faith.

The clerical power for similar reasons was opposed to surgery, and toward the twelfth century there were several decrees forbidding monks and priests to practice medicine or surgery or at least limiting their practice to their own monasteries. These decrees suggest real progress and activity, as otherwise decrees would not have been needed. Before university schools grew up, lay pupils had been received in monasteries for instruction, but this was discouraged also. These decrees were not universally obeyed, and medical monks practiced clandestinely; nevertheless, the general effect of monasticism on medicine was repressive, and not until different influences came to bear did medical art enjoy a revival.

Though it cannot be claimed that much if any progress was made in the scientific aspects of medicine or of nursing during the first ten centuries of the Christian era, there is no doubt that the humane care of the sick was immensely advanced by the release of a great tide of love, brotherhood, and religious zeal, much of which found expression in direct personal service to the sick and needy. Christianity also gave women an opportunity to share in the work of hospitals and other forms of charitable activity organized under the Church. Single women especially had a chance to exercise their administrative and other abilities and to direct their great reserves of emotional energy into useful and productive channels.

Nursing was only one of the many forms of service undertaken by the various orders that developed before and especially after the monastic movement began. The motives that brought men and women into these orders were not always altruistic, nor were special aptitudes and training for such services given much consideration. However, as the Dark Ages came on and secular medicine was almost completely extinguished in the western world, there was little impetus toward advancement in the science and art of nursing or of medicine. This was the age of theological therapeutics, in which orthodoxy of belief, saintly piety, and a reputation as a miracle worker counted for more than medical knowledge or technical skill or even good physical conditions for the sick. There were, undoubtedly, exceptions, as in the monasteries located in beautiful and peaceful surroundings, where patients had the advantage of good climate and sometimes mineral baths and other conditions favorable to health. The main advancement in nursing during this period probably came through the internal organization and operation of monastic institutions and the discipline and training of large groups of sisters and brothers in their cooperative undertakings. These institutions had a great influence on modern hospitals and on the organization of modern nursing services.

SELECTED BIBLIOGRAPHY

Austin, Anne L. *History of Nursing Source Book*. New York: Putnam's, 1957. Ch. 2.

Clay, Rotha M. *Mediaeval Hospitals in England*. London: Methuen, 1909.

Eckstein, Lina. *Women Under Monasticism*. Cambridge: Cambridge University Press, 1896.

Engbring, Gertrude M. "Saint Hildegard, Twelfth Century Physician," *Bull. Hist. Med.*, June 1940, 770-778.

Flack, Hally. "Nursing in Ireland from Pre-Christian Times to the Middle of the Nineteenth Century," *Int. Nurs. Rev.*, September 1931, 428-446.

Gasquet, Cardinal. (Tr.) *The Rule of St. Benedict*. London: Chatto, 1925.

The New Testament.

Nutting, M. Adelaide, and Lavinia L. Dock. *A History of Nursing*. New York: Putnam's, 1907-1912. 4 vols. Vol. I, Part II, Ch. I-III.

Rand, Edward Kennard. *Founders of the Middle Ages*. Cambridge: Harvard University Press, 1928.

Robinson, Deaconess Cecilia. *The Ministry of Deaconesses*. London: Methuen, 1898.

Tuker, M. A. R., and Hope Malleson. *Handbook to Christian and Ecclesiastic Rome*. London: A. & C. Black, 1897-1900. 4 vols. in 3.

Wright, F. A. (Tr.) *Select Letters of St. Jerome*. New York: Putnam's, 1933. Esp. Letter LXXVII.

CHAPTER 4

Aristocratic and Military Influences

DEVELOPMENT OF FEUDALISM AND CHIVALRY

After the downfall of the Roman power in the western empire the social state of Europe was for a long time that of a "melting pot," race clashing with race for supremacy, ancient classic culture and barbaric rawness striving together, each giving and taking something, each contributing to the amalgamating process. The feudal system arose from the redistribution of landed property and was so worked out that the land still remained in privileged hands. A system of protection and military duty bound the lesser lords to the greater and the peasants to the landowner. The older system of chattel slavery was replaced by serfdom of varying grades for the peasant and laborer. Feudalism, with its highborn knights and its vassals, its fealties, homages, and military service, tinctured with religious exaltations and ceremonials, lent itself to the most dramatic possibilities, familiar to all in novels and poems.

Chivalry and the institution of knighthood were outgrowths of feudalism. The knightly orders arose first in France and had their highest development there but were also found in Britain and in other parts of Europe. The ideal, *noblesse oblige*, laid upon the nobly born the obligation of service and especially the protection and defense of the weak. A practical result of this fine idealism appeared in the military-religious nursing orders into which knights and highborn ladies entered that they might meet the needs arising from the Crusades. Before this period individuals of noble birth, including kings and queens, had sometimes retired into monasteries and joined in their activities. The military orders had a good deal in common with the monastic but became more exclusive, class conscious, and autocratic. This in the end was one reason for their decline.

MILITARY NURSING ORDERS OF THE MIDDLE AGES

Three great military and chivalric nursing orders had their rise in those stirring and romantic times and assumed as their duty a combination of war making, charitable relief, and hospital nursing, under devoutly religious forms. Nothing like them has ever been seen, before or since. They were, in the order of their greatest renown, the Knights Hospitallers of St. John of Jerusalem, Rhodes, and Malta commonly called the Knights of St. John; the Teutonic Knights (*Deutsche Orden*); and the Knights of St. Lazarus. Each had provision for a corresponding order of women. The Order of St. John was originally organized for the care of two hospitals, one for men and the other for women, which had been founded at Jerusalem in the seventh century by wealthy Italian merchants. They were dedicated, respectively, to St. John the Almoner and Mary Magdalene. In charge of the sisterhood of women nurses at Mary Magdalene was a noble Roman lady named Agnes, of whom little is known.

In its inception the Order of St. John was secular, and the knights and ladies met at table and in the wards for the sick, but toward the end of the eleventh century, under the direction of Peter Gerard, who was intensely devout, a strictly religious form was adopted, and the knights and sisters renounced the world by taking vows of poverty, chastity, and obedience. Under its second director, Raymond du Puy, who was essentially a

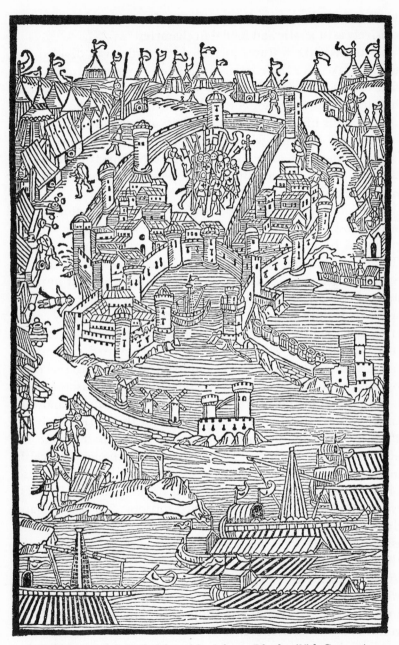

Headquarters of the Knights of St. John at Rhodes (15th Century)

warrior, it took on a markedly military character and became exclusively aristocratic and feudal in character.

As the warlike features increased, the order was divided for utility's sake into three sections: knights or men-at-arms, whose first duty was to fight, yet who were expected to serve in the hospital wards when not engaged in battle; priests who directed the religious life of camp and hospital; and serving brothers or half-knights (*serjeus*) who carried on the regular ward work. These, sometimes called knights-of-grace, came from families that had never engaged in trade or menial work and therefore had some claim to gentility.

The knights and sisters of St. John wore a black habit with a white cross on it. It had eight points, representing eight virtues professed by the order. A red cross was worn by the Knights Templar (not a nursing order). The fame of the Hospitallers of St. John became so great as the result of their excellent nursing and relief work that gifts of land and treasure made the order wealthy. It built hospitals and founded branches in many countries, the English branch dating from the year 1100. A special merit of the order was that it received and nursed the insane, often with great intelligence and sympathy. It was the only one of the military orders that accepted insane patients.

The career of this order was one of great usefulness and distinction until the time of the expulsion of the Christians from Palestine (end of the thirteenth century). From this date its efficiency as a nursing order gradually waned, though its wealth and fame continued to grow. From Jerusalem the central house of the order fled to Cyprus and then to the island of Rhodes, where headquarters were maintained for some 200 years. Again driven out by the Moslems in 1522, the order was given the island of Malta for a headquarters by Charles V. in 1530. By this time wealth and power had corrupted it. Nursing had been gradually neglected, the Sisters of St. John were scattered and weakened, and political activities brought the once famed order into disrepute. It was finally suppressed, but the knights later continued their activities in a very modified form, with branches in several countries, including one recently formed in the United States. The name and best traditions of the order live

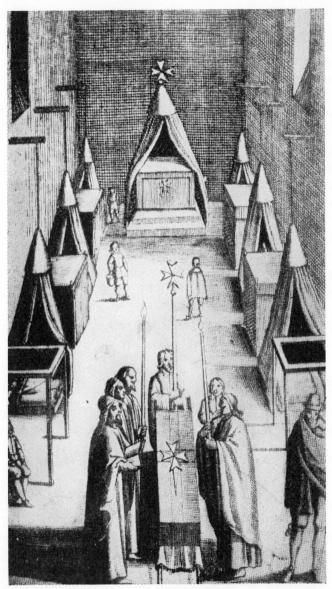

The Great Ward of the Hospital of the Knights of St. John in Valetta, as it appeared in the seventeenth century. From an old German work upon the Order, printed at Augsburg in 1650. The print represents the beds of the sick, with the mosquito-curtains, and the knights in attendance on the patients. In the foreground is a funeral ceremony.

on today in the St. John's guilds and ambulance corps, first-aid-to-the-injured societies, and nursing associations.

At the height of its nursing excellence the hospital regulations worked out by the Order of St. John were adopted by nearly all the city hospitals or *Maisons Dieu* as they arose in Europe. Its influence over medieval hospital management and nursing was therefore very great. Undoubtedly the hospital service of the military nursing orders imprinted a certain military form of organization and discipline upon these institutions, of which distinct traces are still to be seen. The knightly ideals of courtesy and honor, the love of pageantry and ceremonial, the formality and refinement of manner of knights and ladies, must have made a deep impression on hospital life. It is quite probable that certain orthodox hospital ceremonials and forms of etiquette of recent times, notably those of medical rounds and the "standing at attention" of the nurses and junior medical men, have come down to us from the military orders. Their system of marking the various ranks of personnel with different types of uniforms and insignia is perpetuated in Red Cross and similar organizations as well as in hospitals and nursing schools.

TEUTONIC KNIGHTS AND KNIGHTS OF ST. LAZARUS

The Teutonic Knights were founded in 1191 under similar circumstances and on much the same lines as the Order of St. John. Their history is the same, though on a less extended scale, for their branches flourished only in the Teutonic countries. On the whole their nursing service was not so effective as that of the Order of St. John.

The Knights of St. Lazarus specialized in the care of lepers. Tradition carries their origin far back, at least to the days of St. Basil, but their definite organization dates from the First Crusade. Because of the exacting restrictions imposed on lepers, the Knights of St. Lazarus had two divisions, the warriors and the hospitallers. There was also a sisterhood of St. Lazarus for work among women. The order of St. Lazarus had less dazzle of military pomp and glory than the other two knightly orders and a far more sacrificial task in its care of lepers and its struggle with the social conditions surrounding them. Too little is known of its work in detail, probably because of its difficulties. As leprosy, or the ailments classed under that general name, died out in Europe, the order became extinct. In recent times its name and badge were adopted by a modern nursing group in Germany—the "Free Sisters"—of whom more is said in a later chapter.

HOSPITAL WORK UNDER KNIGHTLY ORDERS

The hospitals at Jerusalem under the military nursing orders retained certain aspects of the *xenodochium*. They gave board to the pilgrims (sometimes paying guests) and alms to the poor as well as care to the sick. Asylums for foundlings were a feature of later hospitals under their care. Army hospitals were a specialty of the Order of St. John and of the Teutonic Knights, and these institutions were often filled to overflowing with wounded soldiers. In their work we get the first glimpse of army nursing since the days of the Roman orderly. The hospitallers may indeed be considered as the founders of modern army nursing by professional nurses.

A hint of a kind of visiting nursing service under the auspices of the Knights of St. John in 1725 is given in the "Regulations for the Sick Poor of Malta," in which the following statement is found: "There are four paid maid-servants to wait on the poor, and who make the beds and do anything else that may be necessary." These women as well as the physicians who visited the townspeople and those who dispensed the food were under the supervision of two professed knights, called Commissioners of the Sick Poor, who were appointed by the Grand Master.

Many of the hospitals built by the Knights Hospitallers were of outstanding architectural beauty and were furnished in the most complete way known to their times. At Valetta the patients were served from silver dishes, and linen was provided in abundance. The accounts of their hospital administration show thorough organization. The chief director made rounds with the physicians, and with his assistants supervised all the various housekeeping departments. This hospital continued active up to recent years, and after medicine revived in the twelfth century, a staff physician lectured daily on anatomy and once a week on clinical medicine for the benefit of the younger physicians and nursing brothers. Barber-surgeons, appointed to men's wards, seem to have been entrusted with many procedures now taken over by women nurses. Patients who were needy received clothing and food when they left the wards.

BEGINNINGS OF ORGANIZED RELIEF IN WAR AND CALAMITY

We have pointed out the part taken by the military nursing orders in developing army nursing. The knights of St. John also at an early date brought organization into the work of relief at times of natural calamities and gave an example of efficiency in this type of service in 1783, at the time of an earthquake in Sicily. The account of their services then and the way in which they took charge of the situation reads like a chapter from modern Red Cross relief work. It is therefore not surprising that representatives of the Knights of St. John appeared at the Geneva conference in 1863 to help in founding the committee of the International Red Cross.

ARABIAN INFLUENCE IN MEDICINE

While medical science was stationary or even retrograding in western Europe during the Middle Ages, it was fostered in a remarkable way in the Near East. The Nestorians, a sect banished in the fifth century for heresy, seem to have had a special interest in medical science and in Edessa, Asia Minor, founded a medical school in connection with St. Ephrem's hospital. Thence they went to Persia, taking with them the Greek and Roman classics, and were received with distinction at the Persian court. They built up many medical schools in which the ancient learning of India, China, Arabia, and Persia was cherished and taught with that of Hippocrates and his disciples. A number of famous medical centers of a most cosmopolitan character thus arose where no racial or religious exclusion was practiced and where many Jews and Arabs studied. The term "Arabian medicine" is given to this whole eastern group or school, which for almost ten centuries maintained its leadership over the decaying western branch of medicine, lost in the bogs of the dark ages. The tradition of Greek medicine was thus kept alive and was brought back to Europe when the Arabs conquered Spain.

The Arabs had inherited the wisdom of India, and the Nestorians found that before the Christian era Arabian cities had had hospitals endowed by royal women and named for them. During the 500 years when education was at its most restricted phase in Europe, Saracenic learning, arts, and sciences enjoyed their brilliant period. The Arabs translated the works of Hippocrates and Galen. Though the study of anatomy was discouraged by their religion, they became masters of clinical medicine and trained many skilled physicians. Their chief contribution to medical science was in chemistry and materia medica in which they excelled. Arabian physicians tested the fluids of the body, studied drugs, introduced many new medicinal plants, and showed how to prepare drugs from them. They also kept alive the classical tradition of medicine but had too much respect for the ancients to criticize or add much to what they had written.

Many beautiful hospitals were developed by the Arabs, in which patients were intelligently classified in separate wards. They received lepers and the insane, who were treated with skill and kindness. Some had admirable provision for eye cases and for the blind. They carried on a form of hospital social service by providing needful care for discharged patients who were not quite able to work and had systems of free medical attention for the poor of the cities. Alexandria, Damascus, Baghdad, and Spanish cities maintained such centers of medicine. Cordova alone, in the twelfth century, supported seventeen universities and fifty medical institutions. Jews, who were excluded from other opportunities, studied in these universities and were recognized everywhere in Europe as able physicians. Three of the most distinguished medical scientists of the Arabian school were the Persian Avicenna (980-1037), who translated Aristotle and was the author of standard medical works, Averroës (1126-1198) of Cordova, and Rabbi Maimonides (1135-1204), who served in the court of Saladin during the Crusades. The time came when the Moslem invaders were driven from Europe, but they left an imperishable contribution in their beautiful architecture and their love of learning, shown in their libraries in which the ancient learning of Greece and Rome was preserved for eight centuries. It came back to Europe in the form of a Latin translation of a Hebrew translation of an Arabic commentary on a Syriac translation of the original Greek. Though much garbled, these rediscovered classics helped to rekindle the light of learning in western Europe, and the works of Hippocrates, Galen, and Aristotle were eagerly studied by students at the new universities just founded in Bologna, Padua, and other centers of Europe.

The Knights Hospitallers, who had their roots in feudalism and monasticism and their immediate stimulus in the Crusades, represent a union of diverse and somewhat incompatible characteristics—pride and humility, self-assertion and self-effacement, ostentation and meekness. They soon became more military and less monastic, also less exclusively masculine, as lady hospitallers organized their own branches and united with them in their hospital and first-aid work. The knights set a new standard not only in hospital architecture and equipment but in organization and administration. Personnel were classified according to rank and function, the knights and ladies assuming most of the managerial responsibilities, the clergy and medical attendants having their own duties, and workers of lower rank (but part noble) doing most of the nursing and other practical work. Patients of various classes, not charity cases only, were admitted to these hospitals.

The Hospitallers prided themselves on their voluntary amateur status (serving for love, not gain), but they often had valuable experience in the management of large households, estates, and military units as well as strict upbringing in the system of chivalry which imposed special obligations on those of higher birth. They were taught to do noble deeds, to be courteous and considerate of others, and to give generously to good causes. As they increased in wealth and power, they tended to become more formal and autocratic, to stress pomp and ceremony, and to give less attention to the operation of their hospitals. Nevertheless, they made a real contribution to hospital and first-aid work, and many of their ideas were adopted by the civic hospitals which began to develop with the rise of cities and the decline of feudalism. Later chapters will tell of the Hospitallers' influence on the Red Cross and the conflict between amateurs and professionals which arose when the modern movement for trained nurses began about 100 years ago.

SELECTED BIBLIOGRAPHY

Austin, Anne L. *History of Nursing Source Book*. New York: Putnam's, 1957. Ch. 3, pp. 65-83.

Hume, Edgar E. "Medical Work of the Knights Hospitallers of Saint John of Jerusalem," *Bull. Hist. Med.*, May 1938, 339-466; June 1938, 495-603; July 1938, 677-819.

King, E. G. *The Knights Hospitallers in the Holy Land*. London: Methuen, 1931.

Lamb, Harold. *The Crusades*. Garden City, N. Y.: Doubleday, 1945.

Nutting, M. Adelaide, and Lavinia L. Dock. *A History of Nursing*. New York: Putnam's, 1907-1912. 4 vols. Vol. I, Part II, Ch. IV.

Prestage, Edgar, (Ed.) *Chivalry: Its Historical Significance and Civilizing Influence*. New York: Knopf, 1928.

Schermerhorn, Elizabeth Wheeler. *On the Trail of the Eight-Pointed Cross*. New York: Putnam's, 1940. Ch. III, XII.

CHAPTER 5

Democratic and Secular Tendencies

POLITICAL AND SOCIAL MOVEMENTS

Leaving to one side all the human tragedies connected with the Crusades, those remarkable episodes may be considered as a vast university extension course for great masses of people. New ideas, wider knowledge, and a larger world vision came to medieval society as the Crusaders streamed into Palestine and back again to their western homes. Many narrow conventions were discarded and outworn beliefs exchanged for new, more timely ones. The epoch following on the Crusades was marked by evidences of intellectual growth and popular longing for freedom and progress. Commerce and trade created a powerful middle class. Free cities grew in number and importance, and guilds of artisans and workmen reached a high stage of organization. As the peasants became more articulate, they voiced demands for a redress of grievances, and a free-thinking spirit boldly questioned formal dogmas. The stream of modern democracy took its rise in those wonderful centuries, the twelfth and thirteenth.

This growing tendency was in direct opposition to a type of

formalism, which was at the same time increasing in many of the older orders, even those devoted to nursing. In the military orders it took the form of aristocratic exclusiveness, whereas in the others excessive emphasis was laid upon the great merit of total withdrawal from the world.

ST. FRANCIS'S RETURN TO THE IDEALS OF THE EARLY CHURCH

The newer spirit reacted against the older in the formation of many free secular forms of social groupings for nursing and neighborhood work. The personification of this fresh energy was the youthful Francis of Assisi (born 1181 or 1182), a most lovable, spontaneous, and gentle character, an early Arnold Toynbee (who led in modern settlement work), but more joyous and sunny and perhaps more unconsciously democratic. At a very early age, during an illness, inner promptings turned him with swift completeness to follow literally the teachings of Christ. He therefore left his home (for his family and friends were worldly and pleasure loving, and he had led a carefree life) and went to live among the lepers.

The problem of leprosy had grown increasingly grave since the introduction of the disease into Europe in the fifth and sixth centuries, and attempts to solve it by isolating its victims had had little or no effect. The special genius of St. Francis was shown in his way of attacking the problem. He did not isolate himself with the lepers, nor allow his followers to do so, though one and all were required to live among them. They went back and forth in the world, and by thus bringing leprosy (much of which was really tuberculosis and syphilis) out into the open, as it were, he brought the responsibility home to the entire community, where it belonged, and a beginning was made toward improved social conditions and preventive sanitary measures. His method was very like that used in the modern campaign against tuberculosis.

St. Francis had an immense following, especially among the ardent youth of his age, who became known as Franciscan Men-

dicants, or Gray Friars, and also as Brothers Minor. He insisted
on humility and poverty, but wanted the friars to be joyful and
happy and to live as natural a life as possible, thus leading some
to accuse them of levity and worldliness. They were to work

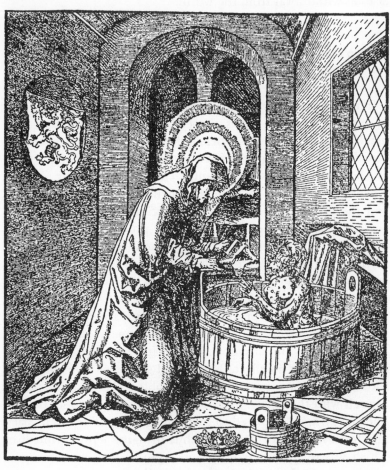

A Royal Saint bathing a leper

with their hands, preach and teach, and convert the heathen.
St. Francis distrusted book learning and emphasized the active,
useful life. After his death, certain friars, such as the scientific
wizard Roger Bacon, studied and taught in the universities.
They were said to have gained much practical knowledge of

medicine, and through their contacts with men and with life they became well informed and worldly wise. Some of them became radical, even revolutionary, and joined actively in the labor movement.

THE POOR CLARES

Clarissa, or Clare, was a charming young girl who had belonged to Francis's worldly circle and who accepted and shared all his ideals. She ran away from her home at night to enter the Church and to put on the garb of a novice. Clarissa then formed and led an affiliated order of young women to help the friars in their work. The brothers undertook to support themselves and the Clarissas or "Poor Clares" by manual labor or begging. In return, the sisters were to mend the brothers' clothes, take care of the little church, and nurse the sick brought to them for special care.

The Franciscan orders were useful and practical during two full centuries. Their nursing may have been very elementary, but it did much good, and the sincerity of the brothers and sisters in carrying out their aim of bringing back the simple, neighborly kindness of the early Church in place of the formal stereotyped charity of the later monastic orders had a great influence on their age.

Later centuries showed a gradual change. The Poor Clares became a contemplative, enclosed order of the most austere type, whereas the friars forgot manual labor in the easier career of begging and were often a general nuisance. But while the spirit of St. Francis remained with them they were a fresh and inspiring example of youthful idealism.

SECULAR ORDERS: TERTIARIES

St. Francis's ideals were most widely represented in the order of Tertiaries, which he founded. In this order the practice of the early Christians was fully revived, for its members were not allowed to leave their homes nor to renounce the world but were to carry their religion into their everyday life and share continually in some unselfish, useful service to humanity. Practical work with the poor, afflicted, and sick was taken up with enthusiasm by the Tertiaries. Such orders still exist in Italy, members volunteering for hospital work, friendly visiting, burying the dead, carrying patients to hospitals, and similar activities. The flexible nature of the Third Order adapted it well to nursing, and it became extremely popular with men and women who were attracted to the care of the sick. Many famous medieval nurses who are now canonized were in their day members of the Third Order of St. Francis, among them Elizabeth of Hungary and Catherine of Siena, a member of the Order of St. Dominic, patterned after that of St. Francis. The demands made upon the Tertiaries for hospital nursing led eventually to the formation of communities and convents, whose members took only simple vows.

As the strictly religious orders, under the pressure of the clergy, inclined more and more to the seclusion of solemn or perpetual vows, new active orders sprang up in many directions which expressed the desire of women for self-organization and self-direction in congenial work without rigid vows. These organizations were not technically "religious" but were imbued with a religious spirit.

THE BEGUINES

The Beguines of Flanders were leaders among these secular orders. They antedated the Franciscan Tertiaries, for their first community was built in 1180, just before St. Francis was born. The organization of the Beguines seems to have been a revolt against abuses that had developed in the double monastery system, for their first spokesman, Lambert le Bégue, a priest of Liége, asserted their claim to live God-fearing lives outside strict church rule and to carry on work separately from men.

The Beguines did not take vows of poverty and promised chastity and obedience only while they remained members of the Beguinage. They could therefore leave and marry, possess property, and earn money. They also continued to a certain extent to share in social and family life. Their work developed according to their own ideas; some made lace, others taught, and many became hospital or visiting nurses. Hospital work was soon one of their chief interests, and, as their communities grew and acquired wealth, they built their own hospitals and administered them. St. Esprit, one of the most famous, which exists in all its beauty today, was founded in 1443 at Beaune in France. Sometimes they provided nursing staffs for hospitals under different control.

The Beguines endured a certain amount of persecution for their freedom of thought and action. They were accused of heresy and of believing it unnecessary "to fast or to obey mortal men." So strong were they in popular esteem, however, that the opposition did them little real harm. They remained numerous and active for several centuries, spreading far into Germany. There are still several communities remaining, notably those at Ghent and Bruges, which are well known to travelers. The Beguines of today do not do as much nursing as their predecessors but respond to special calls. They were, for example, active in World War I.

ORDERS OF THE COMMON LIFE AND SANTO SPIRITO

A similar order of women was the Sisterhood of the Common Life, founded in Flanders in the fourteenth century. These sisters specialized in visiting nursing. On the rolls of a brotherhood of the same name (but not engaged in nursing) appear the names of some of the noted humanists of that day, who correspond to our modern intellectual progressives.

An important secular nursing order of men called Santo Spirito arose in the twelfth century in Montpellier. It was a free brotherhood founded by Guy de Montpellier in 1145 and came to be especially identified with the large general hospitals of towns and cities. From that time on, as towns grew up and became self-governing, more hospitals were taken under the control of the civil authorities or were built anew inside city walls. A related order of women nurses in the Santo Spirito organization, overlooked by historians in their interest in the men's branches, seems to have had a flourishing career for more than a century. The order retained its free character and carried on its work in a great number of cities, especially in Switzerland and Germany, where at one time it had more than 150 hospitals in its care.

It is quite possible that this nursing order of men may have contributed largely to the revival of medicine in the twelfth century, for men engaged in nursing incline naturally toward medicine and often pass into the ranks of medical men. Toward the end of the thirteenth century a papal edict made all the houses of the order subject to the one in Rome. This was the first step toward altering the free form of the brotherhood. Within the next two centuries it became strictly monastic and died out.

THE OBLATES OF FLORENCE

An order of secular sisters, originally called oblates (from "oblation," "dedication," meaning a religious offering or sacrifice) was founded in Florence in the thirteenth century. These sisters have nursed in the chief Florentine hospitals from that day to the present time and have always been distinguished for their excellent work and for the unusually broad professional instruction allowed to them, as compared with that of many other Italian nursing orders.

The history of these important free nursing orders of the Middle Ages suggests a positive incompatibility between the needs of a nursing service and an artificial limitation of the nurse's capacities and training. This was so well understood by prominent women in medieval times that we find numerous examples of such women refusing to be bound by vows because they wished to control their own wealth and be free to conduct nursing work as they thought best. Many entered hospitals which they endowed and in which they spent their lives in service. Among them may be mentioned Elizabeth, Queen of Portugal, and Mlle de Melun, daughter of the Prince of Epinay, both especially distinguished for the practical character of their work.

THE NURSING SAINTS

Whatever the religious belief of modern nurses may be, none needs to feel any unwillingness to accept the title "saint" as conferred upon mortals, for in its symbolic sense it is simply a recognition of a life rich in beneficent service, given as orders of merit are given today. In World War II many nurses were decorated. So, in the Middle Ages, many canonical saints received their titles, sometimes partly, sometimes entirely, for their eminence in the care of the sick, crippled, and blind. It is true that the most prominent nursing saints often had other distinguished deeds to their credit. They organized groups of co-workers, aroused public opinion, were teachers and prophets, guided political events and stimulated social ethics. Modern nurses have also done these things.

Among the nursing saints we have mentioned St. Francis and his remarkable social service. St. Vincent de Paul was a colossal figure, best remembered as the founder of the Sisters of Charity. St. Catherine of Siena, who had a remarkable share in public events, nursed in La Scala Hospital in Siena, where her little lantern was as famous as Miss Nightingale's lamp of later years. St. Hildegarde, doctor as well as nurse, was famed for her scientific learning. St. Camillus was a devoted nurse, greatly beloved. St. Bernard, in the intervals of his public work, treated the eyes, and is shown in paintings as curing the blind. Saints Cosmos and Damian were surgeons. Elizabeth of Portugal, Anne of Bohemia, Bridget of Sweden, Bridgid of Kildare, who nursed lepers, Modwena, who healed epileptics, and Walburga, who studied medicine, all had remarkable gifts and careers in nursing. St. Hedwig, Queen of Silesia, tended lepers, organized hospitals, and carried on many works of charity. St. Roch of Montpellier was devoted to the plague stricken and was said to have healed them with the sign of the cross. Most beloved, perhaps, and sweetest of all the nursing saints was Elizabeth of Hungary,

heroine of the legend of the roses. Similar evidences of extreme
piety, asceticism, and austerity of life are reported for many of
these saints, and they were freely credited with miraculous
powers.

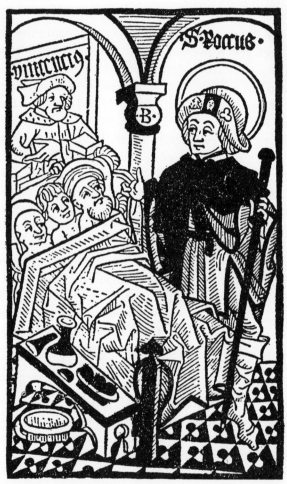

St. Roch, Patron Saint of patients afflicted with Plague

The process of bestowing sainthood upon a nurse has taken
place lately enough for us to see how it is done, as in the case of
Mme de Chantal, grandmother of Mme Marie de Sévigné. After
her death in 1641, an inquiry took place to substantiate her good

deeds. The old peasants from her estates were called to testify to the incidents of her life and told in great detail, and with the most naïve realism, of all the wonderful cures she had brought about by nursing in their cottages and by taking serious cases into her own home.

THE BEGINNING OF CIVIC RELIEF OF POVERTY

Poverty, that social disease which testifies to broken or disregarded natural law in the social organism, has always been the prolific parent of physical disease, as every visiting nurse knows. From the earliest times communities have made efforts, usually futile, to meet this problem. The ancient Jews tried to prevent poverty by their system of redistributing land. Classic civilizations arrived at a caste of poverty, and beggars had certain definite rights. Monasticism carried on an immense system of relief by almsgiving, yet it did nothing to prevent poverty and probably did as much to perpetuate it as to relieve it by doles. However, the whole system of land ownership in the Middle Ages fostered poverty, as it also developed monasticism. Monastic charity was institutional rather than social, as pointed out by Loch[1], who also shows that it was, in spite of its limitations, a step in advance of the older caste system.

The first halting attempts of the civil powers to deal with poverty date from the ninth century. These attempts were quickened in the fourteenth and fifteenth centuries, when the suppression of monasteries, after the Protestant revolts in Germany, England, and Switzerland, threw upon the civil arm the burden of relief which had been carried previously by the monastic orders. England created Overseers of the Poor in 1572. The hospital directors in Paris shared the laicizing tendency by appointing paid secular ward nurses in 1692.

The relation of poverty to disease was long obscured by the profound general ignorance of sanitary laws. The Black Death (1349) carried off, it is said, one quarter of the population of Europe. The first English Sanitary Act was passed by Parliament

[1] Charles S. Loch, *Charity and Social Life* (London: 1910).

in 1388, but the connection between filth and sickness continued to be popularly ignored, though Erasmus, the celebrated humanist and scholar (born c. 1466) pointed it out in his writings. In general, the policy of secular authorities of the later Middle Ages in dealing with poverty was to treat it as a crime and those applying for relief as criminals. The care and protection of children especially lagged under civic guardianship up to the eighteenth century, and the fate of destitute orphans in European countries often made the ancient pagan customs of exposing superfluous infants to death seem kind by comparison.

THE REVIVAL OF MEDICINE IN THE UNIVERSITIES

It is considered that the term "dark ages" must not be applied after the eleventh century, for revivals of intellect and spirit gave a fresh impetus to human progress from that time, and the twelfth century is often spoken of as the period of a true renaissance antedating the Renaissance of the fifteenth century. Groups of students and masters who formed themselves into guilds were the beginnings of universities, and from the tenth century the city of Salerno had been famous for the physicians whose labors culminated in a medical school. The origin of this school has been sometimes attributed to Saracenic influence and again to the survivals of Greek culture in Sicily. It probably owed something to both and also to the Jews, for Jewish physicians were among those who created the medical school. The Benedictine monks of Monte Cassino are said to have shared actively in the building up of this medical and health center, which was situated quite near them on the west coast of Italy. It is believed, however, that secular influences controlled it, since it gave no teaching in theology.

Salerno certainly became an important center of medical learning, and through it flowed that twelfth-century revival of medicine in Europe which produced the famous medical schools in the universities of Bologna, Naples, and Padua, in Italy, and Montpellier, in France. There the works of the Greek masters were studied, and great freedom of scientific inquiry prevailed.

Perhaps the best proof of the advanced liberality, especially of these Italian medical schools, is that their doors were open to women.

In northern countries the progress of medicine was more difficult. There the great universities grew out of the guilds and student bodies, inspired largely by the brilliant intellect of Abelard (1079-1142), but theology long remained dominant in Paris and in English universities, and though the fine arts expanded and flourished there was little freedom for medicine. Surgery, especially, suffered from laws against dissection. Edicts of the twelfth and thirteenth centuries, limiting the surgical practice of the monks, had resulted in the creation of the barber-surgeon caste, which had a long and difficult struggle to gain recognition. Then Louis IX (St. Louis) founded a society called the College of Surgeons, and by 1268 a guild of master-surgeons had been formed which attempted to control the uneducated barber-surgeons and to compel them to limit their practice to minor applications. A bitter struggle followed which resulted in the barber-surgeons agreeing to work under the college-trained surgeons, doing the despised handwork of dissecting and operating while the master did the directing and the lecturing. Finally the barber-surgeons won their freedom to practice independently and it was through them that modern surgery at last came into its own. Many of these men had acquired their skill in the army and, especially after gunpowder came into use, had had extensive experience in the treatment of wounds.

The Italian influence gradually made itself felt in northern universities. The thirteenth century saw many scientific discoveries and felt the stimulus of the experimental method as practiced and taught by Roger Bacon, whereas the dissemination of knowledge was facilitated by the invention of movable type in 1454. The first chairs of medicine at Oxford and Cambridge were established in the fifteenth century, and from this time there was a steady advance.

Before much progress could be made, however, it was necessary to break the habit of looking back constantly to the ancients as the only source of medical wisdom and to turn people's minds definitely toward the discovery of new scientific truth. One of the leaders in this revolutionary movement was the Swiss Paracelsus, born in 1490, a loud, conceited, dissipated fellow, who traveled from country to country, denouncing Galen, burning his books, and advertising his own new discoveries in medicine and chemistry as worth more than all the ancients' lore. In spite of these exaggerations, there was much truth in his teachings and he stimulated a healthy scepticism which helped to pave the way for the new scientific movement in medicine.

Ambroise Paré, who rose from the ranks of the barber-surgeons to become the founder of modern scientific surgery, was born at Laval, France, probably in 1510. One of his contemporaries was Andreas Vesalius, the great Belgian anatomist, who was condemned to death by the Inquisition and was saved only by the interposition of Charles V. The Spaniard Michael Servetus, a fellow student of Vesalius and a pioneer in the study of physiology, was burned at the stake in Geneva by order of John Calvin because he would not recant his unitarian beliefs. Religious intolerance was in the air and neither side had a monopoly of the persecuting mania. In 1578 William Harvey, famed discoverer of the circulation of the blood, was born in England. After being educated in the English universities, he studied at Padua. These men represented the new spirit of scientific inquiry and the new methods of scientific investigation.

The high tide of the Renaissance was now surging over the northern countries. Italy had first felt its sweep, when, after the fall of Constantinople in 1453, scholars and scientists had brought back with them the accumulated treasures of eastern art and learning. The modern era was now beginning, and the darkest age of medicine was over, though a long discouraging period in nursing still lay ahead.

Because of the social changes, the rise of towns, and the great increase in poverty and disease, it became evident that neither the monastic nor the military orders were able to cope with the problems of medical and nursing care. Creative and dramatic leadership was needed to stir the people of these communities to definite action on behalf of their fellow citizens. St. Francis, with his religious idealism and civic spirit, dramatized the need and led the way toward such community activities.

In reviving the simple, direct, neighborly service of the early Church workers, he did a great deal to develop the true spirit of nursing, but he did not see the need to strengthen the knowledge and skill of those who provided it. This was the great lack of the various individuals and groups who were inspired by his example to care for the lepers and other sick and neglected people. The revival of learning had little effect on nursing at this time, and even the most inspired and devoted saints and good neighbors were seriously handicapped without the light of science and adequate technical training.

SELECTED BIBLIOGRAPHY

Austin, Anne L. *History of Nursing Source Book*. New York: Putnam's, 1957. Ch. 3, pp. 84-106.

Chesterton, G. K. *St. Francis of Assisi*. Garden City, N. Y.: Doubleday, 1924.

De Robeck, Nesta. *St. Clare of Assisi*. Milwaukee: Bruce, 1951.

———. *Saint Elizabeth of Hungary*. Milwaukee: Bruce, 1954.

Englebert, Omer. *Saint Francis of Assisi*. Tr. by Edward Hutton. London: Longmans, 1950.

Guttmacher, Alan F. "Ambroise Paré Does a Delivery," *Bull. Hist. Med.*, November 1936, 703-717.

Jorgensen, Johannes. *Saint Catherine of Siena*. Tr. by Ingeborg Lund. New York: Longman's Green, 1938.

Mechelynck, Cecile. "The Beguinages," *Int. Nurs. Rev.*, April 1929, 130-134.

Nutting, M. Adelaide, and Lavinia L. Dock. *A History of Nursing*. New York: Putnam's, 1907-1912. 4 vols. Vol. I, Part II, Ch. V-IX, XIII.

Packard, Francis R. *Life and Times of Ambroise Paré (1510-1590) with a New Translation of His Apology and an Account of His Journeys to Divers Places*. New York: Hoeber, 1921.

Sabatier, Paul. *Life of St. Francis of Assisi*. Tr. by Louise Seymour. New York: Scribner's, 1894.

"Shining Lights," *Nurs. Times*, December 24, 1954, 1431-1434.

Walsh, James J. *The Thirteenth: Greatest of Centuries*. New York: Fordham University Press, 1943.

CHAPTER 6

Dark Period and Dawn of Modern Times

ECONOMIC AND RELIGIOUS MOVEMENTS

The currents of popular feeling which brought about the insurgent movements of the sixteenth century had more than one source. Among the laboring masses there was deep resentment against serfdom and oppression. Intellectual circles criticized and ridiculed the doctrinal absurdities of extreme ecclesiasticism, whereas in deeply religious hearts there was a longing to return to a simpler faith and more sincere observance of religious ceremonials. From the economic standpoint, especially, the dominant church in its then large temporal power had become generally oppressive. Its exactions were felt alike by king and peasant. The Protestant revolt brought to a climax influences that had been previously at work weakening the monastic system, and the changes resulting from the decline of monasticism had a distinct influence on nursing work and hospital organization.

DETERIORATION IN HOSPITALS AND NURSING

While the secular nursing societies of the twelfth and thirteenth centuries were gaining strength, many of the older, more conventionalized orders approached a stage of stagnation. Certain significant events showed this tendency. In 1212 the bishops in council drew up regulations for the French hospitals, including rules for the nursing staffs. It was decreed that all nursing orders were to take vows of poverty, chastity, and obedience and to wear religious garb. It was further decreed that, to economize the gifts of the faithful, the nursing work in hospitals should be performed by the smallest possible number of sisters. The result of this policy of repression and overwork is clearly shown in the history of the nursing sisterhood of the Hôtel Dieu in Paris. It happens that unusually ample records dealing with the nursing service of that famous hospital are available, and these records are written from two opposite viewpoints, the secular and the clerical.

The Sisters of the Hôtel Dieu had evolved from a little group of volunteers who took charge of the sick when the hospital was only a small house containing a few beds and elementary appliances (A.D. 660). The religious order that gradually took shape there never assumed any other duties than ward nursing. It had no diversity through teaching or through embroidery and other household arts. These sisters are distinguished, therefore, as the oldest purely nursing order of nuns in existence. Their first 600 years were probably marked by no more artificial restrictions than were usual in that early time. But under Innocent IV (1243-1254), who was opposed to self-government in women's religious associations, and following the bishop's decree, the Sisters of the Hôtel Dieu were given a rigid rule according to St. Augustine. They became, in effect, a cloistered order, since they could not go beyond the hospital walls except by permission of the clergy.

From the standpoint of the prosperity of the monastic system itself, the growing dogmatism of the clergy was a mistaken policy, for ever since the thirteenth century the trend had been away from the monastic life. With the progress of commerce and trade, the growth of the middle class and the extension of knowledge, it no longer had the same appeal as at an earlier time and there were now other opportunities for self-improvement and service to those in need.

Yet the abrupt change brought about by the sudden closing of monasteries during the Reformation shut many hospitals to the sick poor and threw nursing for a time into a state of utter disorganization. Public authorities were by no means ready to take over such work, nor was medieval Protestantism more liberal in its attitudes. Martin Luther was narrow in his views on women's sphere, and his emphasis on faith rather than works as a means of salvation offered little inducement to men or women to take up self-sacrificing careers. This and the controversial temper of the time helped to account for the marked loss of interest in things charitable and humane.

CHANGES IN ENGLISH NURSING

The altered conditions in nursing brought about by the suppression of the monastic orders were especially striking in England where under the despotic Henry VIII the dissolution of the monasteries was carried out in a very drastic manner. There, it is believed, considerably more than a hundred hospitals were summarily wiped out of existence, with their parent orders, and no alternative provisions made for the sick poor. England did not have secular nursing orders, such as the Flemish Beguines, who worked freely in homes and communities and lived in their own small houses.

The records and history of monastic orders of women in England indicate that, whatever the faults of the system may have been, great sweetness, charm, and usefulness were found in the interior life. In surroundings often of great beauty the nuns practiced housekeeping, horticulture, agriculture, teaching, and nursing. Among those who served in hospitals were found many sisters who were gracious and kindly, well disciplined and practically efficient. Though they lacked the systematic training and knowledge that their professional followers in that country received some centuries later, they showed many of the same personal qualities that are notable in English nurses in modern times. The loss of this system left English nursing in a depth from which secular authorities for a long time did little or nothing to extricate it.

The wealth then taken from the monastic orders was turned into institutions benefiting men only, and thus the possibilities of education for girls, who had been taught in the convents by the nuns, were lost, and nurses for hospital service were drawn more and more from the illiterate classes. The secular authorities now managed all surviving hospitals and staffed them throughout by paid attendants. In some details the English retained the form of the monastic nursing hierarchy. A matron continued to be at the head of the nursing staff, even though she was in effect little more than an untrained housekeeper, and the title "sister" was given as before to the head nurse of a ward. An ordinance of 1699 specified that only the wives of "freemen" should hold the position of sister. The under nurses were of inferior status.

Among the ancient hospitals thus laicized were St. Peter and St. Leonard in York (founded A.D. 936), St. Bartholomew's for Lepers in Rochester (1342), St. John Baptist near Canterbury (1084), St. Giles-in-the-Fields (1117), St. Bartholomew's, founded by the monk Rahere (1123), and St. Katharine's (1148). The three last named are in London.

DECLINE IN SECULAR HOSPITALS

After the Protestant revolt, the deterioration in hospital nursing brought about by such changes continued to spread not only in England but on the Continent. The older system was passing away and the new had not yet unfolded. The political conditions of that period seemed to induce a general apathy and indifference to suffering. The new hospitals erected under city management were mostly cheerless and dreary places, airless and insanitary, very different from the spacious, cloistered, beautiful buildings of the Saracens and the medieval monasteries that had

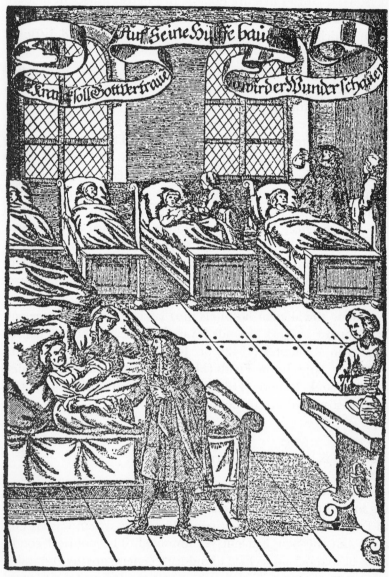

A seventeenth century hospital showing the lay nurses and the physicians on their rounds.

been built in wide country regions, with gardens and fountains in their courtyards.

The medical profession was making some progress toward improved methods of study and treatment, but few trained physicians were available. Though now endowed with a more ample authority in the secular hospitals than in those controlled by religious orders, the physicians had no intelligent nursing staffs to assist them, and the patients were regarded as so much material for experimentation. Their comfort was of little account. The doctors continued to encourage a primitive dread of fresh air; bathing was a luxury, sometimes even tabooed, bleeding and purging and other reducing measures were extensively used, and weak teas, possets, and thin gruels formed the dietary.

The subjection of women increased during these heavy centuries, and superstition was no less prevalent in Protestant than in Roman Catholic countries. Witch baiting and burning continued, and not until 1736 was the crime of witchcraft struck out of the English laws. The deprivation of education for women and girls was deliberate and intentional and was justified by elaborate arguments to prove that such education was not only useless but actually disruptive and dangerous. To add to the general distress of the time, the Great Plague of London struck in 1665, followed by the Great Fire. These disasters, regarded by some contemporary writers as a punishment for sin, called into service nurses who were almost unanimously condemned as worse than none at all.

The secular woman nurse, now at her lowest point, was illiterate, heavy-handed, venal, and overworked. Her time was divided among housework, laundry, scrubbing, and a pretense at nursing of the most rough-and-ready kind. She seldom refused a fee and often demanded it. Strong drink was her weakness and often her refuge from the drudgery of her life. Usually she was a middle-aged woman and often a powerful virago. Charles Dickens, who wrote in the early nineteenth century, has left us an immortal pen picture in *Martin Chuzzlewit* of such persons as Sairey Gamp and Betsy Prig. It is not surprising that the average family of those days dreaded and avoided the hired nurse and dosed itself with homemade medicine, for which the recipes were found in herbals, books containing the family medical traditions well mixed with superstitious notions. The status of the nurse in hospitals deteriorated steadily, as is indicated by the fact that in 1752 the directors of English hospitals made an attempt to change the title "sister" to "nurse" and that of "nurse" to "helper." The power of public sentiment, however, made this attempt useless. Secular men as well as women served in many hospitals and were of an equally low type.

RELIGIOUS HOSPITALS

The sisters of the oldest religious orders suffered also from the general deterioration of nursing standards. The example of overwork indeed had been set by the Church, for the shift of ward work for the nuns, copied sometimes by the secular authorities, was often a rotating twenty-four-hour day. This division of time might have been marked by the observing traveler in Germany and Austria in hospitals nursed by sisters and in vast secular city institutions as late as 1912.

The limitations of the nuns' nursing functions, before the Sisters of Charity appeared, made it impossible for them to be of much real service to patients, and they became increasingly occupied with administrative and housekeeping duties, leaving most of the nursing, such as it was, to servant nurses. They might not care for, nor look at, any parts of the human body except the head and extremities. It followed that they could not prevent bedsores nor keep patients clean. No one knows just when this tradition arose. It may explain much of the persistent effort of women in the Middle Ages to shake off clerical rule and to work under free nursing systems. At any rate, as medical science grew, this tradition of false modesty became more and more untenable for women who had to care for the sick. Then, too, they were continually called away from nursing duties for religious exercises. Possibly this had always been a part of the system of nursing by religious orders, but it was now more clearly recognized as a limitation by some of the clergy as well as by the physicians and the public.

ST. VINCENT DE PAUL —FATHER OF ORGANIZED CHARITY

The upbuilding of modern nursing began with the work of Vincent de Paul and the co-workers associated with him in hospital reform and in the creation of the Sisters of Charity. From the labors of St. Vincent came also the main structure of modern organized methods for dealing with the many-sided problems of destitution and relief. In his long consecrated life we see St. Vincent as a man whose social vision was so far ahead of his time that even yet the majority of his followers have not caught up with him. His life work was a complete whole, and since the Sisters of Charity fitted into this larger pattern we shall deal with them first.

Vincent de Paul was a parish priest, a man of most simple, unpretending character and exceptional goodness and wisdom. He was born in 1576 and lived until 1660, in a period of widespread misery to which war, pestilence, famine, the destitution of religious refugees, and the horrors of industrial slavery all contributed. St. Vincent's study of social conditions, and his reflections, brought him to a most advanced point of view. Indeed, many of his beliefs were then considered revolutionary. He was convinced that poverty could be abolished. Even in this day organized charities have but recently adopted that doctrine, and in his own times, poverty was popularly regarded as a divine chastisement or at least a spiritual discipline. He advocated thorough education for the young, including manual training and the teaching of skilled trades. To deal with beggary, at that time a real pest, he urged that farm colonies be formed and offenders classified according to the work that each was able to do.

Beyond this St. Vincent de Paul would have society as a whole contribute whatever else was needed. He saw that some individuals could never wholly support themselves and believed it was the duty of an organized society to provide for the deficit. To deal with poverty, his plan was to have systematic friendly visiting that the poor might be personally known. Then relief was not to overlap or fail through inadequacy but was to be effective and continuous. The Confraternity of Charity formed in 1617 under his counsel for work on these lines constituted the first societies for organized aid. The women, known as the Ladies (Dames) of Charity, cared for the sick in their homes. To supplement their work, the Daughters of Charity (Sisters of Charity) were organized later with the assistance of Mlle le Gras (Louise de Marillac), one of Vincent's first and most able co-workers. Indeed, Mlle le Gras is regarded as the chief creator of the Sisters of Charity. This assistance was to consist not only of alms but of constructive help.

Vincent's support in bringing about hospital reforms was sought by women who had been his aides in friendly visiting. One of them, especially, Mme de Goussault, had been accustomed to visit the Hôtel Dieu in Paris and had become so keenly conscious of its problems that she persuaded him to extend the visiting service to this hospital. By their efforts an excellent hospital social service department, as it might be called, was developed, first in the Hôtel Dieu and then in other large hospitals of Paris. The close contact of these women with the sick and with the overworked Augustinian sisters impressed upon them the need of reforms in the nursing service.

The Sisters of Charity

To meet this need and others in the simplest way, St. Vincent brought young country girls to live in the homes of the Ladies of Charity and to go with them to work in the homes and hospitals under their supervision. This was so successful that in 1633 a group of these young women was placed in the charge of Mlle le Gras. In a little house on a quiet street in Paris they formed the Order of the Sisters of Charity, perhaps the most widespread and best beloved of all nursing orders.

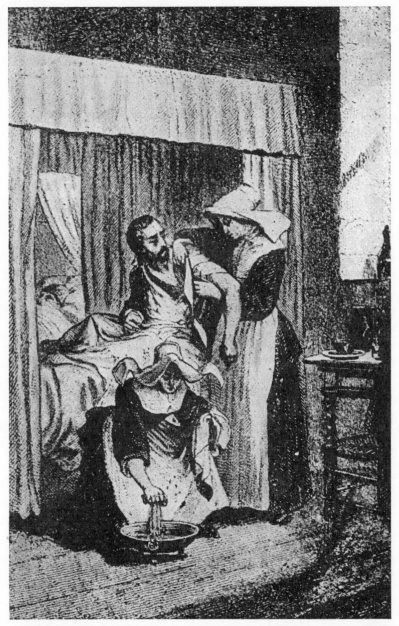

Sisters of Charity dressing a surgical patient (*Les Edifices Hospitaliers,*
C. Tollet, 1892)

St. Vincent's rules for the sisters show how thoroughly he understood the defects of the rigidly organized orders. He would not allow them to take vows or even to make binding promises. They agreed to remain for only a year but could renew this agreement. At the end of any annual contract they might, if they wished, leave and marry. He did not even give them a constitution until they had been organized for twenty years. He wanted them to be properly instructed and gave them most earnest counsel about yielding implicit obedience to the physician. This was radical teaching, for the strictly religious sister obeyed the priest rather than the physician, even sometimes in regard to medical orders.

St. Vincent's advice to the sisters on the necessity for remaining secular, if they were to be useful as nurses, was uncompromising in the extreme. "My daughters," he said, "you are not religious in the technical sense, and if there should be found some marplot among you to say 'it is better to be a nun,' ah! then, my daughters, your company will be ready for extreme unction. Fear this, my daughters, and while you live permit no such change; never consent to it. Nuns must needs have a cloister, but the Sister of Charity must needs go everywhere."

He wished the sisters to be instructed in reading, writing, and arithmetic and suggested that they should form classes among themselves to question one another in the manner of a modern "quiz" on the lectures given them by the physicians. He had no patience with overwork. "Be careful not to overdo," he wrote to Mlle le Gras, "it is a trick of the devil by which he deceives good souls, to entice them to do more than they can and so make them unable to do anything at all."

When the Sisters of Charity had progressed to the point that they were sent to distant parishes as visiting nurses, St. Vincent counseled them not to take more than eight nursing cases at one time. This is just the number that modern visiting nurses later found could not well be exceeded in one day's work, if good nursing was to be done. The sisters brought youth, enthusiasm, and fresh zeal into nursing and became widely popular. Their motherhouses soon encircled the globe. They took charge of hospitals, foundling asylums, homes for the insane, and general parish work. The French army adopted them, and they gave heroic service during the Napoleonic wars. In the early days of the Crimean War, war correspondents, after describing the deplorable conditions in the English regiments, pointed out that an ample staff of Sisters of Charity had accompanied the French forces as nurses and asked why English soldiers could not have similar care.

THE WORK OF JOHN HOWARD

The painful social conditions of the eighteenth century stirred a number of humane men to devote their powers, as St. Vincent de Paul had done, to ameliorating the miserable lives of the unfortunate. Prominent among them was the English philanthropist John Howard (1726-1790), who investigated prisons all over England and in continental countries. Dungeon horrors then unknown to outsiders were recorded and reported by him in writings that made a profound impression and brought about certain improvements. Incidentally, as he came to them, Howard visited hospitals, and also made a thorough examination of European lazarettos. In his book *Hospitals and Lazarettos* his many illuminating criticisms described the nursing conditions very clearly. They were usually deplorable. The only commendations he had to give were for the Sisters of Charity and the Beguines.

The conditions of the indigent insane were perhaps even worse than those of prisoners. The details of the cruel tortures to which they were often subjected under the ignorant supposition that terror, cold, shock, and restraint helped to subdue them are too painful to recite, yet everyone should read in reliable sources the dreadful facts in order to realize how lately we have come out of barbaric darkness and how much still remains to be done, especially in this much neglected field of medicine and nursing.

SOME OTHER EARLY REFORMERS

In the latter part of the eighteenth century several advanced physicians, French, English, and German, began to realize the need for better nursing and wrote textbooks on nursing technique, the management of the sick, and child care. Such books might have helped had the illiterate servant-nurses been able to read them or to apply what they read. However, others, including the intelligent laity and some medical men, did read them and the subject was agitated and discussed.

The Society of Friends has always stood for humane and kindly service to others and for the equality of men and women. Their influence was felt by prominent dissenters, such as John Wesley, who was especially interested in the social aspects of religious work and in medicine. As opposed to the position of the Established Church, chief bulwark of English conservatism, he advocated a wider sphere for women in evangelical and humanitarian work.

The cause of humanitarian reform was greatly aided during the eighteenth century by a movement called the Enlightenment, which culminated in the French Revolution. Radical groups of the century, led by rationalists and intellectuals of France, used both ridicule and reason to undermine the old debasing superstitions that underlay the social order and to advance the ideas of liberty, equality, and fraternity which formed the basis of the new democratic movement. It is true that the French Revolution also led to wild and cruel excesses, but it helped to clear the way for many reforms.

The position of women which began to improve, especially in England, in the early nineteenth century owes much to Mary Wollstonecraft's epoch-making book, *A Vindication of the Rights of Women,* written in 1792. The "rights" claimed by this radical and brilliant woman were, in effect, simply human rights, to be impartially applied to women as human beings. Conservative women were led more cautiously by Hannah More, who in 1788 wrote her *Modern System of Female Education.* She was one of the humanitarian "blue stockings" of England (they) would now be called "high-brows" or "do-gooders") and was sincerely devoted to the welfare and education of the poor. Her aim, however, was rather to make them submissive to their lot than to bring about radical reforms. Neither of these women had anything to do directly with nursing, but they had great influence on public opinion and helped to launch the women's movement with which modern nursing was closely associated.

TWO FORERUNNERS OF MODERN NURSES

More closely identified with practical reforms and with the revival of nursing were Elizabeth Fry, the English Quaker, and Amalie Sieveking of Hamburg, Germany. Mrs. Fry, beautiful, earnest, intensely religious, a gifted speaker, and the mother of eleven children, was a leader in prison reform. Through her efforts among women in Newgate prison, she became widely known as a philanthropist, and toward the end of her life founded a society for visiting nursing, which had its origin in her prison work. The title first used was Protestant Sisters of Charity, later changed to Nursing Sisters.

Mrs. Fry was in close touch with similar leaders of humane thought elsewhere, among them Amalie Sieveking, a single woman of independent means, whose altruism had led her into volunteer hospital service during an epidemic of cholera. She had for a time thought of devoting herself entirely to nursing, but circumstances prevented it, and her life was spent in general philanthropy. Unconventional in her religious views but deeply religious in spirit, she had a gift for wise counsel and was directly concerned in the development of Kaiserswerth, in which Mrs. Fry also had a deep interest. Miss Sieveking formed a society called Friends of the Poor. Its members, who had no formal training for such work, performed a kind of social service which included visiting and a little nursing.

THE FLIEDNERS AND THE DEACONESSES

The beginning of the nineteenth century saw at Kaiserswerth-on-the-Rhine the great modern revival of the deaconess movement of the early Church under Protestant auspices, almost 200 years after St. Vincent de Paul had brought the counterpart of this worker back to the Roman Catholic Church as the Sister of Charity. The mother of the Kaiserswerth Deaconesses was Friederike Münster, born in 1806, just fourteen years before Florence Nightingale, and married when very young to Pastor Theodor Fliedner. He, in 1822, had gone to England to beg help for his little parish and there met Elizabeth Fry, who inspired him by her work in prisons for women. In 1826 Pastor Fliedner and his wife opened a tiny refuge for discharged prisoners. This was the first budding of the vast organization of Kaiserswerth and its branches.

The need for care of the sick poor impelled the Fliedners to open a little hospital in 1836. Pastor Fliedner had seen Protestant deaconesses at work in Holland, and wished the Evangelical Church to have the advantage of such a body of workers as the Sisters of Charity. His wife was even more certain than he just how it could be made a success, and induced a friend of her own, Gertrude Reichardt, member of a family of physicians and experienced in the care of the sick, to enter as the first deaconess. Other young women followed, some from plain families, but all carefully chosen and of blameless life and upright character. When six had entered, the work of the tiny establishment was divided among them in departments. One did the cooking and housekeeping, another the laundry and the linen, another had charge of the women's ward, and so on. After a certain time in each service, they were changed about so that experience would be uniform. They received some theoretical and bedside teaching from physicians, studied pharmacy, and passed the state examination on this subject. Pastor Fliedner taught them ethics and religious doctrine, and his wife, practical nursing.

The Kaiserswerth experiment was successful beyond the fondest hopes of its friends. An extensive hospital grew up there with dependencies and auxiliary buildings, and many related institutions were developed under the wise rule of the Fliedners. One was for the insane, who were treated with great kindness and remarkable intelligence. As the reputation of the deaconesses spread, applications came in from far and near. Groups were placed in other hospitals and sent to other countries. In time, the Kaiserswerth motherhouse developed so many daughter houses that it was like a great tree with its branches.

Friederike Fliedner was the creative partner in working out the training of the deaconesses. She kept a journal in which she recorded all her experiences and framed the principles and methods that this experience showed to be correct. Her journal was never published, and this is much to be regretted, for we have reason to think that it supplied the material used later by many pastors in copious writings on the principles and practice of nursing. As perhaps the first treatise on nursing ethics and the practical training of nurses written by a woman, it would have been a historical treasure. It contained a motto that gives the keynote to Friederike's ideals: "The soul of service must never be sacrificed to the technique." Just before her death, Friederike made some notes on her interpretation of the rules of the deaconesses, which are helpful in understanding their work and character.[1] Friederike died in 1842, and a second wife, Caroline Bertheau, was equally remarkable as a helpmate to Pastor Fliedner and as the head or mother of the deaconesses.

The Kaiserswerth deaconess was not intended to be a narrow specialist but was to be prepared for many kinds of service. She was taught nursing, teaching, the management of children and convalescents (this included occupational work and organized play and recreation), parish visiting, and religious theory, so that she might read and interpret the Scriptures, pray, and instruct.

INFLUENCE OF THE DEACONESSES ON NURSING

Through Florence Nightingale, who had a brief period of training at Kaiserswerth, this institution had a definite influence on the modern nursing system that she established, but as we shall see later the two systems differed fundamentally in their orientation and control. The older one was a modified form of the religious orders of the past, an integral part of a church and under the control of its clergy. The other was a new health

[1] They will be found in the article by D. Disselhoff listed on p. 96.

vocation, independent in organization and more closely allied to medicine than to charitable or church work as such. The line of separation between the two became more marked as time went on, especially on the economic side. Whereas the secular nurse was economically independent and was expected to plan for and in general to control her own life, the deaconess was closely tied to her motherhouse and had much less responsibility for her work or her maintenance. She was not bound for life like the older religious sister, for she might leave and marry. The whole influence of the church, however, was bent toward persuading her to make her career a life work. In sickness and in old age she was cared for. During her working years she was supported but not paid.

The Kaiserswerth Deaconesses, like the Sisters of Charity, brought about a great reformation in hospital service and institutional work generally. They treated patients with loving kindness, as individuals, not as cases. They obeyed scrupulously the directions of physicians, and brought an atmosphere of peace and sweetness into the plainest and dullest wards. The weak point of the system was its unpaid labor. The greater the number of nurses needed, the less could the motherhouse support them all in old age and illness, especially as overwork caused many breakdowns in health. To prevent questionings and dissatisfaction, the pastors who founded deaconess houses after the Fliedners became too repressive and narrow in binding down their pupils to a complete negation of intellectual life and mental initiative. They came to laud self-abnegation, humility, and submissiveness to an absurd degree, and so brought about a reaction which gradually led many young women who were interested in nursing to choose other forms of training that allowed them greater freedom of expression and wider opportunities for education and service.

PROTESTANT ORDERS IN ENGLAND

After the dissolution of the monasteries in England, complaints were heard from time to time of the lack of any worthy career for unmarried women. Not a few observers noted the sad conditions of the sick and bewailed the fact that the Anglican Church had no such body of workers as the Sisters of Charity. The first effort to meet this need was made by Elizabeth Fry in 1840 when she organized her Nursing Sisters. These women, who were of good character, had a short period of experience in Guy's Hospital before going into private houses to care for the sick. They continued to serve in this field up to quite recent times, their training being strengthened as the newer standards developed.

The Anglicans, especially the so-called "high church" group, next developed several sisterhoods which though not devoted especially to nursing included such duties among their activities. Some of their members did useful and courageous work in epidemics which were frequent up until mid-century and later. First of the Anglican orders was the Park Village Community initiated by Edward Pusey in 1845. Its members had no training in nursing but did friendly visiting among the poor and the sick. Next in 1849 came the Devonport Sisters of Mercy founded by Miss Sellon, who did extensive work in epidemics and developed a plan for hospital training. The same year St. John's House was founded as a nursing order of the Anglican Church and for some years its sisters had entire charge of nursing in King's College Hospital, London. It withdrew later and formed a private Institute which terminated its corporate existence in 1918. This sisterhood was in close touch with Miss Nightingale and her work and cooperated with her in several ways. Other groups of a similar type were the Sisterhood of All Saints (founded in 1851), whose head was Miss Byron, and St. Margaret's, founded by Dr. John Mason Neale in 1854. The Anglican orders tended to follow the pattern of the Roman Catholic sisterhoods and at first put little emphasis on formal training in nursing. Their influence was in general highly beneficial because the women who entered them were of admirable character, refinement, and capacity. They set a high standard of personal integrity, intelligence, and devotion wherever they went and began the work of rescuing nursing from the depths into which it had fallen. Some of their members went with Miss Nightingale to the Crimea. They, like the deaconesses, were handicapped by their form of organization and control, their rather rigid regulations and heterogeneous activities, and their lack of sound training in nursing. A freer form was necessary, and this was to be Miss Nightingale's mission.

SOME ADVANCES IN MEDICINE, SURGERY, AND PUBLIC HEALTH

During the first half of the nineteenth century medicine and surgery had shown little evidence of the tremendous strides they were to make in the second half. The prevailing explanation of disease was that it developed spontaneously. The germ theory had not been formulated, though Italian scientists had begun in the eighteenth century to study microscopic forms of life in water and in putrefying materials. Infection and contagion were not understood, and orthodox medical opinion ignored the insurgents who offered new ideas. Oliver Wendell Holmes' illuminating article proving the facts of the contagiousness of puerperal fever had little immediate effect. Still worse was the treatment given to Ignaz Philipp Semmelweiss (1818-1865), who applied his belief in the theory of infection in his work in the Vienna maternity hospitals and actually developed a technique for hand disinfection, with wonderful results to the patients. His professional colleagues, however, opposed him so violently that he lost his position and his mind gave way before he was vindicated. John Antoine Villemin, a French physician, who proved experimentally that tuberculosis was infectious, was also little noticed. He did not, it is true, isolate the bacillus, which might have been conclusive. This was to be the work of Robert Koch, the German medical scientist. The discovery of vaccination and inoculation for smallpox by Edward Jenner and Lady Mary Wortley Montague at the end of the eighteenth century had done something to curb this disease, but without well-organized public health departments such preventive measures had little effect. It was only after Charles Murchison in 1858 had advanced the theory that disease was caused by filth that cities began to install sewage systems and to clean up insanitary conditions.

Surgery was in a worse state than it had been in the late Middle Ages, for the followers of Ambroise Paré had used flame, boiling water, and alcohol in their operations and dressings. The early Victorian surgeons believed that pus was essential to the repair of tissues and applied poultices to wounds. The most virulent forms of sepsis were of common occurrence. This was the more unfortunate, since the discovery of ether and chloroform and their successful use between 1840 and 1850 made possible a much wider use of surgery in the treatment of disease. Definite progress was being made, however, in the basic medical sciences, and the curve of medicine and surgery was soon to take a sharp upturn with the discoveries of Louis Pasteur and Dr. Joseph Lister and other scientific investigators later in the nineteenth century.

There are few bright spots in this long dark period except where the Sisters of Charity, the Kaiserswerth Deaconesses, and similar groups began to revive the older more spontaneous and practical forms of nursing service and to give their members some training for their vocation. At the beginning of the nineteenth century things began to look a little more favorable for social reform. A few philanthropists were taking a deep interest in the conditions under which people lived and the injustices from which they suffered. The early abolitionists labored to wipe out slavery. Sympathy with the victims of the industrial revolution exposed the evils of the factory system and child labor. The novels of Charles Dickens helped to arouse public opinion on many of these social problems, including nursing. We have noted also the work of Elizabeth Fry and others who were interested in prison conditions. Political democracy was making headway in the extension of the ballot to working men. The first claims for woman suffrage were put forth in England and in America. Women pioneers were pressing forward into new spheres of work—medicine, the law, and even the church. Among the first colleges for women were Stephens College (1833) and Mt. Holyoke (1837) in the United States and Queen's College (1848) in London.

This outline of contemporary trends should not lead to the impression that the old prejudices and obstacles had been swept away and that the early Victorians were all openminded on the subject of careers and advanced education for women. "Primness and propriety" represented the prevailing attitude. Orthodox men and women still clung to the legend of "female delicacy" and many vital subjects were taboo. Pioneers in new fields had to put forth superhuman exertions to break through such obstructions, and women who dared to defy established customs had to be distinguished for their intellectual and moral power. This was the type of woman who shortly after mid-century was to take the lead in the fight for nursing reform.

SELECTED BIBLIOGRAPHY

Austin, Anne L. *History of Nursing Source Book*. New York: Putnam's, 1957. Ch. 4, 5.

Bancroft, Jane M. *Deaconesses in Europe and Their Lessons for America*. New York: Hunt & Eaton, 1890.

Baumgartner, Leona. "John Howard and the Public Health Movement," *Bull. Hist. Med.*, June 1937, 409-508.

De Bunsen, Mme Elizabeth S. (Gurney). *Elizabeth Fry's Journeys on the Continent 1840-1841*. London: Lane, 1931.

Defoe, Daniel. *A Journal of the Plague Year*. London: Noble, 1720.

Dickens, Charles. *The Life and Adventures of Martin Chuzzlewit*. Any edition. Ch. XIX, XXV, XXIX.

Disselhoff, D. "The Deaconesses of Kaiserswerth: A Hundred Years' Work," *Int. Nurs. Rev.*, Vol. IX, Nos. 1-4 (1934), 19-28.

Hampton, Isabel A., and others. *Nursing of the Sick 1893*. New York: McGraw-Hill, 1949. Pp. 182-188.

Holmes, Oliver Wendell. *Medical Essays 1842-1882*. Boston: Houghton Mifflin, 1891.

Howard, John. *An Account of the Principal Lazarettos in Europe*. London: Johnson, Dilly, and Cadel, 1791.

Jacobs, Henry Barton. "Elizabeth Fry, Pastor Fliedner, and Florence Nightingale," *Ann. Med. Hist.*, March 1921, 17-25.

Lonsdale, Margaret. *Sister Dora*. Boston: Roberts, 1887.

Maynard, Theodore. *Apostle of Charity: The Life of St. Vincent de Paul*. New York: Dial Press, 1939.

Memoirs of the Life of Elizabeth Fry, with Extracts from her Journal and Letters. Ed. by Her Two Daughters. London: Hatchard, 2nd ed., 1848. 2 vols.

Nutting, M. Adelaide, and Lavinia L. Dock. *A History of Nursing.* New York: Putnam's 1907-1912. 4 vols. Vol. I, Part II, Ch. XI, XIV-XV; Vol. II, Part III, Ch. I-II.

Platt, Elspeth. *The Story of the Ranyard Mission.* London: Hodder, 1937.

Thompson, Morton. *The Cry and the Covenant.* Garden City, N. Y.: Doubleday, 1954.

Whitney, Janet. *Elizabeth Fry: Quaker Heroine.* Boston: Little Brown, 1936.

CHAPTER 7

The Nightingale Revolution in Britain

FLORENCE NIGHTINGALE AND HER TIMES

To understand the remarkable changes in nursing that began about the middle of the nineteenth century one must know the famous woman who started the new movement and guided it almost to the end of her life in 1910. Much had been written about Florence Nightingale, but nothing like a full-sized, well-rounded view of her personality and achievements had appeared until Sir Edward Cook's official biography came out in 1913. In his absorbing and masterly *Life of Florence Nightingale*[1] the founder of nursing is seen against the background of the Victorian age which almost paralleled her own adult life. Among its distinguished figures she stands out as one of the most eminent social and health reformers and humanitarians of the nineteenth century and one of its most fascinating personalities. Later biographers, notably Cecil Woodham-Smith, who had access to previously unavailable materials about the family and personal life of Florence Nightingale, have added important facts and interpretations. We are fortunate today in having these

[1] For a list of this and other biographies and writings, see pp. 120-121.

and several other biographies which show different facets of her remarkably versatile and rather complex personality. We also have access to reprints of many of her writings not available earlier except in special collections. In addition, Miss Nightingale's voluminous correspondence furnishes a key to her phenomenal activities and world-wide contacts. This collection of letters has been catalogued by William J. Bishop, librarian and medical historian of London, who states that in point of numbers alone these letters exceed those of any other famous person. In them she expresses her inmost thoughts and plans for the new system of nursing.

EARLY LIFE AND EDUCATION

Born in Florence, Italy, on May 12, 1820, of well-to-do English parents, and named for that lovely city, Florence Nightingale grew up in a beautiful English home, surrounded by an interesting circle of friends which included several who were prominent in the political, social, religious, and humanitarian activities of that day. She was a highly gifted and rather precocious child with a mind of her own, a social conscience, and a religious nature which led her to seek an outlet for her aspirations and energies in some form of useful service. From childhood she had been roused by the needs of sick neighbors and members of her own family and was drawn to nursing by a compelling interest which she interpreted as a divine call to nurse the sick and to reform nursing. Her revolt against the conventional upbringing of young ladies of her day made her the despair of her mother and governess and at an early age her education was taken over by her scholarly Oxford-trained father who allowed her the free use of his well-stocked library. Under his guidance she became, at the age of seventeen, a highly educated young woman, well grounded in ancient and modern languages and literature, the natural and social sciences, political economy, higher mathematics, and statistics. All these, including the last two which were among her favorite subjects, were to be used to good purpose in her social, sanitary, and nursing investigations and reforms. Indeed, without such equipment much of

Florence Nightingale ~~ Her Times and Contemporaries

	1820	1830	1840	1850	1860	1870	1880	1890	1900	1910

General Events

'21 DEATH OF NAPOLEON
'21 1ST FACTORY LEGISLATION

POLITICAL REVOLUTION IN EUROPE

CRIMEAN WAR '54~56

U.S. CIVIL WAR '61-65
INT. RED CROSS '64

FR.~PRUSS. WAR '70~'71

WARS { CHIN~JAP.'94-'95 / SP.~AMER.'98-'99 / BOER ~ '99-'02 / RUS.~JAP.'04~'05 }

STEADY ADVANCE IN DEMOCRATIC GOV'T.
PARLIAMENTARY REFORM & HUMANITARIAN MOV'T

Queen Victoria — BORN 1819~CROWNED 1837 ~ VICTORIAN ERA ~ DIED 1901

Florence Nightingale — BORN 1820 ~ DIED 1910

Social Reformers and Humanitarians

Elizabeth Fry
Theodore Fliedner
Harriet Martineau
Dorothea Dix
John Stuart Mill
Sir Sidney Herbert
Charles Dickens
William Rathbone
Clara Barton
Henri Dunant
Octavia Hill

Leaders in Medicine and Public Health

Sir Edwin Chadwick
Dr. William Farr
Dr. Oliver Wendell Holmes
Sir John Simon
Ignaz Semmelweiss
William Morton
Rudolf Virchow
Louis Pasteur
Joseph Lister
Robert Koch
William K. Roentgen

the research work she was to do as a health reformer would have been impossible.

Though she went into society and was wooed by highly eligible suitors, she never swerved from her early determination to study nursing. Partly to distract her from this idea, she was sent on a long trip on the Continent and there met a number of interesting and distinguished people who stimulated and broadened her interest in social reform. Wherever she went she studied social conditions, found out how people lived, and noted what was being done to help them. She also visited and inspected hospitals and nursing systems in many countries besides her own and was exceptionally well informed on health matters in general.

Keenly aware of her lack of practical experience, she searched a long time before she found a place for training that would be approved by her family. Her plan to enter an English hospital at twenty-five was vetoed by her mother. The same year she wrote friends in America asking if they knew of a hospital there that would accept her for training. Finally, in 1851, when she was thirty-one, consent was granted for a period of three months at the Kaiserswerth Deaconess Home in Germany under Pastor Fliedner and his wife. Following this introduction, she visited Ireland and inspected some Dublin hospitals administered by Roman Catholic sisterhoods. In 1853 she had made arrangements to serve an apprenticeship with the Sisters of Charity in Paris, but this plan was frustrated by illness and only one month was spent with them studying their organization and discipline. Her excellent grasp of such matters is shown by her published analyses and comparisons (which date from this period) of nursing systems in France, Austria, Italy, and Germany.

After her brief stay with the Sisters of Charity, Miss Nightingale finally overruled her family and took a position in charge of a private nursing home for sick governesses, a semicharitable institution in London. Here she had an opportunity to show her competence as a nurse, her executive ability, and diplomatic skill. About that time, too, she volunteered her services during a cholera epidemic at the Middlesex Hospital where she did actual nursing and learned more about epidemiology. Before the Crimean War started in 1854, she had been looking for a wider field of work in which she would have an opportunity to train nurses. These aspirations as well as her proven gifts of organization and leadership were known to many of her friends, including some physicians. A superintendent's position at King's College Hospital, London, and the possibility of starting a nursing school were under consideration when the call came that was to make her world famous as a war nurse and the widely acknowledged leader of the modern nursing movement.

It is obvious from the foregoing that though Miss Nightingale was largely self-taught she was no amateur when she left for Scutari in 1854. In her youth she had embraced every opportunity to nurse her own relatives and dependents, and these experiences had been frequent and often exacting. Her studies of hospital systems were exhaustive. Her probation at Kaiserswerth was her only formal training, yet in after years she would not have it said that Kaiserswerth had trained her and held that the hospital was the poorest part of the deaconess institution and that the nursing there was crude. These facts show as even more remarkable her extraordinary attainments, for not only in directing others but in all her personal work as a nurse she stands in a class by herself. Her own standards and tests were so much more thorough and exacting than any others of her day that she created an entirely new concept of nursing and nurses.

THE CRIMEAN WAR: CREATION OF ARMY NURSING

Not long after the Crimean War broke out in 1854 distressing reports began to appear about the high death rate and neglected condition of sick and wounded British soldiers. The London *Times* correspondent made an eloquent appeal for help, noting that the Russians and French had their Sisters of Mercy and Sisters of Charity but the English Army had none. Sir Sidney Herbert, then Minister at War, was not only a man of great political influence but an earnest humanitarian of high character and a close personal friend of Florence Nightingale. His appeal to her to go to the front and her offer of her services crossed in the mails and plans for the expedition were soon under way. At that time it was unheard of for a respectable woman, not a member of a religious order, to serve in an army hospital, but all objections were soon overcome, especially since Miss Nightingale was recognized as one exceptionally fitted to take charge of this critical undertaking. In October she left for the East as Lady-in-Chief with a staff of forty nurses, ten of whom were Roman Catholic sisters, eight from Miss Sellon's sisterhood, and six from St. John's House (both Anglican). The others were practical nurses from different hospitals. Though there were obvious difficulties in combining these varied groups in a nursing staff and though a few individuals proved to be undependable or unsuitable, the results they achieved under Miss Nightingale's firm and competent leadership were remarkable.

The nurses landed at Scutari (near Constantinople) on November 4, 1854, and were established in the large barrack hospital. They found the most horrible conditions—a vast hospital with no sewage system, no laundry, no supplies, and no food fit for sick men. The patients, devoured by vermin, were in a most pitiable state of neglect, and the death rate was fifty to sixty per cent. During the time she was in charge, Miss Nightingale organized all the hospitals throughout the Crimea, as well as at Scutari, and some 200 nurses in all passed under her control. Her dominant intellect and character and her exact and wide knowledge of practical detail enabled her to do a truly stupendous piece of work, and she had to do it in the face of every obstacle that official jealousy, red tape, and bureaucratic inefficiency could present.

Though Miss Nightingale systematized a nursing service for the British army in the first demonstration that any country had seen of a trained gentlewoman who was not a religious sister at the head of an army nursing staff, with orderlies as well as nurses under her command, this was not the biggest or hardest part of her mission. Her extraordinary achievement was that she overthrew the long-established method of organizing and administering the medical service of the British army, which was regarded as sacrosanct by the bureaucrats. Turning upon it the searchlight of her intelligence, and backed by the findings of expert sanitarians as well as her own carefully collected facts, she exposed the indefensible blunders that were responsible for the high death rate and wrote Sir Sidney reams of fearless, unsparing criticism, accompanied in every case by constructive recommendations. The nursing and sanitary reforms initiated by her brought the death rate down from more than 400 per 1000 patients to 22 per 1000—a rate never before known in the army even in peacetime. What she learned here of war-office methods provided her with weapons for the campaign she carried on after the war for the complete reorganization of the army medical service.

OTHER SERVICES FOR ARMY PERSONNEL

In the Crimean hospitals Miss Nightingale established not only a well-organized nursing service but laundries and diet kitchens; she brought about the installation of extensive sanitary engineering works and developed a system for the collection of hospital statistics. She also provided supplies, such as clothing, food, equipment, and surgical dressings, whenever the Army system failed, as it frequently did, to furnish them. When the first desperate need to attend to the acutely sick and wounded was over, Miss Nightingale initiated for the first time in any army many of the activities designed to cheer the individual soldier, which have been so marked a feature of recent wars, thus antedating the Red Cross and the first War Camp Community Service. She wrote letters to patients' families, organized a post office and a savings fund for the men, provided rest and recreation rooms for them, fitted up convalescent camps, investigated every detail of the soldiers' health, dietary, and routine, and planned systematic care for their families. Many of these and other plans for active assistance which were begun by her were taken over afterwards by the War Department.

THE QUESTION OF RANK

Miss Nightingale had no official rank until intrigues and jealousies among the army medical staff had so nearly under-

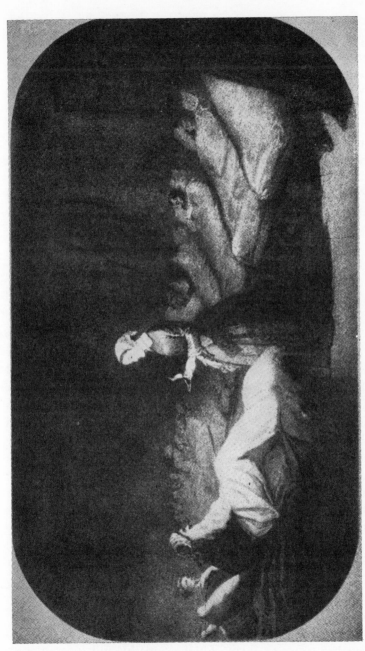

Florence Nightingale, "The Lady with the Lamp," on her nightly rounds in the English military hospital at Scutari.

mined her position that she threatened to resign. The culminating point of this cabal was that in some way a second party of forty-six nurses was sent out from England under Mary Stanley without the knowledge or request of the Lady-in-Chief. They were not to report to her but to a military surgeon who was her chief enemy. The matter was finally adjusted and Miss Nightingale's authority maintained but not without friction and strain which added greatly to her burdens. She at one time wrote of the War Office: "It is profuse in empty praise which I do not want, and does not give me the real businesslike efficient standing which I do want." After this she was given the title "General Superintendent" of the nursing staff, and her authority was defined by the War Office. She could have prevented many mistakes, however, had she been endowed earlier with official status.

Postwar Campaign for the Soldiers' Health

While in the Crimea Miss Nightingale had an acute illness (later diagnosed as amoebic dysentery) which, coupled with her exhausting labors, so depleted her that she never fully recovered her health. However, she refused to return home until the war was over in 1856, and in spite of the warnings of her physicians and the pleading of her friends plunged at once into a long and difficult fight to safeguard the health of her "children" as she called the soldiers. She continued to work at white heat until a Royal Commission was finally appointed in 1857 to investigate the medical service of the British Army. Such an investigation was considered essential by Miss Nightingale and her co-workers in order to prevent a repetition of the Crimean disaster.

The government in power as well as the great majority of the medical profession were vigorously opposed to this inquiry. But Miss Nightingale had powerful support in high places. Shortly after her return to England she was invited to visit Queen Victoria and the Prince Consort at Balmoral Castle in Scotland and, though still convalescent, made the journey in order to present her cause to them. Their sympathy and interest were quickly won. Through them she met the rather formidable Minister of War who, perhaps misled by the frail appearance and modest charm of the invalid and thinking to avoid a long story, asked her to send him some notes on her Crimean experience. Returning home she plunged into the preparation of a bulky volume entitled, *Notes on Matters Affecting the Health and Efficiency of the British Army,* which was completed in six months with the aid of some of her supporters and privately printed. Government officials at once recognizing the powerful impact it would have on the public decided to appoint a Royal Commission to investigate the whole medical and health system in the army and made Sir Sidney Herbert chairman of the Commission.

During the long exhausting weeks which followed Sir Sidney was in constant touch with Miss Nightingale and relied greatly on her astute, practical suggestions concerning tactics, witnesses, and points to be investigated. Her *Notes* provided invaluable source material for this inquiry, but although it was necessary to expose the failures and weaknesses of the old system these reformers put chief emphasis on constructive measures to safeguard the future health and welfare of the Army at home and abroad, in war and in peace.

After the large two-volume Report of the Commission was issued there was a long period of reorganization and reconstruction during which Miss Nightingale served as official adviser to the War Office. Most of the reforms brought about were minutely set forth in her reports and private papers to ministers. She helped to plan new military hospitals and barracks, was active in getting laboratory and other needed equipment for the medical department, and was chiefly instrumental in establishing an army school for new medical officers as well as schools for army orderlies and cooks. All this and much other work was done from her sickroom, where, protected from unwelcome visitors and other interruptions, she carried on what she often called "God's business." Though the intense anxieties and efforts of the campaign for army reform undoubtedly hastened the death of her friend and associate, Sidney Herbert, the chronic invalid survived and for fifty years continued to carry out the pledge she had made in a farewell visit to the Scutari burial grounds—"While I live I fight their cause."

SANITATION FOR INDIA

"The passionate statistician," as she has been called, made good use of this specialty in her battle for soldiers' lives. She insisted on complete reports on the health and living conditions of army personnel at home and abroad and spent many hours poring over government "bluebooks" which furnished this information. From their dry tables she gathered many of the arguments she used to convince government officials of the need for sanitary, medical, and nursing reforms. The exceptionally high sickness and death rates of the British Army in India led her to make an exhaustive study of sanitary conditions in that country. Such investigations carried her as far as the land question, irrigation, taxation, and usury. This vast subject had her constant attention for many years. Largely because of her efforts, a Royal Commission on the Sanitary State of the Army in India was appointed in 1859. She did the lion's share of the work on the Commission's report and wrote most of the brilliant, hard-hitting articles and pamphlets, such as *Life or Death in India,* which informed the British public and especially the administrative officers of their responsibility for the health of the Indian people as well as of their own soldiers. During her whole life she kept watch on Indian affairs and was regarded as an authority on that country though she never visited it.

Her interest in people and in social and vital statistics led her into other investigations concerning the health and social welfare of native races which brought recognition and honor from international organizations of social scientists and statisticians as well as from governor generals and other high officials. But these interests did not in any way deflect her from the purpose that had long held first place in her mind and heart—the reformation of nursing and the establishment of a modern system of education for nurses.

THE NIGHTINGALE CONCEPT OF NURSING

As a result of years of study and of her own wide practical experience, Miss Nightingale had arrived at an entirely new concept of nursing and believed that this field must be opened up as an independent career for large numbers of trained, capable women. She was not opposed to the religious orders. Indeed, she had great admiration for many things in the Protestant and Roman Catholic sisterhoods and borrowed some of their ideas in setting up her new system. She herself was strongly religious and wrote a three-volume work on the subject,[2] but she deplored sectarian divisions and the restrictions often imposed on members of religious sisterhoods. She also attacked superficial amateurishness and continually advised women, often in spicy terms, to fit themselves by hard work and study. Though she recognized the close relationship of nursing and medicine, she regarded them as different vocations. The founder of modern nursing objected to the archaic and sentimental notions of nurses as martyrs, penitents, and ministering angels and to the current concept of "born" nurses, and she rejected entirely the prevailing system in which ignorant and untrained servant-nurses, often of doubtful character, were employed in such service. To her, nursing was a dignified, useful, responsible career for self-supporting women who had the intelligence, training, and physical and moral stamina necessary to face its complex and difficult problems and to fight their own battles.

Although hospital work at that time offered the largest field of opportunity, Miss Nightingale believed that nurses should be prepared to care for the sick at home as well as in hospital and to serve all kinds and classes of people, rich and poor, the mentally disabled, and families and communities as well as individuals. The teaching of health maintenance and the prevention of sickness was to be an important part of their work. A special group of trained leaders was to be prepared to fill the more responsible administrative and teaching posts in nursing schools, hospitals, and district nursing associations. Such

---

[2] *Suggestions for Thought to Searchers after Truth.* Privately printed.

sisters and matrons had to be ready to go where they were needed in civilian or military services in their own and other countries.

THE NIGHTINGALE SYSTEM OF NURSE TRAINING

Miss Nightingale's ideas on the education of nurses were equally modern and, for that day, radical. She believed that schools should be set up for the training of nurses and that they should provide practical experience in nursing as well as a substantial body of knowledge. They must also be equipped to develop the mind and character of the individual nurse as well as her technical skill and practical ability. Such training schools, though independent, should be situated in proximity to hospitals which could be used as workshops or training fields for the young women who were to be recruited for the new nursing army. The whole plan of preparation was brilliantly conceived and outlined in detail. In some respects it was superior to contemporary systems of vocational education for girls and women and even to medical schools which were then changing from the older apprenticeship system and tended to depend too much on theoretical and formal instruction.

After the Crimean War the British people in gratitude to Miss Nightingale presented her with a large sum of money (£44,000), which she accepted on condition that she might use it to found the training school of which she had long dreamed. She had hoped to direct it in person, but her continued poor health made this impossible. It was established in connection with St. Thomas's Hospital in June 1860. Mrs. S. E. Wardroper, who was matron of that hospital and a superior person, was also appointed superintendent of the school, though these positions were under separate boards. Fifteen students entered in the first class. Miss Nightingale, who continued for many years on the training-school committee, kept in close touch with the school and was in effect its superintendent. For many years every detail of management was referred to her and she was personally acquainted with every probationer.[3]

[3] Lucy Seymer, *Florence Nightingale's Nurses* (see p. 121). gives many interesting details concerning the history of this first school.

Her intention was that this first school would train nurses, not for private duty, but to go into other hospitals and there, in turn, to organize, teach, and train. District nurses were to be prepared to nurse the sick poor in their homes. The Nightingale nurses were to be the leaven by which the entire nursing world as it then existed would be reformed. This master plan was brilliantly carried out, as the history of pioneer nursing in other countries shows. The existing system of nursing in civil hospitals was completely revolutionized by the introduction of educated, trained, and refined women. This, however, took time; there was opposition at first, but it gradually died away, and a new era opened in hospital work, which brought with it equally radical changes in district and private nursing.

One especially striking feature of Miss Nightingale's plan for nurse training has been to a singular degree overlooked by commentators and even by nurses. It was, in short, the positive mandate that the entire control of the nursing staff, its discipline and instruction, was to be taken out of the hands of men and lodged in those of a woman who must herself be a trained and competent nurse. Before this school opened, nurses in English hospitals and in others under secular administration were entirely controlled in discipline, routine of work, and training (what there was of it) by hospital directors and medical staffs. Miss Nightingale believed that the right kind of young woman could not be attracted into nursing and that the prevailing low standards of morals and service could not be improved until qualified matrons or lady superintendents could be put in charge and given responsibility for the administration of the school and the nursing service. The school, however, was not to be under the control of a hospital. It was to be established as a separate institution with its own funds and governing body. Coordination of nursing school and nursing service was to be maintained by the matron who would have a position of dignity and authority and of considerable independence.

The matron and her staff of sisters, the Home Sister and the Ward Sisters, were to be responsible for the direction and supervision of the nurses and for their practical teaching and discipline. They were to see that medical directions relating to patients and general hospital regulations were carried out, that proper respect was given to medical attendants and other officers, and that relationships between nurses and other groups would be kept on a strictly professional basis. Though physicians were to be employed to teach certain subjects in lectures and bedside instruction, the educational program was to be planned and controlled by the nursing staff and the governing body of the school. The Home Sister who supervised the life of the probationers off duty held a pivotal position in this plan as did also the Sister Tutor who was added later to give special attention to the supervision of their studies.

The strict system of discipline which was an essential part of the training was influenced by both military traditions and by those of the religious orders. It was designed not only to protect the patients but to safeguard the nurses themselves and to develop their morale and *esprit de corps*. Applicants with superior education and gifts of leadership were selected and trained for the more responsible positions. Though interpreted sometimes in extreme and arbitrary fashion, such discipline did much to establish public confidence in and respect for the new nurses and to convince the skeptics in medical and other circles that the Nightingale plan was not only workable but more efficient and satisfactory than the older system from the standpoint of the patients, the doctors, and all concerned.

The Nightingale Missioners

Though they were bound by no religious vows and represented many different faiths, these nurses had the qualities of missionaries in that they were ready to go to the ends of the earth for their cause. Their profession then had the advantage of being almost the only one that offered cultured women a career that combined prestige, adventure, and the joy of the constructive reformer. In the earlier period of reorganization two classes of probationers were admitted to the Nightingale school and to other schools in England. Social and educational requirements were lower for nurses who were to care for patients in private homes or hospitals and higher for those preparing for leadership who at first formed a special group, paid their own way, and had special opportunities and privileges. As more of the better prepared candidates entered, however, the special probationers gradually disappeared and all students were admitted on the same basis.

THE NIGHTINGALE SYSTEM IN GREAT BRITAIN

Nursing reorganization went on rapidly in the large hospitals supported by voluntary contributions and more slowly, yet steadily, in those called infirmaries that were connected with workhouses under the English Poor Law. The need for change in the infirmaries had been seen earlier by intelligent women visitors to these institutions. Louisa Twining, for example, who with others had observed the care of the sick, endorsed Miss Nightingale's plan when it was put forward in 1860 and later in her capacity as Guardian of the Poor under the Poor Law. Within twenty-five years after the Nightingale school had been founded the old system of nursing in English hospitals by poorly paid, untaught women or by pauper inmates had almost disappeared. Especially notable was the reformation of the immense Liverpool Workhouse Infirmary by Agnes Jones, one of the most remarkable of the Nightingale pioneers, who with a staff of twelve Nightingale nurses volunteered for duty in a dangerous and almost impossible situation. She paid with her life, but the story of her work, which Miss Nightingale wrote under the title, *Una and the Lion,* became a rallying cry for more nursing recruits "to follow in her train." Referring to the flood of current literature on "Women's Work," she observed: "It used to be that people gave their blood for their country; now they give their ink."

Miss Nightingale's Liverpool activities were further extended by William Rathbone, a wealthy businessman and philanthropist, who wrote her for advice on his plan for district nursing. This led in 1859 to the first organization of a district nursing society, the plan of which was copied in many countries. Needing more nurses, he wrote again asking for some from the school in London and was advised to establish a hospital training school in his own city. This he succeeded in doing by interesting the trustees of the Royal Infirmary in the plan and by contributing to the cost of building a nurses' home.

In all such reorganization work the best features of the earlier hospitals were retained and the transition to the new order was gradual. Matrons and sisters had long held positions in these hospitals, but under the new plan the dignity, powers, and responsibilities of their positions were greatly enlarged. Probationers and staff nurses took the place of "old style" attendants in most hospitals, and ward maids were employed for the domestic work. Night duty was established on much the same basis as day duty, and an orderly system of continuous, responsible nursing care was substituted for the old plan by which a night watch was supposed to keep an eye on large numbers of patients or the patients were left alone to look after each other.

New buildings, spaciously planned and efficiently equipped, began to take the place of many of the obsolete insanitary buildings, while others were remodeled with modern plumbing and other conveniences. It was not long before the whole atmosphere of hospitals—moral as well as physical—was changed. The fact that matrons, sisters, and staff nurses may retain their posts during their active lives helps to give these English hospitals the restful, friendly homelike atmosphere that impresses the visitor and also, no doubt, accounts for the inbred traditionalism of a good many of them.

For some years a few (not all) hospitals in London maintained staffs of private nurses much as the motherhouses did, paying the nurses a salary and sending them out to private cases. Miss Nightingale approved of this custom when private duty was to be done, believing it to be best for the nurses and a guaranty for patients and physicians. Although desirable in the transition period, it soon became unwieldy and was gradually given up but not without a final contest between the nurses and the hospitals. A later tendency to merge the new schools with hospitals brought many changes which are more fully discussed in Part II.

FLORENCE NIGHTINGALE AND THE INTERNATIONAL RED CROSS

The founder of the Red Cross was Henri Dunant, a Swiss humanitarian who had seen the horrors of war after the battle of Solferino. He first presented his plan to the Society of Public Utility in Geneva (1863) and ascribed to Miss Nightingale much of the credit for it, saying that what she had done in the Crimea had inspired his idea and fortified his belief in its feasibility. His proposal that societies for relief in war be organized nationally and that permanent headquarters be established in Geneva was adopted in 1864, when the formal treaty was signed by the representatives of several nations there present. To this meeting the English delegation brought a full set of recommendations, prepared largely by Miss Nightingale, many of which were incorporated in the basic principles of the new organization.

National Red Cross societies were thereafter built up in many countries, and older groups, such as the St. John's Ambulance Association and women's associations that had carried on relief work in earlier wars of the nineteenth century, were affiliated with it. Although Miss Nightingale supported the Red Cross movement and was a life member of the Red Cross Committee in Britain she opposed the practice followed by many Red Cross Societies of giving brief courses of training to volunteer nurses who were to serve in times of war and disaster. Largely because of Miss Nightingale's influence the Red Cross Societies of Britain and its dominions employed only fully trained nurses for such missions. After her death in 1910 Red Cross VADs (Volunteer Aid Detachments) were organized in Britain but served only under professional nurses.[4] The American Red Cross adopted similar regulations after the Spanish-American War.

FLORENCE NIGHTINGALE'S FAME AND INFLUENCE

Influenced no doubt by her early studies and travels on the Continent and by her nursing experiences in Germany and France, this leader was a confirmed internationalist. Her Cri-

[4] See p. 173 for further details.

mean adventure extended her knowledge of foreign lands and people and made her name known throughout the civilized world. The glamour it cast over her never faded, but the halo tended to obscure the hard-headed practical qualities and the solid learning that made her the foremost international health statesman of her day. Kings and commoners, generals and governors, scholars and businessmen sought her advice, and her correspondence came from all quarters of the globe. Students from many countries studied at the Nightingale school in London and went back to found schools in their own lands. They and the English "Nightingales" sent out on similar missions were in constant touch with their "Mother-in-Chief" in London (see map, p. 117).

For many years Miss Nightingale had an unparalleled influence in hospital and nursing matters and in general questions relating to health and sickness, and her advice was sought on many other problems. Much of this influence came through her writings, which were widely distributed, often in translation. This was true especially of her *Notes on Nursing: What It Is, and What It Is Not,* first published in 1859. Later it appeared in many different English editions (costing sixpence up) also in French, Swedish, and other languages. Another well known book, *Notes on Hospitals* (1858) was for many years regarded in both civilian and military circles as the chief authority on hospital construction and administration. *Notes on Lying-in Institutions* (1871) dealt with the more specialized problems of maternity hospitals. There were scores of other reports and articles relating to hospitals, nursing, and sanitation, many of them appearing in magazines or in pamphlet form. Her writings and studies on India have been referred to earlier. The list of her articles and pamphlets also contains several concerned with racial questions: "Notes on the Aboriginal Races of Australia," "Notes on the New Zealand De-population Question" (an article on the Maoris), "Sanitary Statistics of Native Colonial Schools and Hospitals," "Deaconess Work in Syria," and similar topics that indicate the wide scope of her social and humanitarian interests.

This "soldier nurse" continued throughout her life to be

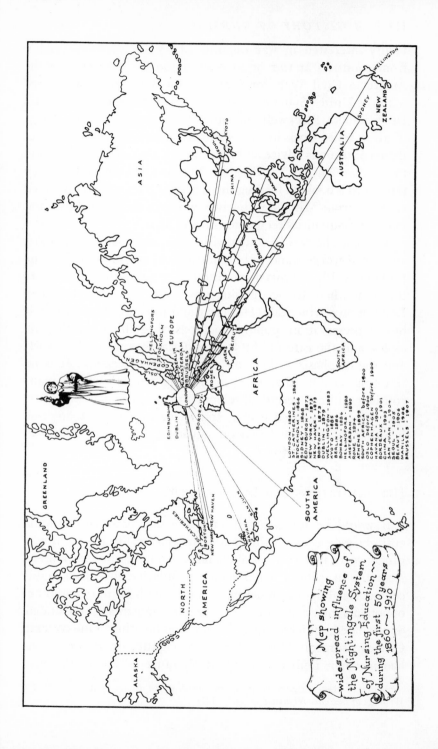

Map showing widespread influence of the Nightingale System of Nursing Education ~ during the first 50 years 1860 ~ 1910

LONDON - 1860
ST. CATHERINES - 1864
STOCKHOLM - 1866
SYDNEY - 1868
EDINBURGH - 1872
NEW YORK - 1873
NEW HAVEN - 1873
DUBLIN - 1879
WELLINGTON - 1883
BERLIN - 1886
BOMBAY - 1886
HELSINGFORS - 1888
AMSTERDAM - 1890
ROME - 1894
ATHENS - 1899
SOUTH AFRICA before 1900
OSLO before 1900
COPENHAGEN before 1900
BORDEAUX - 1900
CHINA - 1901
SAN JUAN - 1903
SEOUL - 1905
BEIRUT - 1906
MANILA - 1906
BRUSSELS - 1907

vitally interested in war nursing. Many appeals came to her from countries at war or in preparation for war. During the American Civil War, for example, she was closely associated with the United States Sanitary Commission through her friend Dr. Elizabeth Blackwell and other women who were in charge of army relief work in the North. In correspondence she gave them continuous advice and sent nursing literature to them and to the War Office in Washington. The Army of the South, which published a book on feeding the sick in army hospitals, included excerpts from Miss Nightingale's writings on this subject and many large-quantity recipes for invalid diets.[5]

At home she was in touch with numerous medical, sanitary, and social workers and public-spirited citizens interested in improving health and social conditions. She wrote timely letters to the press when district nursing was about to be established in London on a wide scale. Her clear and forceful ideas on public health preservation, popular methods of teaching health principles, and the care of children underlay her whole life work, and she emphasized them on every possible occasion. It is interesting to note that even in nursing research which many consider quite a recent development, the Founder, a century ago, was a recognized leader. Indeed most of her nursing and health reforms were based on statistical and other studies in which she was an expert.

HER LIMITATIONS AND INCONSISTENCIES

It would be surprising if such a strong personality should entirely escape opposition and criticism or, in a long life of ninety years, make no mistakes and reveal no serious weaknesses. Actually, in spite of her immense popularity, she was a highly controversial figure. In her many battles with military and other opponents she was accused of being temperamental, highhanded, opinionated, quick-tempered, and domineering. One veteran Crimean surgeon, when asked by a Nightingale admirer if he had met her, replied testily that of course he knew "the Bird

---

[5] Many of these original writings on nursing are to be found in *Selected Writings of Florence Nightingale* (see p. 121).

—much over-rated—certainly no saint—a very interfering woman." Even her friends sometimes found her difficult, especially when she was driving forward furiously with one of her plans for reform. But they were fascinated also by her brilliance and charm, her astonishing vitality, and the very contradictions in her personality. She was both humble and proud, democratic and autocratic, kindly and scathingly critical, an indulgent foster mother and a military martinet. Yet her versatility was such that she managed to harness a wide variety of talents and, in spite of her long invalidism, to achieve distinction in such varied roles as nurse, sanitarian, dietitian, war-office consultant, research worker, statistician, writer and publicist, social worker, hospital administrator, educator, and leader in the women's movement.

Though Miss Nightingale in her youth might properly have been called a revolutionary, she showed in her later life, as many youthful liberals do, a tendency toward conservatism in some matters. For example, she opposed the movement for professional organization and state registration which was designed to control the serious deterioration in nursing standards that developed in the 1880's (see pp. 165-169). Another quaint example of conservatism was her great dislike of the "germ theory." She expressed this at times in the wittiest epigrams and apparently was never convinced that bacteriology was a respectable science. Her fear seemed to be that belief in germs would weaken the doctrine of cleanliness on which she had built many of her nursing and sanitary reforms. We point out these evidences of fallibility because an attitude of uncritical adoration for a great person is unintelligent and Miss Nightingale herself would have been the first to discourage it.

None of these human weaknesses or mistakes reduces in any way the size of this heroic figure or her immense contribution to her own times and to ours. Indeed, as noted earlier, the farther away we get, the greater she appears. Each generation will undoubtedly see her in a different light and will discover new aspects of her life and character. But her influence will go on and we shall see more clearly that she belongs to no country or age or professional group but to the world.

This chapter tells how with the Nightingale revolution in Britain the curve of nursing progress started sharply upward and the modern movement began to spread not only in that country but in many other parts of the world. The story continues in Part II, and it will be seen that there were still many battles to be fought before ignorant untrained servant-nurses were replaced by modern trained nurses and the new vocation became a true profession. Despite many changes, both favorable and unfavorable, the inspiration of Miss Nightingale's example continues to be a precious heritage for the young profession she did so much to create.

SELECTED BIBLIOGRAPHY

Aloysius, Sister Mary. *Memories of the Crimea.* London: Burns, 1897.

Austin, Anne L. *History of Nursing Source Book.* New York: Putnam's, 1957. Ch. 6, 7.

Bishop, W. J. *A Bio-Bibliography of Florence Nightingale.* London: Dawsons of Pall Mall. First volume published, 1962.

Cook, Sir Edward. *The Life of Florence Nightingale.* New York: Macmillan, 1942. 2 vols. in 1.

Cope, Zachary, *Florence Nightingale and the Doctors.* Philadelphia: Lippincott, 1958.

——. *Six Disciples of Florence Nightingale.* London: Pitman, 1961.

Godlee, Sir Rickman John. *Life of Lord Lister.* London: Macmillan, 1917.

Gould, Marion E. "Miss Nightingale's Influence on the Nightingale School," "The Nightingale Training School Today." "The Early Nightingale Nurses." *Nurs. Times.* November 5, 1954, 1227-1228; November 12, 1954, 1254-1255; November 19, 1954, 1286-1287.

Gumpert, Martin. *Dunant: The Story of the Red Cross.* New York: Oxford University Press, 1938.

Haldane, Elizabeth S. *The British Nurse in Peace and War.* London: Murray, 1923.

Hallowes, Ruth M. "The Nightingale Training School, St. Thomas's Hospital, London, 1860-1960," *Int. Nurs. Rev.,* June 1960, 11-16.

Hart, Ellen. *Man Born to Live.* London: Victor Gollanez, 1953.

Henley, Ernest. *In Hospital; Rhymes and Rhythms.* Portland, Me.: Mosher, 1921.

Memorials of Agnes Elizabeth Jones. By Her Sister. London: James Nisbet, 14th ed., n. d.

Newman, Sir George. The Commemoration of Florence Nightingale. *Int. Nurs. Rev.,* October 1954, 4-10. Reprint.

Nightingale, Florence. *Notes on Hospitals.* London: Longmans, 3rd ed., 1867.

——. *Notes on Nursing.* Philadelphia: Lippincott, 1946.

Nutting, M. Adelaide, and Lavinia L. Dock. *A History of Nursing.* New York: Putnam's, 1907-1912. 4 vols. Vol. II, Part II, Ch. I-VIII.

Rathbone, William. *Sketch of the History and Progress of District Nursing from Its Commencement in the Year 1859 to the Present Date.* New York: Macmillan, 1890.

Seymer, Lucy Ridgely. *Florence Nightingale.* New York: Macmillan, 1951.

———. *Florence Nightingale, 1820-1910. Selected Writings.* New York: Macmillan, 1954.

———. *Florence Nightingale's Nurses. The Nightingale Training School 1860-1960.* London: Pitman, 1960.

———. "Mary Crossland of the Nightingale Training School," *Am. Jo. Nurs.,* May 1961, 85-88.

Stewart, Isabel Maitland. *The Education of Nurses.* New York: Macmillan, 1943. Ch. II.

Tooley, S. A. *The History of Nursing in the British Empire.* London: Bousfield, 1906.

———. *The Life of Florence Nightingale.* London: Bousfield, 1904.

Woodham-Smith, Cecil. *Florence Nightingale.* New York: McGraw-Hill, 1951.

CHAPTER 8

Nursing in the New World from Early to Modern Times

EARLIER CONDITIONS AND INFLUENCES

American nursing may be thought of as a stream that had its origin far back in prehistoric times among the Aztecs and Mayas and the Indian tribes whose cultures varied from simple savagery to highly complex and relatively advanced civilizations. Into this stream were poured ideas and customs from many different races and cultures—Spanish, Portuguese, English, Dutch, German, French, and later many others. Among those who founded hospitals and cared for the sick were missionaries and religious refugees, military conquerors, officials of civil governments, commercial adventurers, and ordinary settlers. In hospital, tent, or cabin, they introduced the medical and nursing customs with which they were familiar in their own lands. In the north in New England most of the newcomers were British. These strains were intermixed with Dutch and German in the middle colonies and with French and Spanish in the south. Along the St. Lawrence River in the earlier stages of colonization the French influence predominated, and on the Pacific coast, the Spanish. Religious ideas and institutions, always a potent influence, came from Roman Catholics, Puritans, Episcopalians, Presbyterians, Quakers, Lutherans, Huguenots, Moravians, Jews, and other faiths. Some of these western European traditions and systems of nursing and hospital work can still be traced in the remains of early hospital buildings and equipment which survive in parts of the United States and Canada.

The main stages of nursing history outlined in the preceding chapters can be seen in American nursing. Primitive concepts of disease and methods of treatment were found among the Indian tribes which continued long after America was explored and colonized. Home nursing and doctoring prevailed among the early colonists, in which neighbors assisted, but some communities had among their residents partially trained or practical physicians, barber surgeons, and midwives who were called upon in emergencies. Religious orders traveled with the early colonists and gave valiant and devoted service, though they frequently had little or no experience or training in nursing and medical work. Some nursing orders established hospitals and trained lay workers according to the customs of their countries of origin. The few public hospitals and workhouses that existed in the larger cities employed servant-nurses or pauper attendants, and Sairey Gamp had her prototypes among the monthly nurses and midwives employed by private families and by hospitals. During the Revolutionary War and even as late as the Civil War nursing in military hospitals was done by enlisted men or volunteer nurses, often the mothers, wives, and sisters of the men but sometimes religious sisters or paid practical nurses. The Nightingale system followed the Civil War and appeared in the United States and Canada at about the same time. This chapter gives only a brief outline of the first stage of that movement, a fuller account of which is given in Chapters 11 and 12.

NURSING IN CONTINENTAL AMERICA TO 1700

We know little of the care of the sick among the ancient peoples of this continent. Some historians have found in Central

America and Mexico indications of the development of medicine, nursing, and hospitals that go back to remote antiquity. These records refer to the work of women physicians and nurses, but we have too few particulars to form any opinion of the functions or methods of these workers.

The Indians, it is known, had their tribal systems for the care of the sick which were directed by medicine men (in some tribes also by medicine women) trained in the use of magic and other methods of driving out evil spirits. They and their assistants developed considerable skill in massage, sweat baths, crude surgery, and the use of medicinal plants and foods. Some of this knowledge the Indians shared with the early settlers. It is recorded by the colonists in Jamestown, "these people which were our mortall enemies" aided patients suffering from "cruell diseases such as swellings, fluxes, burning fevers and famine," and brought "victuals in great plentie which was the setting up of our feeble men." The religious sisters who pioneered in mission hospitals taught something of their art to Indian women and undoubtedly learned something from them as well. A religious brotherhood of Indians trained in the care of the sick is mentioned in the history of the second oldest hospital on the continent, Santa Fe, Mexico (1531). The first hospital, in what is now Mexico City, was the Immaculate Conception (later named Jesus Nazareno), founded by the stern conqueror Cortes in 1524, possibly to atone for his cruelties. It was staffed at first by an order of monks or nursing brothers.

Two hospitals established in the early French settlement on the St. Lawrence River have had the longest history of active service in America. From small rude bare cabins in the wilds they have grown into imposing and spacious modern city hospitals which have continued to serve the people of their communities for more than three centuries. The first, Hôtel Dieu of Quebec, which dates back to 1639, was staffed by sisters of the Augustinian Order sent out by the Duchesse d'Aiguillon, a niece of Cardinal Richelieu, who was advised on the project by St. Vincent de Paul. The second is the Hôtel Dieu of Montreal (1642), staffed by sisters of the Order of St. Joseph de la Flèche under the leadership of a lay woman, Jeanne Mance. Both orders, like most of the French orders of that day, were enclosed, and they remain so to this day.

Jeanne Mance stands out among the pioneer nurses of those early centuries not only for her humane activities but for her exceptional ability and force of character and the strong influence she exerted on public affairs. Devoutly religious, of distinguished ability and appearance, highly connected, and economically independent, she felt at the age of thirty-four, an inward call to leave her comfortable home in France to journey to the New World. Like the religious sisters who went with her, she had been deeply moved by harrowing stories of hardship and suffering that had reached the home country in letters from missionaries in French Canada. Though she knew nothing of nursing, she accepted a commission from wealthy friends to build and direct a hospital in Montreal and became not only the founder and administrator of this institution but the guiding spirit, planner, and chief executive of the settlement. Because of her responsibility for fund raising, negotiations with government officials, and the business affairs of the settlement, she did not take religious vows. Soon after the hospital was established she placed at its head one of the nursing sisters, Judith de Bresoles, a highly trained person for that day, since she had skill as a pharmacist and chemist and was a good practical clinician. Much has been written about Jeanne Mance and her remarkable achievements as a colonial administrator as well as an able leader in nursing and relief work. Statues in her honor may be seen at the entrance of Hôtel Dieu and in the public squares in Montreal, where her name is closely associated with Sieur Paul de Chomedey de Maissoneuve as one of the city's founders.

Other French orders, including the Grey Nuns, did notable work in the new world. The Ursulines, a teaching order, undertook active nursing service in the French colony of Louisiana, especially during epidemics of yellow fever, cholera, and smallpox. This order in 1716 agreed to establish a hospital in Louisiana which did not materialize at that time, but in 1737, St. John's Hospital, now Charity Hospital of New Orleans, was founded as a hospital and shelter. A memorial to the authorities

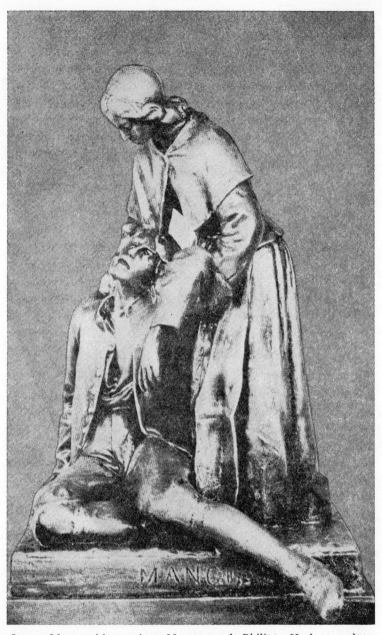

Jeanne Mance with a patient. *Monument de Philippe Herbert, sculpteur canadien, cour d'honneur de l'Hotel-Dieu de Montreal.*

in France from the officials of the colony indicates that among the first to be admitted to the hospital were four or five sick persons.

The first secular hospital in America (later Bellevue, New York) was established in 1658, when traders of the Dutch West India Company built a small shelter in a clearing on Manhattan Island as a pesthouse for infected sailors or slaves. The motive was probably self-protection rather than charity or concern for the sick men, though it is recorded that a nurse was left to care for them. The New Netherland's Register of 1652 notes that a midwife and two sick men's comforters were sent to the colony, the latter with orders "to nurse and doctor the injured, conduct prayer meetings, read the Bible, and look after the welfare and morals of the community." Whether these were the duties of the nurse at the hospital we do not know. With the change in government, the hospital passed out of the hands of the Company and was united with a small poorhouse founded by the Episcopal Church in Manhattan. As the city grew, this expanded into "Old Bellevue," a combination city poorhouse, orphan asylum, house of correction, penitentiary, pesthouse, and hospital for pauper sick, including the insane. In the early part of the nineteenth century all the other parts of this huge unit were removed to Blackwell's Island, leaving the hospital alone at its present site. At a later period, as will be seen, Bellevue became famous as the location of the first Nightingale School of Nursing in America.

HOSPITAL AND NURSING DEVELOPMENT FROM 1700 TO 1800

Through most of this century the "dark period" in nursing continued here as in the older countries. Conditions were especially bad in the big city hospitals, where civic indifference, poor administration, and political intrigues led to many shocking abuses. The Philadelphia General Hospital, founded in 1731 and long known as "Old Blockley" was a notorious example of the public almshouse type of institution. With its dreary

barrack buildings, its filth and squalor, high death rate, con-
glomerate population, indifferent medical staff, and rough ignorant attendants, it was all that a hospital should not be.

Toward the end of the eighteenth century some signs of a revived interest in the care of the sick appeared in the new world
as well as in the old. This was stimulated by the humane influence radiating from the French Enlightenment and the
general decline of superstition and religious prejudice. The
Puritan doctrine of justification by faith rather than by charitable works and the common belief that disease was a punishment for sin had tended to attribute to Providence the high
death rates from epidemics and other preventable diseases and
so to discourage efforts to control them. A few progressive
physicians appealed for better nursing and were supported by
leading intellectuals and liberals such as Benjamin Franklin who
urged kindness and consideration for the sick in the name of
humanity and the public interest. Humanitarian leaders such
as John Howard, John Wesley, William Tuke, Philippe Pinel,
and Elizabeth Fry made their influence felt on both sides of the
ocean, and the humane, tolerant spirit of the English Society of
Friends found an outlet in many practical philanthropies. Since
the Friends were strong in Philadelphia, the City of Brotherly
Love, it is not surprising that the first secular hospital in the
New World to be divorced from workhouse association was
established there. The fact that it was designed for the care of
the sick in body and mind, in the ways then best known to
medical science, is an indication that it was in advance of other
secular and religious hospitals of that day.

The Pennsylvania Hospital was founded in 1751 by Dr.
Thomas Bond and Benjamin Franklin with the support of
public-spirited Quakers, liberal Jews, and other prominent citizens. It was followed shortly after in 1771 by the New York
Hospital, which was established largely by the efforts of a group
of progressive New York physicians. Both of these hospitals
employed paid staffs of men and women nurses who stood out
among hospital attendants of that day as quite respectable and
kindly, though still classed as domestic help and having very
little training. Dr. Valentine Seaman took a forward step when

he organized a series of twenty-four lectures for those employed at the New York Hospital, but the claim made that this was the first training school for nurses in America would seem to be based on a limited concept of the term "school."

Secular hospitals in Canada began to develop about the middle of the eighteenth century, the first one appearing in Halifax, Nova Scotia. With the fall of Quebec in 1759 and the transfer of New France (Canada) to Great Britain, that country came more under British influence, but the religious orders continued their work as before, especially in the French-speaking sections. After the American Revolutionary War (1775-1783), Canada and the United States were divided politically, but, as will be seen, they continued to develop their hospital, medical, and nursing work along nearly parallel lines.

HOSPITAL AND NURSING DEVELOPMENTS UP TO THE CIVIL WAR

With independence won and a republican form of government established, new forces which led to rapid expansion were released in the United States. Wealth increased as many took advantage of the opportunities for trade and speculation and for the immense industrial development made possible by new machinery and the factory system. Immigration, in which Irish, Scandinavian, Italian, and eastern European groups supplied the largest quotas, was increasing at an enormous rate by the end of the nineteenth century. In the large cities slums were developing, with their crowded tenements and sweatshops and high mortality chiefly from epidemics of cholera, yellow fever, malaria, typhoid fever, and other contagious diseases.

With the new settlers came several religious orders both Roman Catholic and Protestant. It was in the South that the Catholic sisters did their most notable work in the earlier part of the century. The Sisters of Charity, founded by Mother Elizabeth Seton in 1809 at Emmittsburg, Maryland, gave special attention to nursing and the care of the poor. Affiliated with the Sisters of Charity of St. Vincent de Paul, its houses soon spread in America. The Sisters of Charity of Nazareth, organized in Louisville in 1812, were also active in nursing, as were the Irish Sisters of Mercy, who arrived in 1842, and the French Sisters of the Holy Cross, who came at about the same time. Many hospitals were built and organized by these and other orders, who also visited the sick in homes and shared in military nursing during the Civil War.

Anglican and other Protestant sisterhoods similar to those noted earlier in Germany, Holland, and England soon began to organize branches in America. Three houses of Kaiserswerth Deaconesses were established in Pittsburgh, Chicago, and Milwaukee, through the cooperation of Pastor Fliedner who visited this country about mid-century, bringing some of his sisters with him. Other deaconess organizations were later introduced in the Episcopal and Methodist churches as well as in the Lutheran. Several orders of Episcopal sisters, patterned more on the Roman Catholic orders than on the Lutheran deaconesses, did nursing and hospital work in the United States. Sisters of the Holy Communion, founded in response to the pleas of Pastor William Muhlenberg of New York, served for thirty years in charge of the nursing service in St. Luke's Hospital of that city. Other Anglican orders were the Sisters of All Saints, Baltimore, Sisters of St. Mary, New York, and Sisters of St. Margaret in Boston, who claim to have been the first in America to train their members as nurses. This, however, was after the first secular Nightingale schools had been established in that part of the world.

Two philanthropic agencies established for the purpose of visiting patients in their homes were the Ladies Benevolent Society of Charleston, South Carolina, founded in 1813, and the Philadelphia Lying-in Charity, in 1828. The first group did some nursing, and in some cases of need provided nurses for patients in their homes. The second joined with the Nurse Society of Philadelphia, founded in 1839 for home nursing and dispensary work. It was supported chiefly by the Friends and aided greatly by Dr. Joseph Warrington, a physician of liberal opinions and philanthropic interests. Following the example of Elizabeth Fry, they appealed to "pious and prudent" young women to work as nurses under their society and arranged a short course of training for them in maternity nursing. A few lectures were given and nurses were required to assist in six cases before they could receive "certificates of approbation" and become eligible for private duty under the general supervision of the society. Fifty nurses were employed between 1839 and 1850. After the opening of a Home and School in 1850, the course was extended somewhat, but since the hospital experience was restricted to obstetrical nursing and the training was not more than three months, (even in 1897 consisting of the care of a few private cases in homes under the supervision of the physician), the claim sometimes made that this was the first *modern nursing school* in America has not been considered valid.

Three other attempts before 1873 to establish nurse training schools were made by women physicians, themselves at this time struggling to find a place in hospital and medical work. The first was in the Women's Hospital of Philadelphia, at which in 1861 a school was announced but was not established until some years later. The second was in the New England Hospital for Women and Children in Boston, where in 1872 Dr. Marie Zakrzewska developed a plan for twelve months of practical hospital experience with a course of twelve lectures to which ladies from the city as well as resident pupils were admitted. The third was planned as a part of the New York Infirmary for Women and Children established in 1859 by two sisters who came from England, Drs. Elizabeth and Emily Blackwell. Elizabeth was a personal friend of Miss Nightingale and a firm believer in her nursing and sanitary reforms. This school would have been the first in America but for the interruption of war work in which the Blackwell sisters took a leading part.

NURSING IN THE WAR OF NORTH AND SOUTH

The war gave an immense impetus to reforms in nursing as well as in medicine and sanitation. When it began in 1861, there were almost no trained nurses in the country. Dr. Henry W.

Bellows, Unitarian minister, issued the first call to New York women to organize for war service. The meeting, held at the Cooper Institute, led to the formation of the Woman's Central Association of Relief, which in turn was followed by the United States Sanitary Commission. The work of the commission was of the greatest importance. It was a Red Cross organization without the name, and so well known in Europe that one wonders why so little recognition of its work was given by Henri Dunant and the other founders of the International Red Cross Society in 1863 and 1864. Dr. Elizabeth Blackwell should have had the honor of leading the work of these Civil War organizations, but prejudice against women physicians was then so great that she withdrew from official responsibility rather than handicap the work. Behind the scenes, however, she was active and influential largely through the valuable advice and suggestions she received from Miss Nightingale. This recognized authority also sent literature on nursing and sanitary measures to government agencies and to some groups in the South. Short intensive courses were given to volunteers in several hospitals which opened their wards to recruits, one hundred being so inducted in Bellevue and at the New York Hospital. Although the South did not have an organization comparable to the Sanitary Commission, groups of volunteer nurses were to be found in its war hospitals, many of whom did heroic work.

Most of the war nursing was done by untrained volunteers, male orderlies drawn from enlisted personnel, and paid practical nurses. It is estimated that two thousand women, from the North and South, shared in such war service, including members of religious orders, Roman Catholic and Protestant. Among these women were such forceful and colorful characters as "Mother Bickerdyke" (Mary Ann Ball), Mrs. Ella Newsome Trader, Sister Anthony O'Connell, and many other well-known persons who left impressive records of their achievements and influence. Several wrote books and articles about their experiences: Mary Livermore, Katharine Prescott Wormeley, Jane Grey Swisshelm, the Woolsey sisters, Louisa May Alcott, and Walt Whitman of the North; and Kate Cumming, Susan Leigh Blackford, Judith Brockenbrough McGuire, and Phoebe Yates

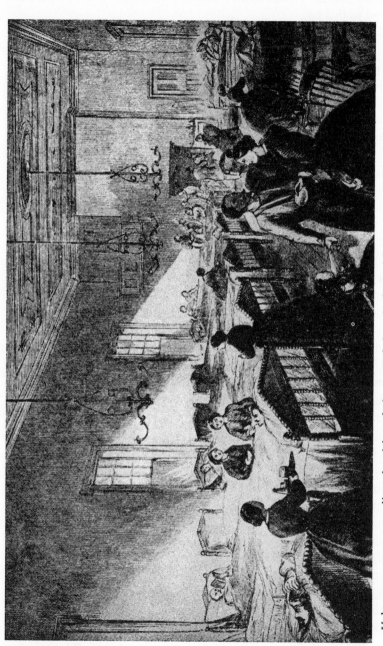

Volunteer nurses attending the sick and the wounded at the United States General Hospital at Georgetown, D.C. From *Leslie's Illustrated Newspaper*, July 6, 1861.

Pember of the South. Other names from both sides could be added to this list.

Early in the war the government appointed as official superintendent of nurses Dorothea Dix, who had aided Dr. W. G. Eliot of St. Louis in organizing the Western Sanitary Commission (1861) along the same lines as the United States Sanitary Commission in the East. Miss Dix was a remarkable woman, a second John Howard, or as Pope Pius IX called her, "a modern Saint Theresa." In the United States she had made a series of investigations into asylums for the insane, and by her forceful and persistent reports and appeals to legislatures had helped to bring into existence laws providing for state hospitals for mental patients. Her character and life-work were alike impressive, but she was not young enough at this time to lead in nursing reform. She did succeed in having the army adopt a fairly systematic plan of regulations for nurses, but her ideas on discipline, dress, and the like were rather severe, even for those days, and she had a definite mistrust of young and pretty nurses.

Clara Barton, who later was to persuade the United States Government to ratify the Geneva Treaty of the Red Cross (1881), served as a volunteer "free lance" during the war and did notable work in the search for missing men. She showed remarkable courage and initiative and carried succor to friend and foe alike, thereby earning the ill will of some extreme patriots. But her war work was not primarily in the care of the sick, and she did not identify herself with those who led in basic nursing reforms. Devoting herself to the ideals of the International Red Cross, she accepted its emphasis on volunteer service with short courses by physicians and brief hospital service as a preparation for war work. Strongly individualistic but benevolent in spirit, a teacher rather than an organizer, she was known chiefly for her service to the Red Cross. Her later connection with war nursing during the Spanish American War is referred to in Chapter 11.

The New York Woolsey family's record of voluntary service in the war and postwar period is surely an exceptional one. Jane, Georgeanna, and Eliza served as nurse administrators during the war, and their mother and sister Caroline worked for shorter periods in war hospitals. Abby Woolsey had a responsible position on the central committee which prepared and sent out hospital supplies and her sister Harriet assisted her. Like Mrs. Preston Griffin and Louisa Lee Schuyler, also of New York, who nursed in the war hospitals, three of the sisters pioneered in introducing modern nursing schools and services in the New World after the war was over. Jane became the first director of the new Presbyterian Hospital in New York, where she was assisted by Abby, leaving a good record as a firm and fearless administrator. Georgeanna and her husband Dr. Frank Bacon were active members of the committee which founded the training school for nurses at the New Haven Hospital (one of the three started in 1873). Abby was for a number of years a valued member of the Bellevue Committee, which initiated the first training school for nurses in America. She not only helped to plan the educational program but wrote *A Century of Nursing*, which recorded current developments in Britain and on the Continent. In addition to nursing activities, Georgeanna and Eliza played an important role in the establishment of the Chaplain Service in the hospitals of the Army of the Potomac early in the war. All were writers in the fields of their respective interests, another sister, Mary, having written war poems which had a wide circulation and were much appreciated by the soldiers in the war hospitals. Even Charles, the only brother, was for a time active on the hospital transports in the East in the work of identifying and classifying patients as they were brought on board, a service that called for some nursing and first aid.

BEGINNINGS OF POSTWAR NURSING REFORM

The first suggestion for a national nurse training program in the United States came from Dr. Samuel D. Gross, an eminent Philadelphia physician who had traveled abroad and had been impressed by the nursing reforms in Germany and Britain. Like many of his medical friends in these countries he saw the need for improvement but felt that control of nursing and nurse training should be left to his profession. After presenting some of his ideas before the newly formed American Medical Association, he was appointed chairman of a committee to prepare a plan for the training of nurses in the United States. His report the following year (1869) proposed that the AMA develop a nationwide scheme for hospital training schools which would be sponsored by county medical societies. The members of these bodies were to help to organize such schools, provide the instruction needed, and otherwise be responsible for their direction. Although it was suggested that homes for nurses in training be placed under the direction of a deaconess or lady superintendent, as in Germany, such appointees were not to have authority in the hospital or to function as the matrons and ward sisters did in the Nightingale system. This report was accepted by the AMA and circulated among its members, but no schools can be traced to its influence. It is probable, however, that some of the medical opposition to the independent Nightingale schools which were established four years later arose from this source.

The Nightingale schools were sponsored chiefly by civic and philanthropic groups in which were many women who had served in the war hospitals and had come back deeply impressed by the need for better nursing and general hospital reforms. The New York group was stirred into action by the graft and corruption of the notorious Tweed Ring and the exposure of hospital and other scandals by the press in the early 70's. This led some influential citizens to organize the State Charities Aid Association (1872) as a means of improving conditions in public hospitals and workhouses. Among the leaders was Louisa Lee Schuyler, who had won distinction for her work in the United States Sanitary Commission, and was widely known for her civic and philanthropic work. Appointed chairman of the Visiting Committee of the State Charities Aid, she, and her co-workers, at once started the hospital visits which were to lead to the founding of the Bellevue School in May 1873. Its story will give some idea of the problems faced in this and other pioneer schools, two of which followed in the same year. These were the Boston Training School for Nurses, connected with the Massachusetts General Hospital, and later called by its name, and the Connecticut Training School at New Haven

Hospital. The Boston school was founded by the Women's Educational Association of Boston and that in New Haven by a group of men and women, among whom were several physicians.

THE FIRST NIGHTINGALE SCHOOL IN AMERICA

The Bellevue story opens with the dramatic meeting of the Women's Visiting Committee in New York and the report of Mrs. Elizabeth Hobson's momentous visit to the wards of this old and then notorious institution. With the help of an interested house surgeon, Dr. Gill Wylie, who suggested that the visitor follow him at a safe distance, she got a shocking picture not only of the neglected patients but of the so-called nurses, most of whom were vagrants or prisoners from the nearby workhouse who had been arrested for drunkenness, immorality, and other misdemeanors. They slept on straw beds laid on the bathroom floor, terrorized the helpless sick, took fees, and were not to be trusted with medicines nor with food brought in by visitors.

The Women's Visiting Committee took action at once, and a special committee was appointed to plan for a school of nursing following the Nightingale pattern. Vigorous opposition was met from commissioners, warden, and a large part of the medical staff of the hospital, but with the support of prominent citizens and a few influential physicians the ladies secured permission to use a small group of wards for their training plan. The hospital agreed to turn over to the Committee the sums paid to former workers; other funds for the nurses' home and school were to be raised by the Committee. As in Britain, the first American schools were separate from the hospitals in which training was given, their obligations for patient care and ward administration being specified in a contract which was signed by both parties concerned.

The always helpful Dr. Gill Wylie made a great contribution to the whole plan by offering to go to Britain at his own expense to get details about the workings of the schools there. Though he did not meet the Founder herself, he saw the system in action and was greatly impressed by the results. Soon after his return he received a letter from Florence Nightingale in answer to the questions he had put to her in writing. This famous letter, which contained a wealth of information, including a frank but tactful exposition on the relations of nursing and medicine, became a guide and charter for the Bellevue School and for others starting at that time. The Bellevue School committee soon won over its opponents by the striking transformation brought about in the wards under its control. Other wards were added as applicants increased, and soon the school took over the care of all ward patients. In addition to their hospital assignments, senior students were often sent out on private duty and a few did some visiting nursing.

OTHER EARLY SCHOOLS AND THEIR INFLUENCE

The Bellevue story was repeated with some variations in Boston, New Haven, Philadelphia, Chicago, Detroit, and other large cities where similar pioneer schools were established. Though most of these schools were connected with public, nonsectarian, general hospitals, it was not long before all types and sizes of hospitals were beginning to set up their own training schools. Among these were several for Roman Catholic and Anglican sisters and Lutheran deaconesses. The Sisters of St. Francis of St. John's Hospital, Springfield, Illinois, opened a school for their sisters in 1886, and in 1889 the Sisters of Mercy in Chicago and the Sisters of Mary in Brooklyn opened their schools to lay nurses as well. The Sisters of St. Margaret (Anglican) developed a training school at the Boston Children's Hospital in 1889. Several other "firsts" were established in this period, such as the first school in a mental hospital, McLean at Waverly, Massachusetts, started in 1879 but not well organized until 1882. The first for men nurses (Mills School at Bellevue, New York), dates from 1888 and the first for Negro nurses (Provident Hospital, Chicago), from 1891.

The pioneer school in Canada, in the small General and Marine Hospital at St. Catharines, Ontario (1873), owes its creation largely to the efforts of Dr. Theophilus Mack. After this came the larger schools at the Toronto General Hospital (1881) and the Winnipeg General Hospital (1887), the first in Western Canada. The Sisters of St. Joseph were the first of the Roman Catholic orders to establish a modern school at St. Michael's Hospital, Toronto (1892). Many others were started before 1900, when most hospitals, large and small, had recognized the economic and other advantages of the new system.

Hospital and nursing reform was carried through its first phase by a group of strong, energetic, intrepid organizers and administrators full of the uncompromising spirit of the reformer. What they did was largely house cleaning on an extended scale. They warred against physical dirt and disorder, against immorality and irresponsibility, political corruption and every form of opposition and hostility, striving to regenerate the moral atmosphere, to banish vulgarity, neglect, and indifference, and to make hospitals safe not only for patients but for nurses. Though these nurse administrators were strict disciplinarians and often distant and severe in manner, the great majority were exceptionally courageous and competent and were honored by the public as well as by the nurses who worked with them. Largely through their efforts, nurses and nursing won the respect and confidence of hospital and medical groups and of the general public. With the aid of lay and medical support, they developed private and visiting nurse services, prepared the first textbooks, set up the first registries and nurses clubs, and got the young vocation started toward professional goals.

EXCHANGES IN NURSING PERSONNEL AND IDEAS

Among these pioneers and pathfinders were many British nurses. Bellevue was opened by Helen Bowden, a Sister of All Saints Sisterhood of the Anglican Church (though she agreed not to use that title or wear the sister's habit at the city hospital). She had received some training in a London hospital and was a strong-minded, capable administrator with a quick temper which was probably more of an asset than a liability in this position. Though not herself a product of the Nightingale system, she was a firm believer in it. In her brief but successful period as Lady Superintendent at Bellevue, this militant sister routed the chief enemies of the nursing school, and with the aid of the first group of recruits cleaned up the worst conditions in the hospital. A similar reform was carried through later by Alice Fisher, distinguished "Nightingale" from St. Thomas's, London, who tackled the notorious "Old Blockley" in Philadelphia and died there as a result of her labors. Physicians and citizens were so impressed by her achievements that they secured several other British nurses for similar positions in Philadelphia hospitals, among them Lucy Walker, whose chief work was done in the Pennsylvania Hospital and Maud Banfield who was hospital superintendent at the Polyclinic Hospital, one of the first to hold such a position. The last two were specially active in the professional organization of nurses and in the new educational movements that started around 1900.

The New York Hospital Training School, founded in 1877 in a well-endowed voluntary hospital, became outstanding under the able leadership of Irene Sutliffe, one of its own graduates. Among its internationally famous alumnae were Lillian D. Wald, Annie W. Goodrich, and Mary Beard, all of whom had exceptionally successful careers and exerted a strong influence on nursing service and education in many countries. The Boston City Hospital Training School also produced a number of noted nurses, among them Lucy Drown and Mary Riddle, fine New England gentlewomen and former teachers who became well-known educators and administrators, and Anna C. Maxwell, who distinguished herself as a superintendent of nurses in several hospitals before she established the Presbyterian Hospital School in New York. From the Massachusetts General Hospital Training School came a long succession of able graduates, such as Sophia F. Palmer, first editor of the *American Journal of Nursing* and leader in the campaign for state registration of nurses, and Sara Parsons, a pioneer in mental nursing, who directed her own school for many years and wrote its history.

RECIPROCITY IN NURSING BETWEEN THE UNITED STATES AND CANADA

The fame of Bellevue attracted many capable Canadian applicants, some of whom went back to pioneer in their own country while others remained in the United States, where hospital and nursing work was spreading more rapidly in the 80's and 90's. Among those who returned to Canada were Mary Agnes Snively, who established the nursing school at the Toronto General Hospital, and Edith Draper, another at the Royal Victoria Hospital in Montreal. Louise Darche, with her English associate, Diana Kimber, developed the first school at the City Hospital of New York, twin of Bellevue and equally formidable at this time for its political corruption and other bad conditions. Isabel Hampton, after organizing the Illinois Training School and the nursing service at Cook County Hospital, Chicago, went to the Johns Hopkins Hospital in Baltimore, where she established its new school, setting what was then an exceptionally high educational standard. After her marriage to Dr. Hunter Robb, she was succeeded by her assistant, Adelaide Nutting, a Canadian member of the first Johns Hopkins class, an ardent educator, and an able administrator who was to become widely known in the nursing world as a leader in the university education of nurses. Lystra Gretter was another who came from across the border and did most of her work in Detroit where she directed the Farrand Training School of the Harper Hospital. This school, founded in 1883, was the first to have an endowment, and under Mrs. Gretter it established (1891) the first eight-hour day for student nurses. With the help of a committee, she also formulated the widely used Florence Nightingale Pledge, one of the earliest written expressions of the ethical principles of nursing. Agnes Deans, a Harper graduate from Canada, is remembered especially for her contribution to the organization of nurses' associations. Other examples of similar interchanges of ideas and personnel between these neighbor countries are given in Chapters 11 and 12.

LINDA RICHARDS—AMERICA'S FIRST TRAINED NURSE

Among the earlier American trained nurses few if any had the wide and varied experience of Linda Richards or contributed more to the establishment of the new system in her own country and abroad. After graduating from the Barton Academy in Vermont, she became a school teacher for a short time, then entered a hospital of the older type to find out what she could about nursing. Hearing in 1872 that the New England Hospital for Women and Children (Boston) was offering a one-year course for nurses, she applied and in 1873 became the first nurse to win a diploma. This, however, was not a Nightingale school, for it was attached to a small specialized hospital directed by a woman physician, Dr. Susan Dimock, whose knowledge of nursing was chiefly what she had picked up in her studies in German hospitals. When word came of the opening of the new Nightingale School at Bellevue in 1873, Miss Richards applied and was appointed night superintendent. Here she learned much about the new system and took an active share in establishing it. From Bellevue she went to take charge of a sister school in Boston, where she was able to straighten out some of its difficulties. Then, seeking a wider knowledge of nursing in Britain, she secured an opportunity to serve and share for some months in the work of two outstanding schools at St. Thomas's Hospital, London, and the Edinburgh Infirmary. In addition to having many discussions with other British nurses, she met and talked with Miss Nightingale and returned a convinced disciple, though fully aware of the need to adapt the British system to American conditions and needs. Instead of settling down in one place, she then went from one hospital to another (twelve in all), organizing nursing schools and services along Nightingale lines. She also succeeded in persuading her own New England Hospital to appoint a nurse instead of a physician as director of the nursing school and service. Not satisfied with all this missionary work at home, she accepted an appointment to Kyoto, Japan, and stayed there five years developing the first Nightingale school in the Orient in a small mission hospital. On her return she pioneered in two new branches of nursing, serving for a short time as director of the Philadelphia Visiting Nurse Society, and then giving her attention to schools of nursing in mental hospitals.

Linda Richards also took an active part in the building of professional organizations of nurses; she was elected first president of the new American Society of Superintendents of Training Schools for Nurses in 1894 and later served on the committee which planned the Hospital Economics course opened in 1899 at Teachers College, Columbia University, New York. In the same year she had the honor of buying the first share of stock of the *American Journal of Nursing,* the first national nursing publication in America owned and edited by organized nurses. Finally, she wrote her autobiography, *Reminiscences of Linda Richards* (published in 1911). It tells much more than her own story and gives a vivid picture of the early years of modern nursing in three different countries.

This chapter has included some reviews of older systems and stages of nursing development as well as the introduction of modern nursing in several parts of the New World. It would be a mistake to assume, however, that most of the struggles of nurses were over when the new system was adopted by more and more hospitals and schools of nursing were beginning to multiply at a rapid rate. Actually, as will be seen in Part II, this was the beginning of a long struggle to maintain good standards and at the same time to satisfy the rapidly increasing demand for trained nurses for the widening field of nursing service. The story of the professional organization of nurses and many other nursing developments in the United States and Canada is continued in Chapters 11 and 12.

SELECTED BIBLIOGRAPHY

Atherton, William Henry. *The Saintly Life of Jeanne Mance, First Lay Nurse in North America.* St. Louis: Cath. Hosp. Assn., 1945.

Austin, Anne L. *History of Nursing Source Book.* New York: Putnam's, 1957. Ch. 8, 9.

Blackford, Susan Leigh. *Letters from Lee's Army.* Ed. by Charles Minor Blackford, III. New York: Scribner's, 1947.

Blackwell, Elizabeth. *Pioneer Work in Opening the Medical Profession to Women, and Autobiographical Sketches.* New York: Longmans, 1895.

Brainard, Annie M. *The Evolution of Public Health Nursing.* Philadelphia: Saunders, 1922.

Brockett, Linus Pierpont, and M. C. Vaughan. *Women's Work in the Civil War: A Record of Heroism, Patriotism, and Patience.* Philadelphia: Ziegler, Mc-Curdy, 1867.

Commager, Henry Steele, and Allan Nevins (Eds.) *The Heritage of America;* Boston: Little Brown, rev. ed., 1951. Readings on Dorothea Dix and Hospital Transports.

Cumming, Kate. *Journal of Hospital Life in the Confederate Army of Tennessee.* Louisville: J. P. Morton, 1866. Rev. ed.: *Kate: The Journal of a Confederate Nurse.* Ed. by Richard Barksdale Harwell. Baton Rouge: La. State Univ. Press, 1959.

Dannett, Sylvia G. L. (Comp. & Ed.) *Noble Women of the North.* New York: Thomas Yoseloff, 1959. Esp. Ch. 2-6.

Deans, Agnes G., and Anne L. Austin. *The History of the Farrand Training School for Nurses.* Detroit: Alumnae Assn., 1936.

Delavan, David Bryson. *Early Days of the Presbyterian Hospital in the City of New York.* Published privately, 1926.

Dock, Lavinia L., and others. *History of American Red Cross Nursing.* New York: Macmillan, 1922.

Dunwiddie, Mary. *A History of the Illinois State Nurses Association 1901-1935.* Chicago: The Assn., 1937.

Epler, Percy H. *Life of Clara Barton.* New York: Macmillan, new ed., 1946.

Gardner, Mary S. *Public Health Nursing.* New York: Macmillan, 1936.

Giles, Dorothy. *A Candle in Her Hand.* New York: Putnam's, 1950.

Goostray, Stella. *Fifty Years: A History of the School of Nursing. The Children's Hospital, Boston.* Boston: Alumnae Assn., 1940.

Greenbie, Marjorie Latta (Barstow). *Lincoln's Daughters of Mercy.* New York: Putnam's, 1944.

Hampton, Isabel A., and others. *Nursing of the Sick 1893.* New York: McGraw-Hill, 1949. Pp. 1-24, 50-53, 88-110, 137-144, 149-158, 204-209.

Hobson, Elizabeth Christophers. *Recollections of a Happy Life.* New York: Putnam's, 1916. Ch. VI. This chapter also in Woolsey, *A Century of Nursing,* pp. 135-172.

Jordan, Helen Jamieson. *Cornell University-New York Hospital School of Nursing, 1877-1952.* New York: Soc. of the N. Y. Hosp., 1952.

[Keller, Malvina W.]. *History of the St. Luke's Hospital Training School for Nurses.* New York: St. Luke's Hospital, 1938.

Leech, Margaret. *Reveille in Washington, 1860-1865.* New York: Harper, 1941. Ch. XI.

McCann, Sister Mary Agnes. *The History of Mother Seton's Daughters: The Sisters of Charity of Cincinnati, Ohio, 1819-1917.* New York: Longman's Green, 1917. 3 vols.

Marshall, Helen E. *Dorothea Dix: Forgotten Samaritan.* Chapel Hill, University of North Carolina Press, 1937.

Maxwell, William Quentin. *Lincoln's Fifth Wheel. The Political History of the United States Sanitary Commission.* New York: Longman's Green, 1956.

Nutting, M. Adelaide, and Lavinia L. Dock. *A History of Nursing.* New York: Putnam's, 1907-1912. 4 vols. Vol. I, Part II, Ch. X; Vol. II, Part III, Ch. IX, pp. 326-436.

Packard, Francis R. *Some Account of the Pennsylvania Hospital.* Philadelphia: Engle Press, 1938.

Parsons, Sara H. *History of the Massachusetts General Hospital Training School for Nurses.* Boston: Whitcomb & Barrows, 1922.

Pember, Phoebe Yates. *A Southern Woman's Story.* Jackson, Tenn.: McCowat-Mercer, 1959.

Richards, Linda. *Reminiscences of Linda Richards, America's First Trained Nurse.* Philadelphia: Lippincott, 1949.

Stewart, Isabel Maitland. *The Education of Nurses.* New York: Macmillan, 1943. Ch. III.

Woolsey, Abby Howland. *A Century of Nursing.* New York: Putnam's, 1950.

Worcester, Alfred A. *Nurses and Nursing.* Cambridge: Harvard University Press, 1927.

———. *Nurses for Our Neighbors.* Boston: Houghton Mifflin, 1914.

Part II

This part covers a relatively short period (1860 to the present) but takes in a large section of the globe, following the spread of the modern nursing movement introduced in Chapters 7 and 8. Chapter 9 suggests some of the general historical events of the century which had a powerful influence on this movement, also some national characteristics and conditions which tended to modify the nursing systems that took shape in different countries and the rate of growth in the movement itself. The next four chapters give a general account of nursing progress in five English-speaking countries which adopted the Nightingale system early and did much to introduce it into other parts of the world. They also took the lead in developing nursing as a profession and in organizing it on a national and international basis. Shorter summaries follow of the modern systems that developed in Europe, Asia, Latin America, and Africa. The last chapter focuses on the main international organizations and agencies that have done much to support and advance the world nursing movement. It notes also some issues and trends in international nursing.

On the maps in Part II only the early centers of the modern nursing movement are indicated.

CHAPTER 9

Plan for a World View of Modern Nursing

THE need for a world view of nursing is more obvious today than ever before. With the globe shrinking rapidly, science creating new and terrible weapons of destruction, and powerful forces threatening to divide nations and peoples into warring groups, nurses and other members of the life-saving professions are becoming more conscious of the need not only for a good scientific and technical preparation but for a wider knowledge of health conditions, facilities, and systems of medicine, public health, and nursing in different countries.

Apart from the growing international responsibilities of nurses, there are many reasons for a broad view that throws light on different nursing systems and stages of development and leads to a better appreciation of the problems of nurses in other parts of the world. Needless to say, the main purpose is neither to consider which country has the best system nor to criticize ways of doing things that are unlike one's own but rather to understand why things are as they are and to lay a better basis for friendship and cooperation among nurses of the world. Though such groups often speak different languages and are at different stages of development, they usually find much that they can share with one another. This is especially true of those who are associated with the modern nursing movement and who have united in international and national organizations to promote the health and well being of all peoples as well as the advancement of their own profession in all parts of the world.

GENERAL HISTORICAL BACKGROUND
FOR THIS PERIOD

As in preceding periods, a brief view of general events and movements is needed to understand what went on in nursing during the last century. Beginning with military events, one is impressed by the increasing numbers of wars. The Crimean War in the 1850's, the American Civil War in the 1860's, the Spanish-American and Boer Wars at the turn of the century, the two disastrous World Wars starting in 1914 and 1939 all led to great loss of life and to increasing participation of nurses in military service. Out of the two world wars came also the League of Nations (1920-1946) and its successor the United Nations in 1945, both concerned with the prevention of war and with international cooperation in the cause of world health. These organizations called for a much wider knowledge of health needs and for more modern systems of nursing in all parts of the world.

During this period many other political changes came about that directly or indirectly influenced nursing progress. Liberal and democratic movements were broadening the rights of citizens and giving them a larger share in public affairs. Labor and socialist movements put special emphasis on the health of working men and women and their families. Colonial empires in Asia and Africa and other parts of the globe were breaking up into nation-states. The Russian Revolution, beginning in 1917, introduced new conflicts and divisions as well as ideologies that were to have a direct influence on nursing in large sections of the world.

When the twentieth century opened, science, chief of the forces of the modern age that were remaking the world, was pouring forth new discoveries and inventions in a steady stream. Miracles of healing and disease prevention were made possible by the astonishing series of bacteriological discoveries starting in the final decades of the nineteenth century and continuing into the twentieth. Death rates from communicable diseases and surgical infections fell spectacularly as infected water and food supplies, insect pests, and other disease breeders were cleaned up and educational campaigns began to reach homes, schools, factories, and the population generally. Discoveries in chemistry and physics brought in a wide array of diagnostic and curative devices—X-ray and radium, hormones and vitamins, drugs such as the sulphas and penicillin, and other developments in physical, occupational, and diet therapy. In hospitals the rapid expansion and development of modern medicine and surgery called not only for new operating rooms and laboratories and greatly enlarged accommodations for public and private patients but also for much larger numbers of modern trained nurses. Soon there followed the new psychiatry and many other aspects of medical science that directly affected nursing.

Before the scientific movement was in full swing, the economic aspects of health and medical care were receiving attention in many countries. Individual and family resources, even when supplemented by philanthropy, did not begin to cover the cost of sickness and accidents in most families. This led to experimentation with different forms of sickness, accident, and old-age insurance. At first these plans were undertaken by trade unions, fraternal societies, and voluntary cooperative groups of various kinds. In the 80's the first definite steps were taken by the governments of Germany and Austria to enact social and health-insurance legislation for low-income groups. Other countries soon followed with similar laws, and before 1914 nearly all European countries and a few non-European ones had some form of national sickness and accident insurance and other plans for social security. In 1919 Soviet Russia introduced its nation-wide system of state medicine, and not long after the Nazi and Fascist governments of Germany and Italy developed their totalitarian pattern of centralized planning and control which brought all medical and related services under the state. A new system of public medicine was beginning to take shape, especially in central and eastern Europe. The western democracies which stood for a maximum of voluntary effort and a minimum of government regulation began to extend their public health departments and to adopt voluntary plans for health and sickness insurance.

Though modern medicine and nursing services were in general nonsectarian and closely identified with civic, governmental, and voluntary social agencies, various religious groups continued to administer and support hospitals and other health agencies and to prepare nurses for these services. Many nurse-missionaries were sent into foreign countries carrying with them modern nursing ideas and systems of training. During this period civil, social, humanitarian, and other agencies were also developing, and a more scientific and social attitude toward disease, poverty, and similar ills was gradually weakening the older dependence on philanthropy and charity.

The campaign for woman's suffrage, which had started earlier, was well under way before 1900 and was making its influence felt in nursing as well as in education, politics, and other areas. Though the vote did not come before the end of World War I, except in a few small countries or states, the suffrage movement did much to stimulate nurses' interest in public affairs and to strengthen international bonds which took definite form in the International Council of Nurses organized in 1900. It also helped to develop nurse leadership and to train speakers and writers who could present their cause to political and other groups.

THE NATIONAL SETTINGS IN WHICH NURSING DEVELOPS

Turning now from the international picture, some national influences that help to account for many differences in nursing systems and stages of development are noted. Among them are the physical features of the country, such as climate and topography, the population and its distribution, the food supply, facilities for travel, and other conditions that have a direct bearing on health conditions and services. Examples that suggest themselves are such sections as Alaska and Labrador, the highlands and islands of Scotland, the mountains of Kentucky, the deserts and jungles of Africa, and the almost inaccessible interior of South America. More important are the people themselves, their personal characteristics, and their occupations, which differ as much as their physical surroundings. They may be racially homogeneous or made up of diverse stocks and strains and speaking different languages. Marked differences may exist also between city and country dwellers, plainsmen and mountaineers, insular and seafaring groups. Demographic statistics often show wide regional variations in birth, death, and sickness rates, the prevalence of mental and physical diseases and defects, educational opportunities, and other factors that directly influence all health services. Equally diverse may be national or regional attitudes concerned with such matters as health and sanitation, the position of women, and religious beliefs and affiliations. National psychology and customs may present more difficulties for a nursing service than a frigid or torrid climate or bad transportation conditions.

To understand national systems of nursing, one needs to know something about the established institutions of the country and the machinery through which the people carry on their corporate activities. The nursing system is part of this machinery and is geared more or less closely with the governmental, legal, economic, and educational systems as well as with hospitals and other agencies concerned with the treatment and prevention of disease and with other organized health professions. As a social service, nursing is directly affected by the class structure of the country, by social divisions based on race, caste, or wealth, by patterns of family and community organization, by religious, charitable, and fraternal groups, and by others concerned with civic and social welfare and living standards. Since most nursing is done by women one should know about the status of women as a class, their place in the social structure, and their role in society. The degree to which scientific medicine, sanitation, and popular education have been developed is of obvious importance, since nursing cannot progress far in a country that is backward in these respects.

Many other points will be noted as different countries are discussed and their experience in developing modern systems of nursing is recorded. To keep these in mind, a simple chart could be drawn up that lists the more dominant national influences in each country under such headings as the land, the people, established institutions, and national psychology and customs.

ASPECTS OF MODERN NURSING TO BE SPECIALLY NOTED

Coming now to a survey of modern nursing in various parts of the world, it is obvious that the whole story cannot be told in this short history. Chief attention is given to the main stages in the development of nursing as an independently organized vocation or profession closely related to medicine but with its own functions and fields of activity and its established place in the economic, social, and educational structure of the countries in which it has developed. Clearly the new ideas must be defined and interpreted for those who are to be responsible for the development of schools, the preparation of nurses and the organization and support of nursing services, also for the recruitment and selection of suitable candidates and their placement in the different fields of nursing open to them. Such opportunities must be expanded as new requirements are recognized and new levels of competence are called for. Problems of many kinds must be met, and the members of the new vocation must find ways of uniting their forces in order to deal adequately with these. The need for a means of sharing ideas and suggestions will soon lead to nursing journals and other publications. Special studies will follow dealing with various aspects of nursing—aims and standards, education, fields of service, legislation, registration, ethics, economics, and many other subjects concerned with the growing responsibilities of nurses and their plans for the future.

All vocations and professions must take stock from time to time to note the conditions of the field and their own accomplishments, to set goals and make tentative plans for the period immediately ahead. National nursing groups in many countries have accepted this responsibility. Alone or in cooperation with medical, hospital, and other associations, they have attempted to analyze the nursing situation and current trends in medical and health services and to make recommendations as a basis for further discussion, experimentation and possible future action. Although such studies do not predict the future, they help to prepare nurses for necessary changes and adjustments.

Since emphasis has been given here to the modern nursing movement, consideration is given also to the influences that helped or hindered its advance or tended to change its direction or to disrupt the unity and cooperation of nurses. Among such influences, the kind of leadership developed is especially important. The historian Arnold Toynbee has suggested that progress toward self-determination and self-articulation is an indication of growth in such groups. He puts special emphasis on the development of creative individuals and minorities who inspire and lead the less creative and dynamic majority to meet new challenges—not automatically, but with new techniques and patterns. This suggests special attention to the development of competent and far-seeing leaders who can mobilize the forces needed to keep the movement advancing, help to steer it in the right direction, and unite the members of the nursing profession and their supporters in meeting the problems of the times in new and creative ways. In addition to individual leaders (who are not always nurses) are various organized groups whose interest and support is essential for nursing progress—local, national, and international.

SELECTED BIBLIOGRAPHY

Bennett, B. A. "Modern Trends in Nurse Training and Nursing Practice," *Int. Nurs. Rev.*, Autumn and Winter, 1949, 11-17.
Chronicle of the World Health Organization. Geneva: Published monthly.

Gsovski, Vladimir. *Nursing Legislation of the World.* Cincinnati: Lawyers Directory, 1947. 4 vols.

Headline Series. New York: Foreign Policy Association. Published bimonthly.

International Nursing Review. London: ICN. Published six times a year.

Lindemann, Edward. "Social Planning for Tomorrow," *Proc. Nat. League Nurs. Ed.,* 1936, 251-258.

Mead, Margaret. *New Lives for Old—Cultural Transformation. Manus.* New York: Morrow, 1956.

Methods and Problems of Medical Education. New York: Rockefeller Found., 1932.

Mountin, Joseph Walter, and George St. J. Perrott. "Health Insurance Programs and Plans of Western Europe," *Pub. Health Rep.,* March 14, 1947, 369-399.

Mueller, Kate Hevner. *Educating Women for a Changing World.* Minneapolis: University of Minnesota Press, 1954.

New York Times.

Perrott, G. St. J. "Voluntary Health Insurance in Western Europe," *Pub. Health Rep.,* May 23, 1947, 733-757.

Pocket Guides. On various countries. Prepared by the Office of Armed Forces Information and Education, Department of Defense, Washington: Government Printing Office.

World Today. Royal Inst. of Int. Affairs. Chatham House, 10 St. James Square, London, S. W. 1, England.

CHAPTER **10**

Great Britain and Ireland

THIS is the logical place to begin a world survey of modern nursing, not only because the Nightingale system first took root here but because the general conditions in Britain[1]—political, social and economic—as well as its fortunate geographic situation, its world trade and far-flung empire, gave it exceptional opportunities to carry the new ideas into many quarters of the globe. Among its people also were many with the qualities that make successful pioneers and promoters of social and humanitarian causes—courage, a strong sense of duty, discipline, self-confidence, determination, and the ability to adapt to the conditions of different countries. Though British women in 1860 still suffered under some traditional handicaps, a few were breaking through the old restrictions and taboos and were finding careers for themselves in different forms of public service. Among those who entered nursing were many with a strong religious or missionary bent who were ready to go to the far corners of the earth to introduce the new system and to build up nursing schools and services on modern lines. As we shall

[1] The terms Great Britain and British are used here for the British Isles until 1937, when southern Ireland became a separate state. A brief section (pp. 188-190) summarizes recent developments in that country.

see, they had many hard battles to fight at home before the young vocation was firmly established and its members were able to meet the rapidly increasing demand for their services and to carry out the educational and other plans set up by the Founder.

EARLY NIGHTINGALE SCHOOLS

Before much could be done to reform and develop nursing service in hospitals and homes, it was necessary to recruit and train nurses. The country had many hospitals, but they, at first, showed little interest in the new system of nursing. The National Nightingale Fund had made it possible to create an independent endowed school with its own nurses' home, under a special committee which employed the nurse administrator and her staff, provided scholarships for probationers, and entered into agreements with hospitals and district nursing associations in which these learners were to receive their practical training. Though St. Thomas's Hospital supplied most of this experience and its matron, Mrs. S. E. Wardroper, held a dual position as director of the school, neither the hospital's trustees nor its medical staff had, in the early period, any direct control over the educational policies or program of the school. The hospital administration was shared by three officers—the medical superintendent who headed the medical staff, the matron who directed the housekeeping and nursing staffs, and the secretary of the hospital board of trustees who had control of financial affairs. All three had direct access to the voluntary committee of management, which represented the trustees and adjusted the administrative problems that could not be settled by the three chief officers. This tripartite plan of hospital administration (frequently found in Britain) tended to strengthen the position of the matron. In many cases she became the chief resident administrator and was responsible for many hospital activities other than those directly concerned with nursing.

The Nightingale School's plan to train two groups of probationers, ordinary and special, did much to attract women of

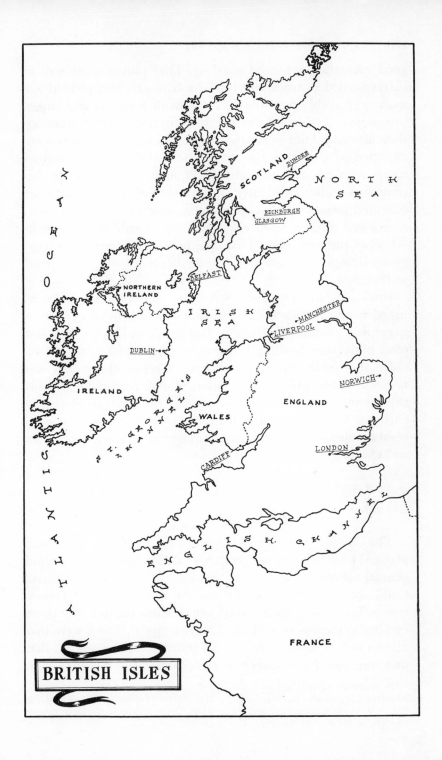

BRITISH ISLES

good education and social standing. They provided the staff of sisters needed to teach and train probationers and to hold the more responsible positions as matrons of hospitals and superintendents of district nursing organizations. After training, they formed a kind of secular sisterhood whose members were expected to go where the matron sent them and to keep in touch with her and the school. Though such paying probationers were eliminated later, the more promising and the better educated members of each class were selected for special experience and training as sisters in the Nightingale School and in others of the same type. This plan provided a tested and tried group from which matrons for new schools at home and abroad were drawn.

During the first two decades thirteen such schools were established in the British Isles, including one each in cities such as Liverpool, Edinburgh, Dundee, Glasgow, and Dublin. In a few cases philanthropists like William Rathbone of Liverpool provided the needed financial support. In others the money was raised by subscription, or probationers were required to pay for their living expenses. There were other variations in plans and patterns, but most of these institutions were real schools with good standards of teaching and training and well selected pupils and teachers.

EARLY DEVELOPMENTS IN DISTRICT NURSING AND ALLIED BRANCHES[2]

The Nightingale School Committee from the start had planned to prepare district nurses as well as hospital sisters and general nurses. In 1859 Miss Nightingale had helped William Rathbone to organize the first modern district nursing association in Liverpool, and it was on her recommendation that three cardinal principles of such work were adopted. These were that district nurses should have special training for their work, that they were not to give alms or material relief, and that they must

[2] A summary of the various branches of nursing established before 1893 is found in the article, "On Nursing," by Mrs. Stuart Wortley in *Nursing of the Sick 1893*, by Isabel Hampton and others, 43-49. Other articles in the same volume are devoted to "District Nursing," The Queen's Nurses," etc.

not interfere with the religious views of their patients. The Liverpool school shortly after made arrangements to transfer some of its probationers to such agencies for experience and instruction and so to prepare leaders for the new district nursing associations that were beginning to develop in other parts of the country. It took time, however, to overcome the older concept of home visiting of the sick as a religious charity or a private philanthropy requiring little or no training and often aiming at saving souls rather than bodies.

Some efforts were made as early as 1861 to coordinate and standardize such societies in London, but it was not until 1874 that a study of district nursing in that city was undertaken by the English Order of the Knights of St. John of Jerusalem. On Miss Nightingale's advice, Florence Lees (then Mrs. Dacre Craven), a brilliant member of the first class at St. Thomas's, was asked to make this study. Largely as a result of her recommendations, the Metropolitan and National Nursing Association was formed (1875) to establish higher and more uniform standards for such work. One such standard was that the trained nurses to be employed in such positions should be educated gentlewomen.

The standards were greatly strengthened in 1887 when Queen Victoria's Jubilee Institute for Nurses was established with part of the funds presented to the Queen by the women of the empire. The Institute prepared nurses for work among the sick poor in their homes, giving a six months' course in London to nurses with hospital training. Some of its funds were used for midwifery training adopting the Metropolitan and National Association as its nucleus. Rosalind Paget (later Dame Rosalind) was the first Queen's Nurse and the first Superintendent of the Institute. Mary Stocks in *District Nursing* states that Queen Victoria took great interest and pride in her nurses and was grieved not to have their care when she was ill because their service was restricted to the sick poor.[3] Independent Associations in different parts of the country were encouraged to affiliate with the Institute, the scheme eventually covering almost all the country, thus setting a national pattern gradually copied in various parts of the Empire.

[3] Mary Stocks, *A Hundred Years of District Nursing* (London: Allen and Unwin, 1960).

The Queen's nurses were soon confronted, especially in the rural districts, with the problem of maternity care. Miss Nightingale considered nursing and midwifery separate vocations and so did not include even obstetrical nursing in the first school's program. Her interest in midwifery reform led her to start a school for midwives, but it was discontinued when puerperal fever broke out in the hospital with which the school was connected. Some district nursing societies employed what they called "cottage" or "village" nurses chiefly for maternity cases, and though these workers sometimes had a brief practical training most of the midwives were untrained and often of a low class. Physicians had done little to improve this situation, apparently believing that the midwife would disappear as medicine advanced. The Queen's Institute, however, considered the trained midwife an essential part of its scheme for better maternal and child care, and after a long and bitter struggle the "Midwives Act" was passed in 1902. An official Central Midwives Board was appointed to set standards of training and certification, the letters C. M. B. indicating the Board's approval. Training schools for midwives were also developed, and many trained nurses, especially those of the Queen's Institute, began to take the course. This led to a close relationship between nursing and midwifery in Britain and in most of the British dominions, a combination that was largely responsible for the greatly improved status of the midwife and for the generally recognized improvement in maternal and infant care. In 1904 when the *Queen's Nurses Magazine* first appeared it became a link between these groups. Revisions of the Midwives Act have been made since its first passage to bring it into line with current trends.

An advance in national health was marked by the comprehensive Public Health Act of 1875, which was followed by a succession of progressive health laws. That year the first industrial nurse, Philippa D. Flowerday, was employed by the Coleman Mustard factory in Norwich. Other employers took up the idea, stimulated by workman's compensation laws and other industrial legislation. School nursing was first introduced in London (1892) by the efforts of Amy Hughes, a later superintendent of the Queen's nurses, and of Honnor Morton, a member of the

London County Council, who had had some nursing training. This step was followed by various acts in the early 1900's providing for the appointment of nurses for services in public schools, as inspectors of boarding homes for children, and in other official capacities under municipal agencies.

Health visitors were early appointed for preventive and educational work in connection with municipal and other health services. These visitors were not required to have nursing training, though they had, in addition to formal instruction, a short period of hospital experience. Later it was found that fully trained nurses made the best health visitors and the great majority then became nurses with extra training. Although Queen's nurses and others who gave bedside care in homes continued to do much incidental teaching, the health visitors in Britain were made responsible for most of the organized health teaching, these two groups thus dividing between them the duties commonly carried by public health nurses in the United States and Canada.

Other Types of Nursing Service and Personnel

Miss Nightingale's great achievement as a "soldier nurse," her reforms in the British Army Medical Service, and her continued influence in the War Office led to the appointment in 1869 of Mrs. Deeble, the first trained nurse to be matron or lady superintendent in a military hospital. During the next decade other nurse superintendents and staff members were appointed to government hospitals at home, and in 1888 Catharine Loch was the first to be sent in charge of a staff of nurses to military hospitals in India. Though such nurses did not have official rank, they had the general status of officers and exercised military authority within their domain. Their duties included the training and supervision of the corpsmen who did most of the actual nursing in military hospitals. In 1902 after the Boer War a reorganization of the armed services opened the way for many more appointments of nurses in both home and foreign service. The Queen Alexandra's Imperial Military Nursing

Corps and the Queen Alexandra's Royal Naval Nursing Corps were the first of a series now attached to the different branches of the armed forces.

Though the International Red Cross was founded in 1864, the British government did not sign the Convention until 1870. Miss Nightingale, who was on the national committee, was in active sympathy with the general purposes of the Red Cross but not with short courses for volunteer war nurses. This influenced the British Red Cross and similar societies in the British dominions to allow only fully trained nurses to serve in war and other serious emergencies. After 1900 courses in elementary nursing and first aid were developed by the British Red Cross, and Voluntary Aid Detachments (VAD's) were organized whose members were to work under qualified matrons and sisters. Similar groups were prepared by the St. John's Ambulance and First Aid Society.

Private nursing had been developed to some extent by Elizabeth Fry's Nursing Sisters (founded 1840). Since this was not considered as urgent a problem as institutional and district nursing, the Nightingale School did not attempt to train private nurses. Though most other modern schools did, this branch of nursing never attained quite the same professional and social status in Britain as did hospital, district, and military nursing. Private nurses were usually organized in clubs or cooperatives under a nurse director who combined the functions of manager, registrar, and house mother. Such homes were sometimes attached to hospitals and run by them as a convenience for their well-to-do patrons and also as a source of income.

The pre-Nightingale systems of nursing soon began to disappear or to recede into the background. The few religious sisterhoods which continued to care for the sick as a rule adopted the Nightingale system of training for their sisters and lay nurses. "Lady Bountifuls" gradually gave up their amateur doctoring and nursing, and some of them became patrons of district nursing. Families continued to care for chronic and minor illnesses at home, but severe cases were sent to public hospitals or private nursing homes, both of which increased in numbers. The worst of the old "Sairey Gamps" disappeared, but there were still large numbers of untrained or semitrained practical nurses and midwives, (often camouflaged by a trained nurse's cap and uniform) many of whom were recruited from discharged probationers or former ward maids and were supplied by commercial registries to the unsuspecting public.

THE MOVEMENT FOR HOSPITAL TRAINING SCHOOLS

In 1876 an article appeared in the *British and Foreign Medico-Chirurgical Review* stating that enlightened physicians everywhere were urging every large hospital and infirmary and every dispensary "to take part in the business of training nurses." This idea took hold quickly, and before long many hospitals, large and small, general and special, voluntary and municipal, were appealing for probationers and calling themselves training hospitals. Actually, the system of training tended to revert to the older apprenticeship system in which trainees, ranked as employees, were paid for their training by their labor and were taught to perform only the duties required in the institutions that employed them. Since many of these hospitals were highly specialized or small, the training received was often quite limited or onesided and included many non-nursing duties. The new scheme also lacked most of the safeguards built up by the old trade guilds to protect the economic rights of employees and apprentices and to ensure proper standards of workmanship and teaching. Low standards of admission, heavy work loads, and long hours prevailed and sickness rates among nurses and probationers increased. Without savings to meet ill health, unemployment, old age, and similar demands, a good many nurses became objects of charity. The whole issue became acute when hospital trustees began to appeal for funds to care for aged and dependent nurses. Another factor was the growing unemployment of trained nurses because of the large number of probationer apprentices and partly prepared nurses. Although nursing services in most hospitals were improved by these hospital schools, the young vocation of nursing got a serious setback from which it did not soon recover.

BEGINNINGS OF REGISTRATION

The first definite suggestion for the organization and legal registration of nurses appeared as early as 1874 in an introduction by Dr. Henry Acland to the well-known *Handbook for Hospital Sisters* by Florence Lees. In 1885 Surgeon General Evatt, in proposing to the War Office a plan for a corps of trained nurses for field hospitals, outlined what he stated was the first definite attempt to incorporate the nursing profession. He urged the group to organize itself, expel its unworthy members, define its curriculum, found a diploma or certificate of proficiency, and develop its own pension fund—in other words, to do as medicine and other professions had done to safeguard the interests of the public and of its own members.[4]

The following year (1886) a newly formed Hospitals Association, whose founder and secretary was Henry C. Burdett of the London Hospital, began to consider a proposal to set up a semicharitable nurses' registry and pension scheme primarily for the use of hospitals of the association. Several matrons were invited to serve on the committee, of which Henry C. Burdett was chairman. When they objected to his proposal to make one year of hospital experience, with or without formal training, the basis for registration and pension privileges and their protests were overruled, they resigned in a body. This was the start of the movement for state registration and professional organization in Britain which soon spread to other countries.

EARLY STAGES OF NURSES' ORGANIZATIONS

The foremost leader in this movement was Ethel Gordon Manson, who had recently resigned as Matron of St. Bartholomew's Hospital, London, to become the wife of Doctor Bedford Fenwick. This intelligent, outspoken, and determined young woman was now a free lance. Her husband, also courageous

---

[4] These and other details about nurses' organizations are found in Nutting and Dock, *History of Nursing*, Vol. III, pp. 30-60.

and liberal minded, was in sympathy with her efforts to organize nurses and to free them from the control of philanthropic and proprietary interests. Mrs. Fenwick at once invited a group of nurse colleagues to meet at her home, where they decided to form a national association to work for a state register of properly qualified nurses. Some medical and lay sympathizers were invited to join them, and in 1888 the British Nurses Association was established with Her Royal Highness Princess Christian, daughter of Queen Victoria, as president, an impressive list of other patrons and members, and a royal charter. This body, which still exists, was the first national nurses' organization (though not made up exclusively of nurses). In 1889 it issued its manifesto calling for three years' training in a hospital and registration by examination.

The next year it appointed the first voluntary registration board as a temporary measure. Dr. Fenwick meanwhile secured a vote by the British Medical Association approving the registration of nurses by act of Parliament, but the request for a special charter was refused because of the influence of Henry C. Burdett (then Sir Henry) who edited *The Hospital* (organ of the Hospitals Association). He and his associates did not oppose registration as much as they did nurses' organizations, which they claimed were in effect trade unions. Hospital boards were advised not to employ nurses who joined such groups and were urged rather to promote pensions, relief plans and other benefits. Many matrons and sisters joined this hospital group. The nurses in the BNA defended registration by legal enactment, claimed that nurses' qualifications could be determined only by medical and nursing experts, stood for the professional and economic independence of nurses, and insisted that they wanted economic justice, not charity or patronage.

Though well supported by some medical sympathizers, the registrationists' position was undermined by an opposing medical faction that got control (1896). By passing a resolution against the proposed measure it struck a blow that only intensified the efforts of Mrs. Fenwick and her supporters. In 1893 this fearless leader who had many of the qualities of her Scottish and French ancestors had become editor of an independent journal, *The Nursing Record* (later renamed *The British Journal of Nursing*), and with this powerful weapon became the spearhead of the registration movement and the target for most of the antagonism it aroused. The commercially sponsored press in general sided with the opposition.

MISS NIGHTINGALE'S POSITION ON THESE ISSUES

What seemed only a local skirmish now became a revolution, probably equal in daring to the first, the more so as Miss Nightingale herself opposed the movement and lent the prestige of her great name to its opponents. When the storm broke she had retired and was out of touch with nursing affairs, but the threat to her life work (as she feared) brought her back with all her old fighting spirit. She believed sincerely that standards would be leveled down by state licensing and that nurses would deteriorate if released from the supervision and control of their schools and given permanent status as registered nurses. Convinced that materialism and individualism had already begun to undermine the spiritual and moral values she had sought to develop, she discouraged even the most reasonable and necessary efforts toward economic self-protection. Apparently she associated professionalism with trade unionism, of which she disapproved, though she had much sympathy with working men and women. The Founder did not oppose the pension scheme but she was against the proposed directory or register of the Hospitals Association as well as the plan of the state registrationists. Her chief argument was that character was nonregisterable and that such a list would "stereotype mediocrity." That she recognized the need for greater uniformity in nursing standards is shown by a letter to William Rathbone in 1891 in which she admitted that registration might be acceptable in forty years after a process of leveling up to the higher standards of the best schools, but she did not say how this should be done.[5]

Her historic paper, "Sick Nursing and Health Nursing," sent to the Chicago World's Fair Congress on Charities, Corrections

[5] Sir Edward Cook, *Life of Florence Nightingale*, Vol. II, p. 364.

and Philanthropy, Section on Hospitals, Dispensaries and Nursing and published in *Nursing of the Sick 1893,* reflects Miss Nightingale's opinions on many of these issues. Though progress was her main theme, and she warned nurses that "no system can endure that does not march," she intimated that some of them were marching too fast and getting off the right track, sacrificing a calling for a profession and practical training in a fine art for academic book learning and "literary lore." In this, as in some other matters, this daring reformer was not consistent because she had insisted that nurses should be truth seekers, that they should aim high, and keep on learning and growing through life.

THE INTERNATIONAL ORGANIZATION OF PROFESSIONAL NURSES

Before Miss Nightingale's death in 1910 trained nurses in her own country and in several others had formed self-governing organizations and had united them in the International Council of Nurses, which was to become an effective medium for carrying forward the modern nursing movement, though not in just the way the Founder had planned. The leader in this new step was the Matron's Council of Great Britain and Ireland, organized in 1894 by Isla Stewart. This was a Scottish Nightingale from St. Thomas's who succeeded Mrs. Fenwick at "Barts," and was her staunch associate in the "cause," in many ways complementing her and helping to moderate her fiery zeal and uncompromising spirit. Before her early death she had organized the first Training School League among the alumnae of her own school and had brought such Leagues together to form the nucleus of the National Council of Nurses of Great Britain and Ireland, also restricted to qualified nurses and entirely self-governing.

In 1899 the International Council of Women met in London, and a section for the discussion of nursing questions was arranged at Mrs. Fenwick's request. Though no action was taken then, some current problems were aired, and several nurses were invited to meet as guests of the Matron's Council, of which Isla Stewart was president. It was at this special meeting that Mrs. Fenwick proposed the plan for the International Council of Nurses, which was enthusiastically supported by her British colleagues and by nurses who attended from the United States, Canada, Denmark, Holland, South Africa, New Zealand, and Australia.

The preamble of the constitution of the International Council of Nurses adopted in July, 1900, admirably expresses its aims:

> We, nurses of all nations, sincerely believing that the best good of our Profession will be advanced by greater unity of thought, sympathy and purpose, do hereby band ourselves in a confederation to further the efficient care of the sick and to secure the honor and interests of the Nursing Profession.

The council's aims and membership requirements further emphasized the principles of self-government under nurse leadership, the determination to develop the nurse as a professional person, an articulate, self-directing human being and a citizen, to improve the quality of nursing service and education, and to raise the ethical, social, and economic status of nurses. Other objectives were added as the organization developed and as the leaders recognized more fully the standards and responsibilities implied in the term "profession."

The History of the International Council of Nurses (1899-1925) by Margaret Breay and Ethel Gordon Fenwick quotes from the Report of the 1901 Congress in Buffalo some remarks of the president, Mrs. Fenwick, which reflect the spirit and ideals of these professional pioneers:

> All nurses who have considered the question intelligently have grasped the fundamental principle that our profession like every other needs registration and control and we claim that this power of control should rest in our own hands, that, in our corporate capacity we must have the right to live and move and have our being, and that it is from our own ranks that the woman must step out to whom the responsibility of guiding our destinies must be entrusted.[6]

[6] P. 22.

At the 1909 Congress in London Isla Stewart in a welcoming address amplified this idea and testified to the success of the new organization:

> The essential spirit of the International Council of Nurses is that of self-government. Nurses who appreciate their profession and take themselves seriously begin to realize that the period of tutelage is past, and that women are now fitted to take up such positions in the world as are now held by many of those here present, and are also capable of governing themselves. We also realize that in professions as well as in individuals the highest and greatest point of perfection is only attained when we do govern ourselves. Under tutelage no one ever attains to the best that is in him. Further, these congresses bring together nurses of all nations and they form a means of communication which widens the nurses' views, deepens sympathy and makes them greater human beings.[7]

The spirit of the ICN was not only democratic and international, it was progressive and liberal. Individuality and diversity rather than uniformity were stressed. Through professional congresses, conferences, and the like, ideas were exchanged and a remarkable degree of solidarity and fellowship developed. The ICN did much to reinforce and support the national groups in their struggle for better conditions and sounder preparation for nurses.

The death in 1956 of Lavinia Dock, Honorary Secretary of the ICN from 1900 to 1923, makes it possible for this *History*, of which she was chief author, to record the important part she played in organizing and developing the ICN. She wrote the preamble and much of the constitution and by-laws and helped to form the ICN's basic policies which have stood the test of time. She also kept up an active correspondence (chiefly by hand) with leading nurses in many countries who were struggling to free themselves from motherhouse and medical control and to develop as self-governing individuals and organizations. At her own expense she visited many of these groups to help them in their organization and other activities, and in these as in her other voluntary contributions to nursing and health

[7] P. 59.

work she was widely recognized as an exceptionally sympathetic and selfless leader, highly intelligent, vocal, and fearless, and blessed with a keen sense of humor.

SOME "FIRSTS" IN NURSING EDUCATION

The professional group took the lead in the effort to strengthen the theoretical foundations of nursing. This need was recognized also by some of the more conservative nurses, especially after the Lister revolution in surgery brought a heavier load of technical duties that called for more scientific knowledge. The first preparatory course (which was also the first established connection between a hospital training school and a college) began in 1893 when a three-months' course in theory was set up in St. Mungo's Medical College, Glasgow, for young women who were to enter the Glasgow Infirmary for the practical part of their training. This plan was worked out by the matron, Mrs. Rebecca Strong, who belonged to the Fenwick group, and by Professor (later Sir William) MacEwan, a Lister disciple and famous surgeon, who was connected with both institutions and encouraged the idea of professional education and registration for nurses. Though the original plan of a prehospital course (during which students paid their own fees and maintenance) was not continued long, it stimulated other experiments in Britain and America. During the next few decades preparatory courses of various types were organized, often in a separate building or wing of the hospital, such units being called in Britain preliminary schools. The first of this type was set up at Tredegar House by the London Hospital, whose matron, Eva Lückes, was a leader of the antiregistration group.

Meanwhile in 1893 Margaret Huxley, a well-educated niece of the famous biologist and one of the leaders of the advanced wing in nursing, started a cooperative plan to centralize the formal instruction of nurses in five of Dublin's training schools in an arrangement with the Dublin Metropolitan Technical School where the lectures were given. Though recognized as a step toward a more uniform and systematic teaching program, this plan was not widely adopted elsewhere. Another scholarly nurse and teacher, Marian Gullan, became the first fulltime sister tutor in Britain. As head for many years of the preliminary school which was opened at St. Thomas's Hospital in 1914, she helped to raise the educational standards of the Nightingale School as well as to dignify and strengthen the position of the nurse teacher. She also did much to develop in 1918 the first course for this group at King's College for Women, part of London University.

WAR CONDITIONS LEAD TO A NEW TYPE OF ORGANIZATION

The struggle for state registration, which had continued up to 1914, was suspended during the first world war. Both military and civilian hospitals were soon filled with sick and wounded and Voluntary Aid Detachments (VAD's) organized by the Red Cross were in great demand. The fact that these volunteers often had more liberties and even more varied opportunities for service than the regular staff nurses and probationers began to have a serious effect on morale and on the number and type of applicants to schools of nursing. To stimulate public support of trained nurses and hospital schools and to induce more well-qualified candidates to enter, Sir Arthur Stanley, Honorary Treasurer of St. Thomas's Hospital and Dame Sarah Swift, a former matron, called together in 1916 a representative group of matrons, hospital trustees, and physicians to discuss the serious situation. They decided to form a new organization called The College of Nursing, which would have the prestige, dignity, and influence enjoyed by similar British organizations which carried on activities of an educational and professional character and held a charter conferring on them special rights and privileges. This new professional organization was to deal with matters closely affecting the status and welfare of trained nurses, to improve their service and preparation, and to promote postgraduate education in this field. Other important objectives were a uniform standard of training, state registration for nurses, and self-government for the nursing profession. Though the members of this group were all trained nurses, the executive council was composed of both lay and professional appointees who were nominated and elected by the members. Sir Arthur Stanley was the first president, and many influential hospital, medical, and lay persons held positions on the council during the earlier years.

The claim that the college was self-governing and that it represented the nursing profession of Britain was vigorously attacked by leaders of the pioneer organizations referred to earlier, and their position was supported by some influential nurses from other countries associated in the International Council of Nurses. Nurse members of the college increased, however, assumed more active leadership, and won support of many influential lay persons. Generous gifts from wealthy patrons helped to finance a fine headquarters and residence club in the heart of London, in which a library, classrooms, and conference rooms as well as business and other offices were established. Regional centers were developed in other parts of England, Scotland, and Ireland, with paid staffs to carry on their professional and educational activities. Refresher courses were organized, and other activities—social, recreational, and economic—were brought into the program. Among them was an affiliated student organization. *The Nursing Times,* which became its official organ, was developed into a weekly journal, professional in character. Queen Mary and other members of the Royal Family became patrons, thus adding to the prestige of the association.

STATE REGISTRATION AND ITS RESULTS

By the end of the war the College of Nursing had a large membership of nurses representing most of the country's leading schools and hospitals and, with the aid of influential political and legal experts, it set up its own plan for nurse registration in

England. Mrs. Fenwick and her colleagues in the National Council of Trained Nurses again mustered their forces and went into action, both organizations campaigning for their own Parliamentary bills. The government finally proposed a compromise measure which was accepted in 1919. Similar laws were then passed in Wales, Scotland, and Ireland, with three general nursing councils to administer them. By providing an opportunity for both groups to collaborate in setting minimum standards and planning registration procedures, it was hoped that differences would soon be overcome. Under the wise impartial leadership of Ellen Musson (later created a Dame of the British Empire), for many years chairman of the statutory body for England and Wales, an excellent organization was set up, and for the first time schools of nursing and their students began to be regulated by nationally recognized educational requirements.

In the new plan provisions were made for separate registers not only for medical and surgical nursing but also for specialties such as fever nursing, mental disease, mental deficiency, and for the nursing of sick children. Obstetrical nursing was not included, but many state-registered nurses qualified as midwives obtaining the Certificate of C. M. B. (Central Midwives Board). The entrance requirements in schools were raised and their programs improved. Courses were offered to graduate nurses preparing for teaching. In the more outstanding schools the senior leaving certificate leading to university matriculation was required for admission. The great majority of nurses who filled administrative and teaching posts had such qualifications.

With the growing demand for sounder theoretical instruction, preliminary courses were strengthened and short blocks of concentrated teaching were introduced in the second and third years. The block system was widely adopted, being preferred as a rule to concurrent classes and lectures which tended to disrupt the practical experience. Bedside practice continued to receive chief emphasis in basic courses, and to many British nurses this was "real" nursing. District nursing and health visitors' work were considered specialties for which postgraduate courses were provided for Queen's nurses and for others engaged in home and community services.

INTERNATIONAL RELATIONSHIPS
AND READJUSTMENTS

Early in 1919, after the Armistice, several national Red Cross societies which had been active during the war joined in arranging a medical conference in Cannes, France, out of which came the organization of the League of Red Cross Societies. This is more fully described in the last chapter, but the contribution of this body to the better education of its own and other nurses should be noted here. With its support, a course was set up at Bedford College, London, at first for international nurse students preparing for public health nursing service adding later those qualifying for administrative and teaching positions in schools of nursing. Most of these students were awarded Red Cross scholarships for one year of study. The College of Nursing in Britain collaborated in the project, and the British Red Cross contributed a beautiful residence at 15 Manchester Square, which became a symbol of friendship and unity among its students and alumnae. During the period of its existence (up to 1939) this international center attracted nurses from many parts of the world. Though their educational and professional backgrounds varied widely and the numbers admitted yearly as well as the general scope of the programs were necessarily limited, students reported many tangible and intangible benefits from the whole experience, including friendships established and the informal exchange of ideas and viewpoints.

By 1923, when the International Council of Nurses began to reorganize after a wartime period of relative inactivity, the College of Nursing had become the largest and most active nursing association in Britain. According to the original constitution of the ICN, it was ineligible for membership, an issue that threatened at one time to divide international nursing into two camps. Fortunately, a compromise was reached through which eligible nurse members of the college might enter the National Council of Nurses of Great Britain and Ireland as a group and thus be represented in the ICN. Thereafter this group began to take an active part in this association and its distinguished president, Dame Alicia Lloyd-Still, Matron of the Nightingale School in London, became president of the ICN in 1933. She and Mrs. Fenwick were closely associated in the planning of the Florence Nightingale Memorial which was jointly sponsored by the ICN and the League of Red Cross Societies.

Like the indomitable leader of the first nursing revolution, the chief living leader of the second continued until her death at ninety (1947) to stand guard over the causes for which she had fought. With the aid for many years of her devoted colleague Margaret Breay, she also edited and managed the *British Journal of Nursing,* and presided over the meetings of the National Council of Nurses of Great Britain and Ireland which she represented in the ICN. Though in her later years inactive in nursing affairs, Mrs. Fenwick lived to see many of her ideas widely accepted and her great contribution to nursing acknowledged even by many who had earlier opposed her. But the new generation was not much interested in the old battle slogans or leaders. Nursing was entering a new era in which the main issues were no longer state registration or the right of nurses to organize and govern themselves. The acute scarcity of nurses was threatening standards of hospital and health services, and the economic situation had reached a critical stage which called for public as well as professional investigation.

STUDIES AND PLANS LOOKING TOWARD REFORMS IN NURSING

Around 1927 a number of studies began to throw some light on the causes of the trouble. The first was *A Draft Report on the Nursing Profession* by the Labor Party, which in Britain concerned itself with all kinds of economic and social problems directly affecting the public welfare. The party tried to find out what was keeping large numbers of eligible young women from entering and remaining in nursing. The picture revealed was that of a sick industry with all the familiar contributing factors— long hours, low salaries, poor living conditions, and often autocratic management. Chief among the measures recommended was the unionization of nurses, the great majority of whom considered such efforts unethical and incompatible with their vocational and professional ideals.

The next study was sponsored (1932) by a well-known medical journal, *The Lancet,* which appointed a commission to look into the shortage of nurses and to recommend remedies. This commission was composed chiefly of prominent physicians, hospital trustees, matrons, educators and representatives of the public. The study was made by a woman physician who interviewed many persons besides student and graduate nurses and discovered some of the reasons why large numbers of eligible girls were not entering or remaining in nursing. The report noted the disappearing sense of "a call" to nurse the sick, the competition of freer, less exacting, and more remunerative occupations, the persistence in nursing schools of older ideas of discipline and education, and the basic conflict between the needs of nurses for an education and the needs of hospitals for nursing service. Although the findings attracted some public attention, more than this was needed to bring about the basic changes called for.

A little later two books appeared, one *A Criticism of Nursing Education* (1937) by Dr. Harold Balme, physician and educator, and the other *A New Deal for Nurses* (1939) by G. C. Carter, a free-lance nurse with a university degree in economics. Both went much deeper than the two preceding studies in attacking the traditional system and in revealing the unsound economic practices and weaknesses of the apprenticeship system of training which kept nursing on a craft basis and prevented its development as a real profession. The assumption that traditional administrative and disciplinary practices were justified on religious, moral, humanitarian, or educational grounds was criticized and the need for a radical reorganization was definitely and clearly stated. Though many leading nurses resented such criticisms and continued to defend the existing system, a growing number joined the group that called for reform.

The next study made in 1938-1939 was sponsored by the government and conducted by the Interdepartmental Committee on Nursing Services which included representatives from the Ministry of Health and the Board of Education as well as major groups directly concerned with nursing problems. Its *Interim Report,* which appeared near the outbreak of World War II, began by recognizing nursing as a national service comparable in public importance with teaching and deserving a similar economic and professional status. It recommended a national plan for salary negotiations between representatives of employers and nurses for the purpose of setting up satisfactory salary schedules in accordance with the prevailing compensation for other types of responsible skilled service. Public grants for approved schools were also urged, these to be used specifically for education. The training and certification of assistant nurses was suggested to provide for the care of chronic and convalescent patients. Other recommendations included a central agency for recruitment, improvement of conditions that kept out many applicants, and the raising of educational standards for admission. This positive program was endorsed by responsible government agencies as well as by leading representatives of hospitals, nursing, and medicine. Action was postponed, however, by the onset of World War II.

THE WAR PERIOD AND PLANS
FOR RECONSTRUCTION

For the next six years (1939-1945) the struggle for survival had precedence of everything else. Civilian nursing problems were especially complicated and difficult because of extensive bombing, the evacuation of cities, the destruction and dislocation of hospitals and nursing centers, and the high rate of civilian casualties. The fact that there was no breakdown in nursing services during these dangerous, exhausting, and harrowing years was proof that British nurses had not lost their steady, stouthearted spirit, good discipline, devotion to duty, and practical competence. Like their people in general, they were at their best when times were worst.

Relations between nursing and governmental agencies were

definitely strengthened in wartime. Nurses held responsible positions not only in the armed services, the Red Cross and civilian organizations but in the Health and Labour ministries, in the Colonial Office, and in international bodies concerned with the health and welfare of peoples of occupied countries. Public officials and distinguished citizens gave much more attention to nursing questions during the war. One important recommendation of the Interdepartmental Committee was the creation of a Salaries Committee under the chairmanship of Lord Rushcliffe, a former Minister of Labour to draw up a revised national salary scale for all categories of nursing service, including students, assistant nurses, and aides. Finding that the last two groups were employed in large numbers on salaries that were little if any less than those of trained nurses the latter's salaries were raised. This move was well supported by the press and the public generally. Many tributes to nurses and honors for national service demonstrated the strong position this group held in the affection and esteem of the public.

Nurses' organizations were active in the war effort and also in planning for the postwar period. The Royal College of Nursing Committee on Nursing Reconstruction was commonly called the Horder Committee after its distinguished chairman, Lord Horder, the King's physician. It prepared and issued a series of monographs dealing with standards for nurse training schools, postregistration nursing education, the assistant nurse, and the social and economic conditions of the nurse. Its recommendations went much further than those in preceding studies in urging a general strengthening of educational programs. Also apparent was a greater awareness of the total health needs of the population and the public demand for changes to meet these needs. One such change authorized by the Nurses' Act of 1943 was the legal recognition of the state-enrolled assistant nurse whose functions were more restricted than those of the graduate nurse. She was required to have two years' practical experience in addition to one year of training before being enrolled by the General Nursing Council of England and Wales and receiving her certificate. Hospitals soon began to employ large numbers of such workers.

THE NEW NATIONAL HEALTH ACT

The nationalization of Britain's medical and health services has been attributed by many to the postwar Labor-Socialist government, but the fact is that it was one of a long series of social and health measures initiated by liberal and conservative governments and was supported by all parties and by the great majority of the population. The wartime coalition government had sponsored a study by a nonpartisan committee under Sir William Beveridge's chairmanship, from which came the famous Beveridge Report—*Social Insurance and Allied Services* (1942). This plan, designed to provide for the major risks and hazards of the entire population "from womb to tomb," as one wit phrased it, was the basis for the National Health Service Act of 1946, which after much discussion and some adjustment went into effect in 1948. Supporting it was the strong sense of national unity arising out of the shared activities and sacrifices of the war and the determination of all classes that facilities for health, education, and other essentials of a good life must be made available to all.

Much had been learned under the stress of war about the weaknesses in the existing system, and some progress had been made toward the unification of hospitals and other community health agencies and the coordination of their personnel. The aim of the new act was to provide a much more comprehensive and better integrated system to meet the medical and health needs of the entire population. It was to cover all disease and age categories as well as the social and emotional factors of sickness and the building of positive health. Obviously, all this could not be done at once. The idea was to create a broad framework within which the details could be gradually worked out, meanwhile maintaining existing services on the highest level possible.

All but a few hospitals, clinics, nursing homes, day nurseries, and similar community agencies, with their endowments and other resources, were incorporated into the national scheme, and the great majority of practicing physicians, surgeons, dentists, nurses, and other health personnel accepted appointment under the government, though a few chose to continue in private practice. These and similar professional groups participated with the government ministries and with representatives of the general public in planning the scheme and in operating it. The Act divided the whole country into regions and subdivided them into areas. Regional boards and area committees were then appointed which were to be largely responsible for over-all planning and local problems of reorganization and adjustment. In addition, there were national committees which gave special attention to all the major problems concerned with the various clinical services and the professional and technical specialties involved in the total scheme.

Nursing Under the National Health Service

The official *Report of the Working Party on the Recruitment and Training of Nurses,* published in 1947, provided a general guide for the reorganization of nursing. This working party was appointed to consider the size of the force required and to suggest how best to recruit, train, and distribute it. Under the chairmanship of Sir Robert Wood, an educator, were two widely known nurses, Daisy C. Bridges and Elizabeth Cockayne, a medical officer of health, a psychologist, and, in an advisory capacity, representatives of health, labor, pensions, and other governmental departments concerned. Many of the current issues in nursing were studied, much valuable information compiled, and plans for reorganization drawn up. By taking a few steps at a time the new scheme was introduced without any breakdown in essential services or in educational programs. The question of nurse supply, however, remained acute. This led to an intensive recruitment campaign for trainees and graduates, but though enrollment was increased the wastage continued high, especially in the younger age and lower educational brackets. More exacting measures were then tried to attract those with suitable qualifications, and plans were made for a better utilization of existing nurse power, including married and retired nurses, and the training and use of assistant nurses and other ancillary groups. Another approach was made in functional studies designed to differentiate essential from nonessential nursing duties and to economize the time and energy of qualified nurses by a redistribution of functions.

The Act recognized two main categories of nurses, midwives, and other health personnel—the institutional and the domiciliary. Private nurses, as such, were not included in the national scheme, but special nursing at public expense was made available in serious cases. With the overcrowding of hospitals and shortage of nurses more families had to depend on the services of district and other visiting nurses. In spite of these and other difficulties, nursing service and morale were well maintained, especially in the hospitals with competent staffs and well-established standards.

CHANGES IN NURSING EDUCATION
AND REGISTRATION

Under the new scheme it was hoped that many of the accumulated weaknesses in the old system of nursing education could be eliminated. Some progress was made in this direction. The Nurses' Act of 1949 set up area or regional nurse training committees and for the first time Treasury funds were made available for nursing education. These funds, however, were limited and did not cover the practical part of the training which was still tied in with the hospital economy. Some of the smaller and more specialized institutions that had formerly conducted their own schools of nursing were combined to provide a wider range of experience and better balanced programs. Central preliminary schools which are part of the more comprehensive training schemes are evolving into central schools of nursing that provide all the organized instruction offered in the three-year program and employ their own sister tutors and lecturers with a principal tutor in charge. The salaries of such teachers are paid from educational funds, and their position is now more independent. The matrons and ward sisters of the various hospital units still have full responsibility for the students' practical experience and ward teaching and for many other aspects of the students' life. This division of responsibility has been a major issue between the two groups directly concerned, though both recognize the importance of coordinating and strengthening the teaching in classrooms and wards.

As to the registration machinery, some changes have been made in the makeup and functions of the General Nursing Councils. For example, these councils now have less responsibility for inspecting and approving schools, determining standards of nursing practice, preparing the official syllabus, conducting examinations, and the like, but are expected to advise the national ministries now concerned with these problems. Such ministries employ qualified nurses as regular members of their staffs and have on their councils representatives of all the main branches of nursing as well as educators, physicians, and other non-nursing experts who are concerned with certain aspects of nurses' preparation.

Though the need for postbasic education had been recognized, little provision was made for it in the government plan. Meanwhile, this program is carried on by voluntary organizations such as the Royal College of Nursing, which has three main educational centers in London, Edinburgh, and Belfast and offers one- or two-year diploma programs in administration and teaching in cooperation with universities in those cities. Edinburgh University was the first in Britain to found a Nursing Studies Unit which awards Nurse Tutor Certificates and is an integral part of the university. It has also established the first research fellowship in nursing and some doctoral degrees have been conferred.

Recent reports of British nursing in the literature indicate that new attempts are now being made to develop a more comprehensive basic nursing program. One, in London, "an integrated nursing course," four years in length, is designed to qualify the graduate as a state-registered nurse competent as a hospital and domiciliary nurse, a midwife, a Queen's nurse, and a health visitor. An experimental course in Scotland, two years in length, is arranged to bring about a better correlation of the various aspects of the student's experience. At the end of an additional year of planned practical work, the nurse will be eligible for a place on the State Register. Another experimental four-year program is being established at the Hammersmith Hospital in London, in cooperation with Battersea College, which combines previous three-year diploma programs, public health programs, and the first part of the midwifery program. The entrance requirements have been increased for this course to "school leaving" and two more years of schooling. After the completion of this program, the nurse will be eligible not only for general practice, but, with six months' more preparation for the course of the Central Midwives Board. Successful candidates receive permission to use the additional letters S.C.M., the present designation of qualified midwives.

CHANGES IN ECONOMIC AND PERSONNEL POLICIES

With the nationalization of health services it was necessary to reconsider the whole question of nurse employment. As noted earlier, the trend in nursing in Britain had been toward the adoption of a uniform system of salary schedules, retirement pensions, and hours, such decisions being reached by negotiations between organized nurses and employers. These agreements are now extended to cover the country as a whole. The Whitley Council plan, which had been used in many other occupations, was adopted as a basis for such negotiations in nursing. Difficulties were met at first in securing recognition for nurses' ethical codes and other professional obligations. For example, some public officials with labor backgrounds did not see why nurses insisted on a "no strike" policy and opposed the "closed shop." This became a national issue when one county council required all nurses as a condition of employment to belong to a union authorized to represent them in collective bargaining. Such an order violated the principle of voluntary membership in a professional organization which the British professions in general considered essential to their dignity and freedom. The local nurses protested and won their case with the support of their own and other professional groups and the public press.

Another issue on which nurses themselves were divided was the introduction of representative councils (similar to those generally used in other forms of employment) in hospitals and health agencies. Under this plan all grades and types of personnel, including student nurses, were expected to elect a council representative to meet periodically with the hospital administrator to discuss matters affecting conditions of work and the personnel policies of the institution. Some nurses felt that the use of such "grievance machinery" tended to undermine the authority of the matrons as well as the professional status of nurses. Others saw it as a way to relax the traditional system of hospital discipline and to give nurses the opportunity that other workers had to present their problems and to make constructive suggestions on matters affecting the institution as a whole.

The general trend in Britain favors a more democratic system of administration in hospitals and nursing schools. Well-known hospital schools that charge fees still attract larger numbers of applicants and are able to maintain higher standards of selection and education, which give their nurses an advantage in competing for the higher posts. But since financial aid is now available from national scholarship funds many promising candidates who formerly would have been unable to attend such schools can now do so and can also take advanced courses. At the start of the new plan the tendency was to stress quantity rather than quality of candidates, but the need for broadly prepared nurses in many important positions was soon recognized and more attention is now given to higher qualifications.

RECENT DEVELOPMENTS IN PROFESSIONAL ORGANIZATIONS AND STUDIES

In the beginning there were some who feared that bureaucratic control might limit the autonomy and freedom of the health professions, but although the government and the general public now have a larger share in deciding how such services are to be planned, maintained, and administered the actual practice of medicine, dentistry, nursing and other healing arts remains in the hands of the experts in these fields and the organizations that represent them. The nursing profession is well represented on most of the important bodies concerned with health services and is frequently consulted on matters in which the rights and interests of its members are involved. Organized nurses are not only free to criticize and to make recommendations but are constantly asked for information and opinions on many questions relating to their own field and the health service as a whole.

While these changes were going on nurses decided to re-examine their cumbersome and complicated professional structure. The representatives of the two major national associations began to study and realign their overlapping functions and to coordinate their activities. The National Council of Nurses of Great Britain and Northern Ireland (a federation of sixty-two affiliated societies including a number of training school leagues or alumnae) was recognized as the official body representing the profession in its relationship with the national government and with international bodies such as the International Council of Nurses and World Health Organization. The Royal College of Nursing decided to divide into two distinct departments—one a professional membership association and the other an educational agency serving not only the nurses of Britain but many who came from different parts of the empire as well as Europe and elsewhere. To extend and support its educational program and staff, the college carried on a successful fund-raising campaign. Lucy Duff Grant, who was its president during this period of reorganization and was later elected president of the National Council, was able to do much to readjust the functions and relationships of these two bodies and to coordinate their activities.

Nurses were also forced to re-examine the entire concept and system of nursing, including its aims, functions, patterns of organization, methods, and procedures. A series of pamphlets issued by the Royal College of Nursing provided a basis for some of these adjustments, especially those in the educational and economic phases of nursing. Further studies were initiated by some of the government ministries, notably the Ministry of Labour and National Service, of which Bettina Bennett was Principal Nursing Officer. Her interest in nursing research led to the use of new techniques in psychological tests, functional analysis, and work organization. Some of these studies were aided by such voluntary agencies as the Nuffield Trust, the King's Fund, and other foundations, and several service institutions and their staffs cooperated. The realization that more nurses should have special preparation in research was one result of these studies.

The different government nursing services, such as those related to the army, navy, and air force, continued much as before. However, the Colonial Nursing Service under Florence Udell became much more active during the postwar period when it shared in the general international plan for aiding underdeveloped countries to establish national health services and schools. Many of these activities are referred to in later chapters.

No attempt has been made here to evaluate the new National Health Service in Britain from the standpoint of general patient care and the reactions of the medical, nursing and other professions involved as well as those of the general public. There are many arguments pro and con and even those who are most favorable to the new system admit the need for many changes. It is hoped that the references suggested in the bibliography will be helpful in rounding out the brief account given in this chapter of the plan as a whole and the issues that the British medical and health professions have had to meet in recent years in putting it into effect.

MODERN NURSING IN IRELAND

A large section of this island severed its relations with Britain and became an independent republic in 1937. During the earlier period of about sixty years southern Ireland's nursing history was much like that of the rest of Britain, except that Roman Catholic orders, especially the Irish Sisters of Charity and Sisters of Mercy, had a much larger share in hospital work. Sixteen of the Sisters of Mercy had gone with Miss Nightingale to the Crimea, and Sister Mary Scholastica of that order was the leader in 1891 in establishing a training institute along Nightingale lines to prepare both sisters and lay nurses. Its head was a secular trained nurse, B. M. Kelly. The next year a similar school was opened by the Sisters of Charity. Both had been preceded in the 80's by schools for lay nurses in two old Dublin hospitals. One at Madam Steevens Hospital of many traditions was headed by Miss Franks, the other at Sir Patrick Dun's by Margaret Huxley.

Opportunities for secular nurses developed slowly partly because nuns held most of the administrative positions in hospitals and economic resources for other services were limited. Many Irish nurses found work in Britain or the United States, where they often remained. Later when an active branch of the Queen's Nurses was developed in Ireland with district and school nursing and midwifery services, more positions were opened for nurses at home. One of the foremost leaders in this field was a nurse-midwife, Lady Hermione Blackwood, daughter of Lady Hariot Dufferin who had done much for nursing in India. After 1937, when the new state revised its health laws and services, it employed large staffs of nurses and midwives and focused attention especially on infant and maternal health and on tuberculosis, since these were the areas in which sickness and death rates were exceptionally high. The Irish Sweepstakes Fund, which has helped to rebuild and modernize many of the old hospitals, did much to improve conditions in nurses' homes and schools as well.

The first professional organization for nurses (1925) was a branch of the National Council of Great Britain and Ireland. Margaret Huxley, a Dublin matron and a pioneer in the council's work, was for many years president and chief leader of this branch, whose journal was *The Irish Trained Nurse and Hospital Review*. Though the relationships of such lay nurses and the religious sisters were cordial, the nuns did not join actively in professional organizations until after the separation, when the National Council of Nurses of Ireland was organized and the sisters became more active. The new Council, which was created by federating two associations of general nurses and others representing matrons, mental nurses, and a guild of Catholic nurses was accepted as a member of the International Council of Nurses in 1947. Largely through its efforts, a nurses' registration law was passed and the General Nursing Council of Ireland was set up to administer it. The Nurses' Act of 1950 amalgamated this council and the Midwives Board and extended the new body's functions to include postregistration education.

Though Ireland did not adopt a national health service such as that of Great Britain and Northern Island, increasing political pressure led to a more comprehensive and better organized plan for the nation's health. According to reports in the late 1950's, health authorities were then employing, outside hospitals and other institutions, a much larger staff of nurses which included public health nurses, dispensary midwives, and district nurses (in addition to those who remained under District Nursing Associations). Most of these nurses had midwifery training and attended a large proportion of normal deliveries, especially in rural areas. Several Dublin hospitals, such as the old Rotunda of worldwide fame, gave midwifery training to Irish nurses and often to those of other countries. Postgraduate courses in district nursing, tuberculosis nursing, and similar branches are also available in Ireland. Nurses seeking special preparation as matrons, sister tutors, and health visitors have gone, as a rule, to one of the three branches of the Royal College of Nursing in London, Edinburgh, or Belfast. Since the government has increased nurses' salaries and improved general conditions of service, a much larger proportion of these workers now find positions in their own country. Private nursing here as in Britain seems to employ a relatively small number of trained nurses.

This chapter has pointed out some of the highlights in the development of modern nursing in the country where the new movement began. British leaders and systems have been widely influential in all parts of the world. Sometimes they taught as much by their mistakes and conflicts as they did by their successes, but no one who has followed their record and known their stalwart nurses could fail to admire their spirit of independence and the generous sharing of their ideas and experiences with others. A pioneer in nearly all phases of nursing service, education, organization, publication, legislation, ethics, and economics, Britain's nursing history provides a valuable record of achievement and of continuous adjustment to new conditions and needs. The recent period following the introduction of the new National Health Service has been one of special difficulty requiring an extensive reorganization of medical and nursing services and calling for many other changes in all phases of health care.

SELECTED BIBLIOGRAPHY

Abel-Smith, Brian. *A History of the Nursing Profession.* London: Heinemann, 1960.

"The Act in Operation," *Nurs. Times,* September 30, 1950, 999-1000.

Beaulah, Lois. "Early British Midwives," *Nurs. Times,* September 4, 1954, 946-948.

Bennett, B. A. "The Evolution of the Nursing Profession in Britain," *Nurs. Mirror,* May 13, 20, 27; June 3, 1960, 587-590; 681-683; 778-779; 867-868.

———. *A Guide to Professional Nursing: Nursing, Midwifery, and the Allied Professions.* London: Faber & Faber, 1951.

Beveridge, Sir William. *Social Insurance and Allied Services.* New York: Macmillan, 1942.

Blair-Fish, Hilary M. "The Royal College of Nursing, 1916-1950," *Nurs. Times,* April 1, 1950, 332-336, 338-343.

British Information Services Reference Division. *Health Services in Britain.* New York: Rockefeller Plaza, 1954.

Cockayne, Dame Elizabeth. "The Evolution of the Nurse to Meet the Needs of Today," *Nurs. Mirror,* May 22, 1959, vii-x, 604.

———. "Ten Years of Nursing in the National Health Service," *Nurs. Times,* July 4, 1958, 762-763.

Dan Mason -Nursing Research Committee. *The Work of Recently Qualified Nurses.* London: Comm. of Nat. Florence Nightingale Memorial, 1956.

Department of Health for Scotland. Nuffield Provincial Hospitals Trust. *Report on Experiment in Nurse Training Conducted in Glasgow Royal Infirmary 1956-1961.* Glasgow: Dept. of Health, 1961. Mimeographed.

Dixon, Nancy M. "Modern Trends in District Nursing," *Nurs. Times,* November 15, 1952, 1133-1134.

"Edinburgh University—The First Research Fellowship in Nursing," *Nurs. Times,* March 28, 1953, 311.

"Fifty Years of Progress," *Br. Jo. Nurs.,* April 1954, 39-41; June 1954, 67-69.

Haggo, M. M. "Joint Nursing and Midwives Council for Northern Ireland," *Nurs. Times,* September 27, 1957, 1085, 1091-1092.

Hampton, Isabel A., and others. *Nursing of the Sick 1893.* New York: McGraw-Hill, 1949. Pp. 24-43, 43-49, 67-73, 111-119, 158-164, 172-175, 201-204.

Heaton, Hilary M. "Nursing Education in England," *Methods and Problems of Medical Education,* 147-158. New York: Rockefeller Found., 1932.

"Industrial Nursing Organization in Retrospect," *Nurs. Times*, November 22, 1952, 1152-1155.

International Council of Nurses. *National Reports. 1933*, 5-7; *1947*, 5-8; *1949*, 1-5; *1957*, 38-41, 51-52; *1961*, 40-41, 94-97.

Lancet Commission on Nursing Final Report 1932. London: The Lancet, 1932.

Menzies, Isabel E. P. "Case-Study in the Functioning of Social Systems as a Defence Against Anxiety—A Report on the Study of the Nursing Service of a General Hospital," In *Human Relation Studies Towards the Integration of the Social Sciences*, May, 1960, pp. 95-121. "One of a number of projects undertaken by Tavistock Institute of Human Relations and Associated Workers."

Merry, Eleanor J., and Iris Dundas Irven. *District Nursing*. London: Bailiere Fundall & Cox, 2nd ed., 1955. Ch. I-IX.

Ministry of Health, Department of Health for Scotland, Ministry of Labour and National Service. *Report of the Working Party on Midwives*. London: HMSO, 1949.

——. (1) *Report of the Working Party on the Recruitment and Training of Nurses*. London: HMSO, 1947. (2) *Working Party on the Recruitment and Training of Nurses Minority Report*. London: HMSO, 1948.

"A New Development in Nursing Education," *Jo. Roy. Br. Nurs. Assn.*, September 1956, 139.

Nuffield Provincial Hospital Trust. *Observations Submitted to the Ministry of Health on the Ministry's Working Party's Report on the Recruitment and Training of Nurses*. Oxford: Oxford University Press, 1948.

——. *The Report 1948-51*. Oxford: Oxford University Press, 1951.

——. *The Work of Nurses in Hospital Wards*. London: Nuffield Lodge, 1953.

Nutting, M. Adelaide, and Lavinia L. Dock. *A History of Nursing*. New York: Putnam's, 1907-1912. 4 vols. Vol. III, Ch. I, pp. 1-115.

Parsons, H. C. "Progress of Nursing Education in this Country," *Nurs. Times*, March 13, 1954, 281-284.

"Royal College of Nursing—The Council, Its Standing Committees, Scottish Board, and Northern Ireland Committee," *Nurs. Times*, June 22, 1956, 569-575.

Royal College of Nursing. *Memorandum on the Report of the Working Party on the Recruitment and Training of Nurses*. London: The College, 1948.

——. "The National Headquarters in London," *Nurs. Times*, April 5, 1952, 335-344.

——. *Observations and Objectives*. London: The College, 1956.

Seymer, Lucy Ridgely. "The Nursing Profession 1852-1952," *Nurs. Times*, July 19, 1952, 704-706.

Stocks, Mary. *A Hundred Years of District Nursing*. London: Allen & Unwin, 1960.

Working Party Report on the Recruitment and Training of Nurses. Comments Submitted to the Minister of Health by the Ten Group. Croyden, Surrey: H. R. Grubb, 1953.

CHAPTER 11

The United States of America

Since the first stage of modern nursing in this country was included in Chapter 8, this will begin about 1890. The new movement was then well started in several eastern cities, in which the influx of new citizens of different nationalities had produced many social, economic, and health problems. The country was also emerging as a world power and taking on new international responsibilities. These and other influences, such as advances in medical science and in women's status and education, were reflected in the expanding nursing movement and in the efforts of nurses themselves to unite for more effective leadership in this new field of service.

SOME CHANGES IN THE ORIGINAL NIGHTINGALE SYSTEM

Though the basic principles of the Nightingale system had been adopted in America and many of the early leaders had been trained in Britain, it soon became evident that some changes were needed in the British system to adapt it to the conditions and needs of a new country in which class divisions were less marked and there were few wealthy families. The result was that all probationers were admitted on the same basis and after a short period of probation were classed as pupil nurses, put on a small allowance, and given head nurse and other responsibilities when they showed ability for such assignments. Here there were few paid positions for nurses even in the large hospitals, and the new system was being introduced so rapidly that the better qualified students often went directly into charge positions on graduation. The majority, however, became private nurses, and in comparison with their British and other European sisters were free lances with little or no direct supervision or control. The better schools nevertheless kept in touch with their graduates, helped to organize registries and clubs for them and often residences in the larger cities. Though the Roman Catholic sisterhoods and the Lutheran Deaconesses soon began to adopt the new system of training for their own members in hospital work and also for lay nurses, this group was small in comparison with the total number of schools and nurses.

During the earlier period a few efforts were made to introduce other systems of nursing from Europe but with very little success. One such experiment was made by Dr. Alfred Worcester at Waltham, Massachusetts, where he organized a school modeled on *La Source* in Lausanne, Switzerland (pp. 314-315). Though similar in some respects to the Nightingale school in London, this endowed school had no hospital connection in its early years and nurses in training got their practical experience chiefly in private homes. Such schools also were at first administered by medical men with nurses serving under them. Another plan sponsored by Clara Barton, who herself had received only brief training in Germany, was started in a small Red Cross hospital in New York before 1900. Here, under a German physician and nurse, Red Cross nurses were prepared for service in war or disaster. This was given up after the Spanish American War when its weaknesses were revealed. By that time also the regular hospital schools were multiplying and had won the support of hospital trustees, superintendents and the general public. The map shows only the early centers.

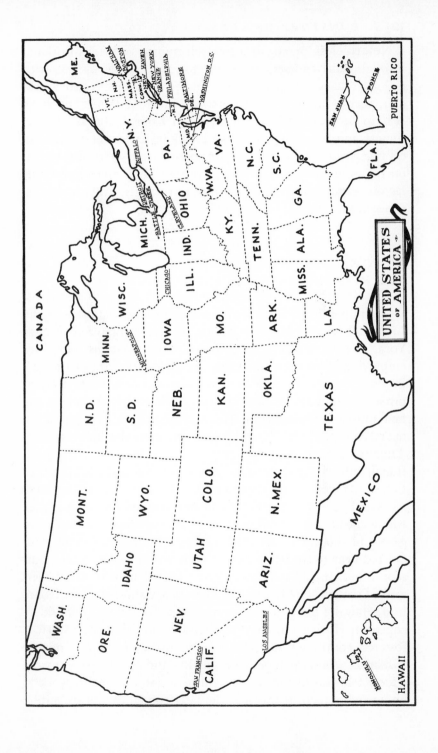

Nevertheless, practical nurses, self-trained or briefly initiated through short courses, continued to practice side by side with trained nurses. At first it was assumed that this group would disappear as more trained nurses became available, but as in Britain its ranks were often recruited from discharged probationers and ward maids. Commercial registries tended to encourage such deception and correspondence courses also traded on the popularity of the trained nurse. These were important factors leading to the movement for nurse registration which began around 1900.

TRENDS IN VISITING NURSING
AND RELATED BRANCHES

Beginning in 1886, visiting nurse societies similar to the Liverpool District Nursing Association were organized in New York, Boston, Philadelphia, Buffalo, and Chicago and were employing a few trained nurses chiefly for the care of the sick in their homes. In 1893 a new approach was made by two nurses, Lillian D. Wald and Mary Brewster, who started the first nurses' settlement, on Henry Street, New York, as a cooperative and partially self-supporting neighborhood service. Their work soon branched out into a wide variety of recreational, cultural, and social as well as nursing and health activities. Many friends and lay supporters shared in the Settlement's work and became interested in the new concept of health service which encouraged the initiative and independence of those who gave and those who received nursing care. Nurses came from far and near to study the new experiment at Henry Street, and soon other nurses' settlements were started in Richmond, Virginia, Orange, New Jersey, San Francisco, California, and Honolulu, Hawaii. Though this form of organization was not widely copied in visiting nursing, the friendly and democratic spirit it fostered continued to influence the work of visiting nurses. Lillian D. Wald's magnetic personality and creative vision were widely felt also in the whole field of social and health work at home and abroad. It was she who later coined the term "public health nursing" to cover a wide variety of nursing activities under public and private agencies which were becoming more active in promoting health and preventing disease on a community-wide basis.

In 1902 Miss Wald also introduced in New York City a plan for school nursing she had observed in London. By offering to give the city the service of one of her nurses (Lina Rogers) during the trial period she succeeded in having a staff of school nurses appointed by the City Health Department. This staff soon grew and covered all the public schools of the city, and in a short time the plan spread into other states and countries. In 1909, after a talk with Dr. Lee Frankel of the Metropolitan Life Insurance Company, Miss Wald and he created a plan for the home visiting of industrial policy holders by Henry Street nurses in New York. This scheme was later extended to many parts of the United States and Canada and was copied by some other insurance companies there and elsewhere. It was later modified when other health organizations developed but its influence was great, especially in industrial nursing.

In 1912, also at Miss Wald's suggestion, the American Red Cross started a national scheme for a rural visiting nurse service which continued for some years but was discontinued as municipal and state health programs expanded and there was less need for voluntary agencies. The Children's Bureau, organized the same year, in the Department of Labor of the Federal Government was another of Miss Wald's inspirations. It began an active nation-wide program for the health of mothers and babies which had a marked influence on the conservation of child life and welfare and the development of nursing throughout the country. Though many nurses and lay associates contributed to all these activities, Miss Wald's initiative and her remarkable skill in securing support for new ideas and plans made her one of the most influential health workers of her day and one of the most widely known in America and other countries.[1]

Other forms of specialized nursing services began as early as 1895 when industrial nursing got a start at the Vermont Marble

---

[1] More details will be found in her biographies and writings. See Bibliography, pp. 235-238.

Works, Ada Stewart being the first nurse employed to care for sick employees. Such programs soon increased in factories, stores, and other industries, many stimulated by industrial legislation and the advance of preventive medicine and health insurance. The discovery that tuberculosis was a preventable and curable disease led in the 1890's to special sanatoria (the first in this country at Trudeau, New York). The Los Angeles City Department of Health was the first to employ a nurse (Elizabeth Bush) to visit such patients in their homes. Agnes Talcott, who succeeded her, did much to establish this work on a firm basis. Shortly after, in 1903, the New York City Board of Health put nurses on its staff for the same type of service. The organization of the National Association for the Study and Prevention of Tuberculosis (1904) led to the employment of many other institutional and visiting nurses and to special preparation for such work. Another new field closely allied to both public health nursing and social work was opened up in 1905 when the first medical social service department was established at the Massachusetts General Hospital, Boston, by Dr. Richard Cabot and two nurse associates, Garnet Pelton and Ida M. Cannon. This new work was similar in many ways to that of the almoner in British hospitals.

Early in the 1900's nurses were undertaking studies that led to reforms in the care of mothers and babies. Among them were two by Elizabeth Crowell on the foreign midwife and Caroline Van Blarcom on ophthalmia neonatorum, both sponsored by the New York Committee for the Prevention of Blindness. These studies resulted in a plan for the inspection of midwives by Board of Health nurses, a school for the training of such workers at Bellevue Hospital (continued from 1911 to 1935), and an active campaign for sightsaving backed by medical and nursing organizations. Some nurses in both institutional and public health work at that time began to advocate the preparation and use of nurse-midwives in America, especially in areas in which medical care was lacking, but this movement was not sufficiently well supported by physicians, nurses, or the public to make much headway. A few schools for nurse-midwives were developed later, and although the nurses so qualified were relatively few in number (around 400 in 1950) they made a notable contribution to maternal and infant care not only in the United States but in several other countries. The names of Anne Stevens, Louise Zabriskie, and Hazel Corbin in New York and Mary Breckinridge in Kentucky are outstanding among nurse leaders of this movement. Mary Willeford, on Miss Breckinridge's staff, was the first nurse to receive a Doctor of Philosophy degree for her study of *Income and Health in Remote Areas* (1932). This was from Columbia University.

Specialization along clinical lines continued as new demands in orthopedic, psychiatric, and other clinical specialties increased. Some nurses qualified as technical specialists in X-ray and laboratory work, physical therapy, anesthesia, and the like, and many took special preparation to fit themselves for positions in doctors' offices where they became expert assistants to busy medical practitioners. Susan Tracy, a nurse, at Adams Nervine Hospital, Boston, was one of the first to develop courses in occupation therapy, then considered a phase of nursing care especially important in mental cases.

BEGINNINGS OF PROFESSIONAL ORGANIZATION

While these developments in nursing education and service were going on, American nurses had been organizing themselves in professional groups. The first steps were taken when the graduates of Bellevue led (1889) in forming an alumnae association, a plan soon followed by other pioneer schools. The chief purpose was to foster fellowship, mutual support, and school loyalty and to provide economic and other assistance in case of need. They also did much to train the leaders and workers who were to develop the larger professional organizations that soon took shape. Isabel Hampton apparently was the first nurse in the New World definitely to propose and push the idea of a national nurses association. She had suggested the plan and even the name in 1890 in a letter to a friend.

Before definite action was taken an opportunity for conferring with other nurses on the subject came at the meeting of the

1893 Congress on Charities, Corrections and Philanthropy in Chicago during the World's Fair. Through Dr. John S. Billings, a liberal-minded physician who was chairman of the Section on Hospitals, Dispensaries, and Nursing, Isabel Hampton was made chairman of the Nursing Committee of this Section and also asked to present a paper on "Nursing Standards." Before the meeting, Mrs. Fenwick who was in charge of exhibits, came over from London and conferred with Miss Hampton and her associates, Adelaide Nutting and Lavinia Dock at the Johns Hopkins Hospital. Her stirring account of the nurses' battle in Britain convinced this alert and able trio that steps must be taken at once to organize nurses in the United States and Canada. This led to plans for a meeting of representative nurses of these countries following the Congress in Chicago. Forewarned that the antiregistrationists in Britain, headed by Henry Burdett, were to attend the Congress and present their views and that Florence Nightingale was to have a paper opposing registration, Miss Hampton arranged for several papers representing other views. In her own paper on "Educational Standards" [2] she urged the need for stronger controls and greater uniformity in training-school programs and educational facilities, citing the chaotic situation in American schools in support of her plea. Other papers were prepared by leading nurses of the United States and Canada, such as Louise Darche, Irene Sutliffe, and Edith Draper, who vigorously supported the idea of professional organization. The delegates of these two countries who had been invited to remain over the following day to discuss the matter then took immediate action and launched the American Society of Superintendents of Training Schools for Nurses as a binational organization.

Although siding with the British Nurses Association on the issues of organization and registration, the Superintendents' Society went farther than any nursing group had then gone toward full self-government. It restricted its membership to qualified nurses who directed schools of acceptable standards, thus becoming, in effect, an accrediting agency for schools of nursing in the United States and Canada. Instead of electing

[2] *Nursing of the Sick 1893,* "Educational Standards for Nurses," pp. 1-12.

the same officers year after year, it rotated such positions among its members, thus providing for more democratic leadership and more nurses with experience in professional affairs.

By 1896 this group was ready to proceed as planned with the creation of a second organization for the rank and file of the profession, which was called the Nurses Associated Alumnae of the United States and Canada and elected as its first president Isabel Hampton (then Mrs. Hunter Robb). This attractive, dynamic, and able leader continued until her tragic death in 1910 to take an active part in organization work. Though she always insisted that nurses could and should manage their own professional affairs, she realized the need for the understanding and cooperation of medical, hospital, and lay groups in working out plans for the improvement of nursing schools and services and was exceptionally successful in interesting such groups and in interpreting the viewpoints of leading nurses on professional issues.

THE CAMPAIGN FOR STATE REGISTRATION

Although their leaders hoped that these two voluntary organizations would be able to check the multiplication of mediocre schools, it soon became evident that stronger controls were needed. Between 1880 and 1900 the total number of nursing schools in the United States had risen from 15 to 452 and their graduates proportionately. A large number of these schools operated in small hospitals, standards were highly variable, and complaints about poor nurses and nursing services were growing. In 1899, when the International Council of Nurses was formed in London, American nurses supported the plan to make state registration a primary objective.

Shortly after, Sophia Palmer, a prominent member of the Superintendents Society, in a public address urged that New York State pass a law requiring supervision of all its nursing schools by the University of the State of New York and the licensing of all nurse practitioners after a theoretical and practical examination. She claimed that nurses should have a place on such examining boards comparable to that which physicians had on their boards. The same year one of her friends and supporters, Mary E. P. Davis, was appointed chairman of the Nurses Associated Alumnae Committee on Periodicals, which succeeded in forming a joint stock company to launch *The American Journal of Nursing* (1900) under Sophia Palmer's able editorship. The *Journal* gave great impetus to the registration movement and was indeed indispensable in the twenty-year fight for state laws. Since in the United States such laws were the responsibility of the individual states (not of the Federal Government), it was necessary to develop state organizations to conduct the campaigns for registration. This as well as the need for legal incorporation of the Associated Alumnae led to the withdrawal of Canadian alumnae societies in 1901. A little later the Canadians formed their own national associations and began to develop provincial branches similar to those of the various states.

Four states—North Carolina, New Jersey, New York, and Virginia—secured nurse registration laws in 1903, and by 1923 all of the forty-eight states had enacted similar laws which varied a good deal in minimum standards and other details. These laws were permissive, not mandatory, and most of them gave nurses very inadequate representation in the administration of the law and on examining boards. Largely by the persistent efforts of state and national organizations legal controls were gradually strengthened, standards were raised, and examinations were made more effective and uniform. A definite advance began when the first full-time nurse inspector, Anna Alline, was appointed (1907) in New York State, primarily to help the schools meet and maintain acceptable standards. Such paid appointees were soon at work in most other states.

State registration, though far less effective than nurses had expected, brought definite improvements and some degree of uniformity in nursing school programs. For example, a three-year training in a hospital became the accepted standard for the majority of schools even in states like New York where the required minimum was still two years. Experience in the four major clinical branches—medical, surgical, pediatric, and obstetric nursing—was required by most laws, and where clinical facilities were lacking hospital affiliations were arranged to meet the requirement. By such affiliations nurses in America avoided the special registers set up in Britain for those who qualified often in one clinical field only. Here also obstetrical nursing (not midwifery) was a requirement for all R. N.'s. Registration did not eliminate all weak schools, and minimum standards, once accepted, were hard to change. Moreover, vigorous opposition was met not only from commercial hospitals, registries, correspondence schools, and similar agencies but sometimes from the better schools that wanted more freedom to experiment. New laws were often bitterly contested by such groups, and some fierce legal battles were fought.

The struggle for state laws, however, did much to strengthen and unite the young profession. Some nurses revealed exceptional ability in dealing with legal problems and in public speaking, lobbying, and vote getting. Many of them gained an intimate knowledge of the realities of political life and when women got the vote in 1920 could speak with conviction on the obligations of citizenship. Moreover, war experiences had made them aware of the need for political influence in safeguarding the position of nurses in the Army and Navy and making it possible for them to function effectively in such organizations.

THE SPANISH-AMERICAN WAR
AND POSTWAR DEVELOPMENTS

When the war with Spain broke out in 1898 the Army was unprepared, especially for tropical warfare in which epidemic diseases often caused ten times more deaths than bullets. No plans had been made to use regular trained nurses, and when Clara Barton's Red Cross nurses failed to provide for the army's needs it advertised for contract nurses. Among those who responded, the majority were untrained and often quite unsuitable, especially for positions calling for administrative responsibility. Serious lacks in nursing organization and discipline as well as appalling death rates brought public protests. Mrs.

Robb, president of the two-year-old Associated Alumnae, was then authorized to offer the services of that body to the army to establish a more efficient system and to supply competent nurses for key positions, but this offer came a day too late. The Daughters of the American Revolution had volunteered and their vice-president, Anita Newcomb McGee, a physician with no previous administrative experience, had been appointed in charge of the Army Nursing Service.

Leading nurses were accused of petty jealousy when they criticized this appointment, but they had a quarter century's experience in civil hospitals to support their position. Moreover, they could point to the remarkable results accomplished in the British Army by the introduction, three decades earlier, of qualified nurse administrators in charge of all military nursing services. Though the American Red Cross under Clara Barton's direction continued to oppose such a system, influential members of the New York Chapter finally were able to apply sufficient pressure in Washington to secure the appointment of Anna C. Maxwell of the New York Presbyterian Hospital and some other experienced nurse superintendents who had volunteered to go with their own trained staffs to the worst of the typhoid camp hospitals.

Their remarkable demonstration of what good nursing could do to save lives brought high praise from officers in command, but this came too late to have much effect on the appalling mortality of the Spanish-American War. Immediately after the war, however, the Associated Alumnae with the backing of influential citizens, took the issue to Congress and on Dr. McGee's own recommendation a bill was passed in 1901 authorizing the organization of the Army Nurse Corps to be composed of fully trained nurses under an able nurse director. The first appointee to that post was Dita M. Kinney. In 1908 the Navy Nurse Corps was created along similar lines. In 1909 the Associated Alumnae's offer to provide from its members a Red Cross Nursing Reserve was accepted and a contract to that effect was made. These trained nurses were to serve with volunteer auxiliaries in disaster service as well as to provide extra army nurses in time of war. Under the skillful leadership of Jane A. Delano, a distinguished graduate of the Bellevue Training School, this plan, which set up a completely new pattern in organized nursing and Red Cross relationships, was successfully carried through before World War I. Largely because of her efforts, professional nurses and Red Cross volunteers began to work together in greater harmony and effectiveness.

Other postwar developments in which both military and civilian nurses shared had to do with the introduction of modern nursing in the former Spanish colonies that were taken over by the United States, some for shorter and others for longer periods.[3] Such experiences helped to widen the horizons of American nurses and to prepare them for their international responsibilities which began to increase steadily from 1900 on.

ADVANCES IN THE EDUCATION
OF GRADUATE NURSES

Though American hospitals had begun in the early '90's to offer postgraduate courses of the apprenticeship type, this work did not help much to prepare nurse administrators and teachers. Later in the decade the Superintendents Society appointed Mrs. Robb, who was herself a teacher, chairman of a committee to look into the matter. Their search for a suitable place for this preparation led them to Teachers College which was affiliated with Columbia University, New York. Its progressive, open-minded dean, James E. Russell, consented to try the experiment, provided the Superintendents Society would assist with financial and teaching aid. An eight months' fulltime program, called the Hospital Economics Course, was then drawn up and approved. In the fall of 1899 the first two students entered, one of whom, Anna Alline, was retained as a part-time assistant on a small salary. The committee continued to take an active part in raising funds and providing lectures on nursing subjects until 1907, when Adelaide Nutting, who had been connected with the project from the start, was persuaded to accept a fulltime professorship in institutional administration in which was in-

[3] For details concerning nursing in Cuba and Puerto Rico see pp. 233-234, 419.

cluded the course in hospital economics. With an exceptionally wise and farsighted director and a permanent status in the college, growth was rapid, especially after 1910, when through an endowment by Helen Hartley Jenkins, wealthy trustee of Teachers College, the Department of Nursing and Health was created. This included a program for public health nurses in cooperation with the Henry Street Visiting Nurse Service. The same year a program for nursing school instructors was established and others were added as new specialties developed.

Created by the binational Superintendents Society and by an educational institution which attracted students from many lands, this department was from the first international in character. Nurses from Canada, Britain, Finland, Japan, and Germany as well as from the United States studied at Teachers College before 1910, and soon many other countries were represented. Similar graduate nurse programs then began to develop in other colleges and universities in the United States and Canada. The initial one-year programs were strengthened and expanded, and nurses began to qualify for bachelor's and higher degrees, which were increasingly recognized as a requirement for leadership in professional fields. Despite predictions to the contrary, it was soon evident that deeper and wider knowledge did not spoil nurses but led as a rule to increased interest in nursing and to more intelligent and effective service.

Connections with the university world had a profound influence which went far beyond the individual nurses who studied or taught in such institutions. Liberal-minded educators interested themselves in problems of nursing schools and often gave invaluable support and advice. Thoughtful nurses, observing that many of their troubles resulted from antiquated concepts of administration and education, which sharply conflicted with modern scientific, social, and democratic principles, began to revise their ideas on such matters as military discipline and the apprenticeship system. They saw the need for a better balance between theory and practice, the science and art of nursing, and the processes of education and of training. They also began to define their aims and policies more clearly and to study their problems more objectively in the light of fundamental principles and the wider experience of experts in related professional fields.

CHANGES IN THE BASIC EDUCATION OF NURSES

During the period after 1900 the influence of newer educational viewpoints was reflected in a number of experiments and innovations. In 1901 the Johns Hopkins Hospital School of Nursing, then under Adelaide Nutting's leadership, developed the first preparatory course in North America. This was a well-balanced six-months' program of theory and practice, which gave priority to the learning needs of students and compared favorably with many collegiate programs in the level of its teaching, attention to serious study and well-organized laboratory and ward practice. Warnings from head nurses and others that probationers would be ruined by too much theory proved unfounded. Drop-outs were reduced, time was saved, and better qualified applicants were attracted into the school. Other schools soon followed in organizing preparatory or preliminary courses, many of them shorter and less carefully planned but still an improvement on earlier probation periods. Between 1901 and 1910 several detached preparatory courses were tried out at Drexel Institute, Philadelphia, Pratt Institute, Brooklyn, and a few other places. Most of these courses were discontinued in a short time, but the one at Simmons College, Boston, continued, and now receives affiliating students for the teaching of the sciences. A collegiate school later evolved through the public health nursing course for graduates, begun by Anne Strong.

In 1909 a three-year basic nursing program was developed at the medical school and hospital of the University of Minnesota, Minneapolis, through the sympathetic interest and influence of Dr. Richard Olding Beard, Professor of Physiology at the Medical School, and Dr. Louis Baldwin, Superintendent of the University Hospital. Under Louise Powell's able direction and with their continued support, this school made a secure place for itself in the university, and within a few years a number of similar connections were developed. The next step was taken in 1916 when five-year degree programs were introduced with about equal emphasis on general and nursing education. The degree was at first optional, and the majority of students in such schools enrolled in the three-year diploma program. Soon, however, nursing, like teaching, home economics, library, and secretarial work, found a permanent place in many American universities, which were much more flexible than those in Europe in combining general academic and professional studies.

This upward trend in a few schools did not prevent a lowering of educational standards in others, chiefly because of the multiple creation of hospital schools of all varieties and a growing shortage of suitable applicants. The newly organized American Hospital Association of the United States and Canada, meeting in 1908, urged a return to the two-year course and a little later proposed a plan for three grades of nurses and of training schools, each having different requirements and certificates. Though organized nurses opposed both proposals, this had little effect.

The wide variation in existing standards was shown in *The Educational Status of Nursing* (1912), the first comprehensive and critical survey of schools of nursing in the United States or in any other country. This study was sponsored by the Federal Bureau of Education and directed by Adelaide Nutting, then secretary of the Superintendents Society, who prepared the questionnaire and interpreted the results. Of the 1100 schools responding, the great majority were rated as mediocre educationally and essentially utilitarian in purpose. It was noted that the few excellent schools which had attained a professional or near professional level had no lack of applicants, whereas the poor schools complained of a chronic shortage attributed as a rule to too high educational requirements. The report recommended that standards be raised not lowered, that schools of nursing secure independent financial support, and that they become educational institutions in fact as well as in name. This was radical doctrine in 1912 but it was not long before support came from many leading nurse educators, also from parents who preferred collegiate preparation for their daughters. Such programs did much to raise the professional status of nursing and to attract desirable applicants.

REORGANIZATION AND EXTENSION
OF NURSES' ASSOCIATIONS

Meanwhile, nurses had decided to expand their organizational structure and activities, differentiate the functions of each group, and develop state and local branches. In 1911 the Nurses Associated Alumnae became the American Nurses Association, with a program focused on the problems of nursing practice and legislation, the ethical and economic status of nurses, and other issues affecting the profession as a whole. The next year the *American Journal of Nursing* became the property and official organ of the ANA and continued to grow in influence and professional quality under the courageous and capable editorship of Sophia F. Palmer and her successor Mary M. Roberts.

The American Society of Superintendents of Training Schools for Nurses, which also had outgrown its name and early organization, in 1912 became the National League of Nursing Education. Its membership was enlarged to include teachers and supervisors of nurses, directors of public health nursing, members of state boards of nurse examiners, and all nurses whose work was directly concerned with education. Building on the solid foundation laid by the pioneers, it developed its own state and local branches and soon expanded its activities to cover a wide range of interests growing out of its original concern with better educational standards. By this time the goal of uniform standards was seen to be impractical as well as detrimental to progress because it was so frequently interpreted in terms of the minimum requirement for state registration which varied from state to state. The League decided that its function was to help schools of nursing to move forward as rapidly as possible toward a professional status comparable with that of schools of education, social work, and schools of other similar professions. Since the apprenticeship system was now recognized as the chief obstacle to further progress, special attention was given to better financial support for schools of nursing, sounder educational programs and where possible closer relationships with higher educational institutions which would stress education as the primary object of such schools.

The League's Education Committee, under Miss Nutting's chairmanship, began in 1914 to prepare a series of guides for schools that accepted this professional objective and were ready to make the necessary effort to advance step by step to a higher level. Starting with some studies aimed at shorter hours for students of nursing and the elimination of noneducational activities, the committee next prepared and issued (1917) in book form *The Standard Curriculum for Schools of Nursing,* which included administrative as well as teaching recommendations. This was the first of three successive editions prepared and issued by the League, the other two coming out in 1927 and 1934. The number of League studies dealing with all aspects of nursing education and practice grew rapidly and had an important influence on the development of better standards in the United States and abroad.

The National Organization for Public Health Nursing, created in 1912 with the aid of the two other national organizations, concentrated its efforts on the building up of soundly organized voluntary and official agencies for home and community visiting nurse services. It was the first to include such agencies in its membership and to admit qualified non-nurse members. The first president was Lillian D. Wald; other prominent officers were Mary Gardner, widely known as a pioneer in visiting nursing and author of a standard book on public health nursing, and Ella Phillips Crandall, who had directed the first public health nursing program at Teachers College and who now became the first fulltime executive secretary employed by a nursing organization in the United States. The NOPHN went ahead rapidly in promoting the cause of public health nursing and the better preparation of public health nurses.

It would be difficult to overestimate the influence of this group in broadening the social concept of nursing, emphasizing its preventive and educational objectives, strengthening community contacts, and supporting the League in its plans for better education. One of its major projects was the evaluation and listing of approved postgraduate courses in public health nursing. Its official organ, the *Public Health Nurse* (later changed to *Public Health Nursing*), had been started in 1909 as the *Visiting Nurse Quarterly* and presented to the new national organization by the Visiting Nurse Association of Cleveland. Though these three national associations, commonly known as the ANA, the NLNE, and the NOPHN, had different functions, they had many purposes and interests in common and worked closely together, especially after the opening of an official headquarters in New York (1921) brought them under one roof. All the organizations then began to employ permanent paid staffs, though much voluntary work was still done by their officers and members.

The National Association of Colored Graduate Nurses had come into existence in 1908 at the suggestion of Martha Franklin, a white nurse friend of Negro nurses, who was elected its first president. Its purpose was to work for better standards of admission and training in schools for this group, to break down discrimination where it existed, and to develop leaders from its own ranks. Though the first Negro nurse, Mary Mahoney, was graduated (1879) from a school for white nurses at the New England Hospital for Women and Children, Boston, public opinion in the United States was not ready at that time to proceed with a nonsegregation policy. None of the three national nurses' associations in the United States had ever excluded individuals on the basis of race, religion, national origin, or sex, but a few state branches refused to admit Negro nurses, and the low standards of many schools for this group had disqualified a good many of their graduates. The NACGN attacked these problems with great courage and vigor, and with the active support of the other national nurses' organizations they were able later (1951) to dissolve and to merge their members and functions in the two new groups then consolidating. Much credit for this remarkable achievement should go to Mabel K. Staupers for many years executive secretary of the NACGN and president at the time it was dissolved. Further details about these organizations and their activities will be found in Mary M. Roberts' *American Nursing,* Chapters 38-42.

WORLD WAR I—NURSING ISSUES
AND SPECIAL PROJECTS

In the United States, as in Britain, this war offered the greatest test that professional nurses had yet met. Though the Army, Navy, and Red Cross nursing services had been organized before 1917, initial confusion and conflict could not be prevented. Differences soon developed between the Red Cross and organized nurses on the use of nurses' aides for service abroad. This question was finally decided by government authorities who ruled that only trained nurses could be sent to France with the army, but the feeling aroused did not subside for some time. It was soon apparent that the supply of nurses was insufficient for both civilian and military needs, and some prominent medical, hospital, and lay spokesmen began to insist that the admission and graduation requirements of schools of nursing be drastically cut as a war measure and even that legal requirements be waived at this time. Highly publicized campaigns were started, urging that tens of thousands of "subnurses," "housekeepers for the sick," and other briefly prepared persons be recruited for nursing in homes and hospitals.

Fearing war hysteria and warned by the experience of Britain, three leading nurses in New York formed an Emergency Committee on Nursing immediately after the call for national defense was issued. These nurses were Lillian Wald, Annie W. Goodrich, and Adelaide Nutting, who served as chairman. This committee, which immediately conferred with officers of nurses' organizations, directors of leading nursing schools, and women's colleges, presented a plan designed to deflect some of the better qualified war volunteers into nursing schools, where they would gradually replace nurses released for the army and, if the war continued, would be prepared to serve as graduate nurses in much more responsible positions than would otherwise be open to them. With the promise of a selected group of schools that they would shorten the usual three-year course by about eight months for college graduates with good science backgrounds, the committee's announcement was sent out at once and met with an excellent response. This plan was followed by many others, all of which were designed to safeguard as much as possible the existing standards of nursing service and education and at the same time to meet the exceptional demands that war had brought.

This committee was soon enlarged and appointed to represent nursing in the Government's Medical Council for National Defense. Though it was well supported by organized nurses and by a number of medical, public health, and other influential persons, there were some conflicts with other official agencies, including military and Red Cross groups responsible for nurse supply. This whole story, which is fully discussed by Mary Roberts in *American Nursing,* is omitted here. We note, however, a few war projects that led to new educational patterns which influenced nursing policies in the future.

One was the Army School of Nursing established at Walter Reed Hospital, Washington, with branches in other military hospitals throughout the country. Planned largely by its first dean, Annie W. Goodrich, it bore the mark of her creative imagination and gift for organization and demonstrated what could be done by a large-scale central school, financed entirely by the Federal Government, to provide student experience in military as well as civilian institutions. Another project that showed courage and bold initiative in utilizing existing agencies and in enlisting the support of influential groups was the Vassar Training Camp, which was financed partly by a wealthy trustee of Vassar College, Mrs. John Wood Blodgett, and took the form of a centralized preparatory course in nursing developed on the college campus in the summer of 1918. The alumnae of Vassar and other women's colleges recruited more than 400 college graduates who received three months' initial preparation. Most of them then transferred to cooperating schools of nursing to complete a somewhat shortened and accelerated wartime program.

The Student Nurse Reserve also set an important precedent for mass recruitment in a national publicity campaign and the establishment of a central clearing house for sifting applicants and providing channels through which they and nursing schools with vacancies could get in touch with one another. The final report of the chairman, Adelaide Nutting, which summed up the committee's work and the conclusions reached as a result of the whole experience, is a fearless and outspoken document. It spared neither nurses themselves nor those responsible for their preparation and appealed to the public for better understanding and support of the education and service of such workers.[4]

OTHER INFLUENCES OF THE WAR ON NURSES AND NURSING

While these struggles were going on at home, American nurses on active duty were meeting not only the dangers, horrors, and discomforts of war service but many frustrations and conflicts. These conditions arose chiefly because American nurses had no military status. Army matrons and sisters from Britain and her dominions had a dignified and assured position resulting from long-established regulations of the British Army which gave them relative military rank with full responsibility for teaching and directing orderlies and corpsmen and handling other administrative problems as heads of wards and nursing services. The fact that American nurses could not assume such responsibilities under their army regulations seriously undermined their morale and their effectiveness, and though nothing could be done during the war the nursing profession shortly after decided to attack the problem directly. With help from legal and other advisers and the added support of the Votes for Women Amendment (passed 1920), they appealed to Congress for changes in the status of army nurses. After a long battle in which they met determined opposition from the majority of medical and military officers but strong support from former enlisted men and many other citizens, the nurses won their case and were given relative rank. Julia Stimson, then Superintendent of the Army Nurse Corps received the rank of major and other army nurses corresponding ranks down to second lieutenant. It was not until World War II, however, that nurses got

---

[4] Detailed accounts of all these activities may be found in various references listed in the Bibliography, pp. 235-238.

full rank in the armed services on the same basis as men officers. These questions of professional and military status were important, not primarily because of the social and economic factors involved, but because it was impossible otherwise to function properly in a military organization. As the vanguard of many other women workers, including physicians, who were to serve their country in military service, nurses established several other precedents from which all women workers in the army service profited.

When demobilization came many nurses found it difficult to locate themselves in suitable positions or were restless and uncertain about their future. Some wanted to change their fields of work or to study or otherwise better their conditions. During this period the Red Cross Nursing Service gave invaluable support and help. Its director, Jane Delano, who was popular with both lay and nurse members, had done much to inspire and help those in service. She had died in France at the end of the war, and Clara D. Noyes who had succeeded her secured Red Cross assistance in financing a nursing headquarters in New York to serve as a clearing house for nurses then demobilizing. By 1921 such a headquarters had become indispensable, and nurses' organizations took it over, enlarging it as their work grew. The ARC was generous also in providing scholarships, chiefly for advanced study in public health nursing. This field was now expanding as a result of the war, and many state and local health boards as well as industrial concerns and voluntary agencies were employing larger nursing staffs.

IMPORTANT POSTWAR STUDIES AND THEIR RESULTS

The need for changes in nursing schools and services had been highlighted by the war and by recent developments in medical and health work. As a result, several important studies were initiated, in most cases by nurses, though medical, hospital, educational, and lay groups were represented on many of the committees concerned.

The first of these studies was the result of a conference called by the Rockefeller Foundation in 1919 to discuss medical proposals for the training and employment of health visitors in the United States, based on the war experience in France. One suggestion, which was to substitute such workers for public health nurses in many positions, was opposed by Miss Wald and other nurse leaders at the conference. At their suggestion the Foundation agreed to finance an impartial investigation. Dr. C.-E. A. Winslow, a distinguished sanitarian and educator, was appointed chairman of the committee and Josephine Goldmark, a trained investigator and economist, directed the three-year study. Since the committee decided to cover the whole field of nursing service and education, all the major branches of nursing as well as medical and lay groups were represented on it. After a thorough survey of the situation, the committee decided against the proposal and recommended instead that the existing system of nurse education be strengthened so that graduate nurses could better combine health teaching with nursing service.

The recommendations went much farther and included the preparation and licensure of attendants, who were to have about nine months' training and to take over some of the less responsible duties of nurses. The basic preparation of nurses was to be about two years and four months, with an optional period of eight months added to provide special preparation for public health nursing and head nursing. The report, entitled *Nursing and Nursing Education in the United States,* also urged the development of more university schools of nursing offering broad, general education as well as professional preparation and giving more emphasis to the social, preventive, and curative aspects of nursing. These recommendations were based on the fundamental principle that all nursing schools should be real schools, with education their primary purpose and with financial support, clinical facilities, qualified educational staffs, and other necessary provisions to carry out that purpose.

Though the report was widely discussed and supported by many leading nurses, very few schools voluntarily shortened their courses, and the majority of nurses opposed the plan for trained attendants. The chief arguments were that such workers would be "half-baked nurses" who would compete with professionals and that any course less than three years would be over-crowded and superficial and would "let down" those who had stood so long for higher standards. A quarter century later, when the shortage of nurses was more acute and auxiliary workers were employed in many hospitals, the proposals of 1923 were more favorably considered, and the training of both attendants and nurses' aides was widely approved.

One immediate outcome of the report was the establishment of an experimental demonstration school at Yale University, endowed by the Rockefeller Foundation and having the same independent status as other professional schools in the university. Under its first dean, Annie W. Goodrich, and her associate, Effie J. Taylor, who succeeded her, this school did much to demonstrate what a real professional school of nursing should be. It was followed by a similar one at Western Reserve University, Cleveland, endowed by Frances Payne Bolton, and organized by Louise Powell, who had helped to build the first basic collegiate school in the University of Minnesota. Both these institutions attracted much attention from nurses of other countries as well as from those at home.

Another project which started a few years later reflected the influence of Abraham Flexner's study of medical colleges in 1910, in which those that survived examination were graded: A (excellent), B (good), or C (mediocre). Since this had resulted in a drastic reduction of C schools and a rapid rise of B to A ratings, it was hoped that a similar study of schools of nursing would have the same results. The Committee on the Grading of Nursing Schools was composed of representatives of nursing, medical, and hospital organizations, with some educational and lay members. Dr. William Darrach, a well-known surgeon, was its chairman, Dr. May Ayres Burgess, a psychologist and statistician directed the study, and many other experts, chiefly nurses, shared in the eight-year program. Nurses' organizations contributed liberally to the cost.

Two reports were issued during the eight years of this study: the first, *Nurses, Patients, and Pocketbooks* (1928), an analysis of nurse supply and demand, showed that training schools and trained nurses had multiplied about fifty times in forty years.

It was found that there was a surplus of general nurses in the larger centers and in the less exacting types of service but a serious shortage in the more specialized and responsible positions and in rural areas. The second report, *Nursing Schools Today and Tomorrow* (1934), showed a great preponderance of small schools with limited clinical and educational facilities, highly varied standards in theoretical and practical programs and a marked gap between the upper and lower groups of schools on many essential points. Two definite advances credited to the study were the wide acceptance of an eight-hour day for student nurses and of a four-year high school preparation for admission. The essentials of an *acceptable* school were defined, and each cooperating institution was told where it stood on certain items. Partly because hospitals and schools were then disrupted by the depression, the results were not made public. The committee recommended, however, that the National League of Nursing Education undertake the accreditation of nursing schools following surveys which were to be based on comparative studies and trends rather than on fixed criteria.

The main points were then outlined in an important pamphlet, *Essentials of a Good School of Nursing* (1936). This and other publications of the League, including the 1937 edition of *The Curriculum Guide for Schools of Nursing,* give a general idea of the changing concepts of nursing education during that period. The National Organization for Public Health Nursing prepared its own important suggested curriculum for those entering that special field and moved toward closer cooperation with the League on educational questions.

In 1933 a new organization, the Association of Collegiate Schools of Nursing, was formed. It was composed of schools (both basic and postgraduate) that were of a collegiate type and were integral parts of accredited colleges and universities. By defining objectives, standards, and policies and by providing a means for comparative study and experimentation (individual and collective), it was hoped that those responsible for such schools would make the most of the resources available in higher educational institutions such as the broader range of knowledge available and freedom to experiment with different plans and patterns. Results tended to justify these hopes and to encourage the development of such schools in many colleges and universities throughout the country.[5]

SOME EFFECTS OF ECONOMIC AND SOCIAL CHANGES IN NURSING

During the depression, beginning in 1929, many private and some public hospitals were forced to close their doors or to limit their services. There was also a marked reduction in schools of nursing and in the number of their graduates. To help relieve serious unemployment among nurses, many hospitals employed larger graduate staffs, often on subsistence salaries, while other nurses were employed as visiting nurses and paid from relief and other public funds. Private nursing declined sharply and thereafter took second place numerically, with public health nursing a fairly close third. In the hospital and health fields as a whole the wider use of national, state, and local tax funds in health and welfare services and the rapid growth of voluntary insurance plans for financing hospital and medical care were results of the depression. Despite strong opposition to socialized medicine in the United States, conditions in the "hungry thirties" and the war years that followed led to increasingly heavy state and federal subsidies for health and social welfare.

During this period the American Nurses Association began to make more comprehensive and continuous studies of employment conditions and trends, personnel policies, and the distribution of nurses. Community Councils were organized to study nursing service needs and working conditions. Economic hazards in such fields as private nursing also received much more careful attention. The eight-hour day in nursing services became more general after it had been tried as a device to spread the work during the period of acute unemployment. These and other common problems led to closer relationships among nurses in various fields and among members of the medical and health professions generally.

[5] More details on these organizations and studies will be found in Roberts, *American Nursing*, and Stewart, *The Education of Nurses,* Ch. VI.

WORLD WAR II (1939-1945)—NURSING PROBLEMS
AND PROJECTS

When war in Europe again seemed imminent, the three
national nursing organizations and representatives from the
American Red Cross and the nursing agencies of the Federal
Government formed a Nursing Council for National Defense to
plan for joint policies and activities and to speak for the profession as a whole. Later this council was enlarged to include the
six national nursing organizations[6] and representatives from
such organizations as the American Hospital Association. After
the declaration of war, this voluntary group became the National Nursing Council for War Service. Though the official
Health and Medical Committee of the Office of Defense, Health,
and Welfare had a subcommittee on nursing, there was little
overlapping of functions, and the two groups worked together,
especially on the problem of nurse supply. This problem was
much more serious than in World War I because of the longer
duration and wider scope of the war effort and the much larger
forces engaged in war industries as well as in military and civil
defense.

Nurses were now more conscious of the need for reliable
statistical and other information as a basis for such planning
and proceeded at once to make an inventory of nurse power
(including professional and practical nurses and nurses' aides).
They then considered the additional persons to be recruited
and trained as well as the best use of existing resources. As
military quotas increased, a serious deficit threatened, and
a system of priorities was devised whereby quotas would be
assigned to states and local communities. Regional committees
of professional and lay workers helped nurses and employers
to make decisions about nurse assignments and replacements
involving military versus civilian needs. When later a draft of
nurses was debated in Congress, other measures were employed,

---

[6] American Nurses Association, National League of Nursing Education, National
Organization for Public Health Nursing, Association of Collegiate Schools of
Nursing, National Association of Colored Graduate Nurses, and American As-
sociation of Industrial Nurses.

including short courses for nurse teachers and supervisors as well as refresher and in-service programs for older nurses and aides. Programs for students were also accelerated.

At this time, a committee of the National Nursing Council, with the aid of the United States Department of Education, prepared a request for federal funds to enlarge the facilities for nurse education. After much delay, the first appropriation of more than a million dollars was voted (1941), the administration of which was assigned to the United States Public Health Service under Surgeon General Thomas S. Parran, who had vigorously supported the proposal. Pearl McIver and other capable members of the USPHS nursing staff put the plan into immediate operation. Another precedent was set with this vote of Congress which made substantial federal funds available for schools of nursing, most of which were not under government control.

The next step (1943) was the Cadet Nurse Corps, authorized by the Bolton Act, named for Representative Frances Payne Bolton, long a friend of nursing, who had sponsored the plan. A sixty-million-dollar appropriation was voted at this time and later increased. The details of this project are to be found in *The United States Cadet Nurse Corps,* prepared under the direction of Lucile Petry, its chief nurse officer. With the aid of a high-powered recruiting program, liberal scholarships and subsistence grants, and an attractive uniform, 170,000 cadets were enrolled in 1125 schools between 1944 and 1946, comprising ninety per cent of the total enrollment in basic nursing programs for those years. This was a remarkable achievement, considering the competing appeals for women war workers at this time and the difficulties met in expanding the teaching, clinical, housing, and other facilities needed for these enlarged quotas.

SOME ADVANCES DURING THE WAR AND POSTWAR PERIOD

Though nursing services and educational programs were on the whole less efficient and stable because of the rapid turnover and other abnormal conditions of wartime, definite and permanent gains were made. Some resulted from the efforts to economize nurse power, accelerate educational programs, and improve the preparation of hospital and nursing school staffs. Federal and other scholarships were available also, and later the G. I. Bill of Rights provided substantial assistance to men and women who had served in the armed forces. The better salaries of the Veterans Administration also gradually brought about an improvement in those paid in civilian hospitals.

Among the notable advances were the trend toward integration of the races in basic nursing education and the commissioning of Negro nurses in the armed services. Coeducation of men and women and the admission of married nurses in civilian and military nursing services were other breaks with tradition. A more cordial relationship gradually developed between professional nurses and nonprofessional workers (the term "subsidiary" being dropped). In nursing education the need for additional fields for clinical practice was recognized and the expansion of the hospitals of the Veterans Administration and other government agencies opened up new facilities for such experience.

Toward the end of the war a restudy was made of the whole situation in nursing by the National Nursing Council for War Service. A five-year plan was evolved and its results later published in *A Comprehensive Program for Nation-Wide Action in the Field of Nursing*. The American Red Cross Nursing Service and other health agencies participated in the plan, which covered five areas: Nursing Service, Nursing Education, Distribution of Services, Standards and their Implementation, Information and Public Relations. It also included the work of all nurses, both professional and practical.

After demobilization it was expected that gaps would be filled in civilian hospitals and nursing agencies and that prewar standards of service would be restored. But, in spite of the large wartime increases, the shortage of nursing personnel and the instability of services grew worse instead of better. Student recruitment fell off sharply, volunteer aides melted away, and many graduates dropped out permanently or temporarily to study, rest, retire, marry, or go into other work. Hospitals which had increased their admissions seventy-five per cent between 1936 and 1946 because of hospital insurance plans, higher birth rates, and other causes were having to reduce their patient intake and in many cases to close wards because of lack of nursing and domestic staffs. In some large institutions the quality of nursing service had deteriorated so much that little more than custodial care could be given by the relatively untrained and shifting war personnel. Before nurses could catch their breath, medical, public health, and hospital planners were announcing that hospitals must double their capacity in the next few years to care for expanding hospital and public health needs. Few of them anticipated any difficulty in filling the quotas of nurses needed, and some again proposed a lowering of standards for registered nurses.

Meanwhile, practical nurse preparation and licensing were being actively promoted by the National Association for Practical Nurse Education, formed for this purpose during the war under the leadership of professional nurses such as Hilda Torrop, its first president, and with the backing of influential medical, lay, and nursing groups. By 1947 half the states had made provision for licensing practical (or vocational) nurses, and an approved list of schools offering courses of nine to eighteen months was prepared. In 1949 another association, the National Federation of Licensed Practical Nurses, was organized, with state branches to bring together those who met acceptable standards. Professional nursing organizations now recognized more and more their responsibility for assisting in the teaching, supervision, and licensing of practical nurses, and in 1947 a joint committee of the National Association for Practical Nurse Education and the six national professional nursing organizations issued a pamphlet entitled *Practical Nurses and Auxiliary Workers for the Care of the Sick,* which defined the role of each group and set forth standards for qualifications and preparation. Teaching of home nursing, child care, first aid, and in-service training of various groups were also increased. One of the indirect results of the war and the depression, also of the increased contacts between countries at that time, was the influx of nurses from abroad who came to study or to find work and who often remained in the United States for longer or shorter periods.

MORE RECENT STUDIES AND TRENDS

The pyramid structure of nursing services now had a base of informed citizens who were more capable of safeguarding family health and a graduated series of occupational groups beginning with paid aides and topped with professional nurses. The lines between the groups were not yet clear, and before the National Nursing Council for War Service disbanded it secured, by the efforts of its secretary Elmira Beers Wickenden and others, the cooperation of the Carnegie Foundation in financing a study to clarify the situation. Dr. Esther Lucile Brown, research specialist of the Russell Sage Foundation and author of several monographs relating to the professions, made this study. Her report, published in 1948 under the title *Nursing for the Future,* brought to a focus ideas and trends which had been developing over a period of years. The evidence indicated that the demand for nursing service would increase and that the responsibilities of nurses would increase with it. Dr. Brown visualized the eventual development of two main groups of nurses, professional and practical, the practical to work under the leadership of the professional and the professional to be upgraded and substantially reduced in numbers. An educational structure was suggested to complement the service pattern. After much discussion, a Joint Committee on Implementation of the Brown Report was appointed and later renamed the National Committee for the Improvement of Nursing Services (Marion Sheehan, Chairman). Its first report, *Nursing Schools at the Midcentury* (1950), was made with the assistance of the United States Public Health Service and the voluntary cooperation of ninety-seven per cent of the state-accredited schools of nursing.

Another project undertaken at about this time was the establishment of the National Nursing Accrediting Service, which coordinated all existing national agencies concerned with the approval of nursing education programs. An interim list of schools was published, pending the establishment of a more complete accrediting program. In line with the recommendations of the Brown Report to fit nursing education into the general educational pattern of the country, nursing educators conferred with representatives of higher educational institutions. The rising costs of collegiate education were of increasing concern to administrators and to prospective students alike, and the question of financial aid from public funds for nursing education was widely discussed. Although the general problem of financing nursing education remained unsolved, some progress was made. Many schools of nursing were put on a collegiate basis, and regional planning, such as that exemplified by the Southern Regional Education Board project, was introduced to make the best use of existing facilities.

One of the most recent developments has been the cooperation between representatives of junior and community colleges and of nursing educators in experiments to try out a combined academic and technical curriculum qualifying graduates for state registration as nurses. Such a project was initiated in the Nursing Education Division of Teachers College, Columbia University, under the direction of R. Louise McManus and Mildred Montag, and in other places as well. Additional pilot studies in this area were financed by the W. K. Kellogg Foundation. These programs are no longer considered to be experimental and the numbers are increasing.

The Division of Nursing Education at Teachers College had earlier sponsored a study to determine the proportions of the total nursing personnel of the United States which should be allocated to professional and practical nursing. This study, directed by Dr. Eli Ginsberg, was published under the title *A Program for the Nursing Profession.* Its estimates of a 2 to 1 ratio of practical and professional nurses for the country as a whole indicated a trend in the thinking of many hospital and nursing executives faced with the problems of nurse supply.

REBUILDING NURSES' ASSOCIATIONS

The changes in services and education described above involved many changes in organized nursing. In order to meet the challenges of the depression and the war, nurses' organizations had modified their structure and activities, and after this period a four-year study was made which resulted in the report, *New Horizons in Nursing* (1950). Represented in this study were the National League of Nursing Education, the American Nurses Association, the National Organization for Public Health Nursing, the National Association of Colored Graduate Nurses, the Association of Collegiate Schools of Nursing, and the American Association of Industrial Nurses. Some of these were primarily concerned with nursing service and nursing education in which the interest and cooperation of the public and of allied professions were essential. Others dealt with the problems of nurses as professional practitioners and their responsibilities for improving their own efficiency and the welfare of their members. Some also combined corporate members (schools or agencies) with individual nurse and non-nurse members, whereas others admitted only graduate nurses. One important factor was ANA membership in the International Council of Nurses which required that all national members be self-governing associations whose officers and voting members were fully qualified nurses.

After studying and discussing the issues, it was finally decided to have two organizations: one, a somewhat reorganized American Nurses Association, composed entirely of nurses and speaking for the profession, and the other the National League for Nursing, to include nurses and non-nurses, individual and corporate members, representing all those responsible for the sound development and support of nursing services and nursing schools. The proposals of the Committee on Structure were adopted with some modifications in 1952. The two associations, under their newly elected presidents, Elizabeth K. Porter (ANA) and Ruth Sleeper (NLN), immediately proceeded to take the necessary steps leading to the reorganization of state associations and of headquarters offices and staff in New York. More than 1000 student nurse delegates also met to appoint temporary officers and committees to prepare the constitution and bylaws for a national association which later decided to become a unit under the Coordinating Council of the ANA and the NLN. The process of reorganization took some time and while not entirely satisfactory to all concerned the new plan did much to bring the groups together.

PROBLEMS RELATED TO FUNCTIONS, ETHICS, ECONOMICS, AND PERSONNEL

The constantly changing functions of nurses had led to a number of studies which included a five-year project, begun in 1950 by the American Nurses Association with the cooperation of the National League for Nursing. The results, published in 1958 under the title *Twenty Thousand Nurses Tell Their Story*, showed the many changes in functions and the new groups of workers since earlier studies, such as the *Activity Analysis of Nursing* (1930), made by Ethel Johns and Blanche Pfefferkorn.

Earlier reports had been made also on ethical principles and conduct to supplement the widely used textbooks by Harriet Lounsberry and Isabel Hampton Robb. Ethical codes in the form of pledges for particular schools of nursing had been prepared by Mrs. Lystra Gretter and Mrs. Cadwallader Jones. An ethical code had been adopted by the American Nurses Association in 1940, and in 1950 it was revised and adopted as "A Code for Professional Ethics." Compared with earlier statements, it gave much more consideration to social and economic issues and to interpersonal and group relations. It also indicated that professional nurses were assuming much more responsibility for determining the scope of their own field and functions instead of leaving such questions to the judgment of medical, hospital, and other individuals and groups.

Economic conditions, including hours, salaries, and the like, also presented persistent and difficult problems. Pioneer nurses had been handicapped by the earlier concept of nursing as a form of religious or charitable service and by their own reluctance to use measures to protect their interests in the fear that such efforts might be regarded as unethical or unprofessional. After 1935, when the National Labor Relations Act (known also as the Wagner Act) affirmed labor's right to organize and bargain collectively, some professional workers decided to try to solve their problems through their professional organizations by using them as bargaining agents. The California State Nurses Association was the first to work out such a plan under the leadership of the executive secretary, Shirley Titus. In 1946 the American Nurses Association endorsed such action and encouraged state and local branches to adopt similar measures. By 1952 more than half the states had adopted the ANA Economic Security Program, though not all included the plan for collective bargaining.

Other problems having to do with nurse supply, service, and morale came up for discussion and study. Changes in methods of supervision, teaching, and placement and increasing emphasis on better personal and professional relations improved some situations. Old-time registries were converted into professional counseling and placement services, administered chiefly by state and local branches of the American Nurses Association. The Department of Measurement and Guidance, later the National Nursing Accrediting Service, helped schools and state boards to select better qualified students and provided a means by which the methods and results of the basic preparation could be compared on a nationwide as well as a statewide basis.

TRENDS IN NURSING LEGISLATION AND NATIONAL HEALTH SERVICES

Nurses had long recognized their responsibility for improving standards of nursing practice by legal recognition of schools and licensure of practitioners and had done much to bring about improvements in the laws and in state supervision of schools which made reciprocity difficult. A national examination had been discussed, but when many states adopted the examinations for state registration prepared by the Department of Measurement and Guidance of the National League of Nursing Education this helped to solve that problem. Other steps in legislation were the establishment of an office and representative in Washington to keep in touch with proposed federal legislation that would affect nursing and to work for legislation that would make federal and state funds available to nursing schools. Although organized nurses tended to favor a larger degree of public support for nursing schools, the American Medical Association opposed what it interpreted as a trend toward state control, and the American Hospital Association in general tended to discourage any measures that might weaken the existing system of hospital schools of nursing.

In 1952 the President's Commission on the Health Needs of the Nation recommended an extension of prepayment plans, both voluntary and compulsory, for medical care and a closer coordination of federal and state programs to provide more effective health protection for the whole population. Members of the various professions concerned were not in entire agreement on the issues. The American Nurses Association refused to support the American Medical Association's campaign against what it called socialized medicine because the majority of its members believed that the existing system of financing medical and health services and education as then organized was inadequate.

PUBLIC AND PROFESSIONAL RELATIONS AND PUBLICITY

In recent years nurses have been more conscious of the need for improved relations with the public and with other professional groups. Toward the end of the war, Edward L. Bernays, an eminent public relations expert, was employed to make a study of public attitudes toward nurses, the results of which were published in the *American Journal of Nursing*. They showed that although the American public in general thought well of this group few were informed about nurses' activities, contributions, or problems. It was obvious that the nursing profession itself had been remiss in this respect. The study led to better publicity and the employment of specialists to help collect, present, and distribute suitable information and to interpret nursing to the general public and to the allied professions. Much more emphasis is now given to what is called the "image" of nursing and nurses in the minds of the public, of patients and co-workers, of student nurses and of the profession in general.

NURSING LITERATURE, JOURNALISM, AND RESEARCH

It would be impossible in this short history to give an adequate idea of the great increase in text and reference books and the wide variety of other nursing literature. The most significant fact is that nurses themselves are now producing a large proportion of this literature individually or through their organizations. The development of special library services, including employment of trained librarians, has also done much to further the wider circulation and more effective use of nursing literature.

When schools of nursing were started the most urgent need was for nursing text books. The first written by an American nurse (in 1885) was Clara Weeks' *Text Book for Nurses*. She was followed by Isabel Hampton, Diana Kimber, Lavinia Dock and a constantly increasing number of other nurses who have made a reputation as authors.

Nurses have also qualified as journalists and have been very successful in this field. Special recognition should be given to such pioneers as Sophia Palmer and Mary M. Roberts who established the *American Journal of Nursing* on a firm basis and made it one of the leading professional journals in the country. Recognizing that more than experience was needed for such a task Mary Roberts secured special preparation in journalism as well as in nursing. Under her leadership the American Journal of Nursing Company was formed which later expanded to include *Nursing Outlook* (official organ of the National League for Nursing) and *Nursing Research* medium for the publication of valuable studies and surveys on nursing subjects. In her honor a Mary M. Roberts fellowship fund has been contributed by the Journal Company which provides one fellowship yearly for a nurse candidate who is preparing for this type of work.

As to nursing research there are many indications of the growing interest in this field and of the increasing need for nurses with special qualifications and training in it. The first major contribution toward such preparation was made by graduates of the Nursing Education Department of Teachers College in 1939 to provide the salary of a part-time Research Associate, Dr. Genevieve Bixler. This was followed in 1952 by a grant from the Rockefeller Foundation to establish the Institute of Research and Service in Nursing Education whose first director, Dr. Helen L. Bunge, was a nurse. This and other centers of nursing education are building up such programs on a permanent basis in order to prepare the nurses needed to conduct surveys and studies in this field and to train other nurses.

NURSING IN OUTLYING PARTS OF THE UNITED STATES

Up to this point attention has been given to the block of forty-eight states that lies between the Canadian and Mexican borders. Some differences in the timing and sequence of nursing developments can be noted between the East and West and between the North and South, but the general trends were much the same and the increasing mobility of nurses tended toward unification. When we come to outlying parts, which include Alaska in the far north, Hawaii in the Mid-Pacific, and Puerto Rico and the Virgin Islands in the Caribbean area, the differences are more marked, not only in physical environments and in racial, cultural, and social conditions but in some aspects of nursing development. This applies also to many islands scattered over the surrounding seas and oceans which are under the general administration of the United States Government. Only the first three areas are considered here.

ALASKA

Alaska, which became the forty-ninth state of the Union in 1959, is situated in the far northwest. It covers a large territory, part of which reaches into the Arctic Circle, and has a sparse and scattered population, including settlements of Eskimo, Aleut, and American Indian peoples. These groups are especially susceptible to tuberculosis and other infectious diseases. Small hospitals and health centers have been established by the Indian Bureau, the United States Public Health Service, and in some cases by missionary organizations and the American Red Cross. Doctors and nurses in outlying areas travel by boat, plane, and dog sled to reach their patients. In the larger cities there are modern community hospitals and health services but only one school of nursing at the time of writing and that is for practical nurses. Most of the professional nurses come from the United States, but there are a few from other countries. Qualified nurses have organized state and local associations and recently have secured membership in the American Nurses Association. From this and other nursing organizations they have received much advice and help. Already a law governing the practice of nursing has been passed, and a small publication, *The Alaska Nurse,* has been launched to keep the scattered members in touch with each other and with recent nursing developments.

HAWAII

Hawaii, the fiftieth state (also in 1959) is the largest of a group of islands in the Mid-Pacific area. In addition to its native population, which was originally of Polynesian stock, it is inhabited by a wide variety of ethnic groups which were attracted to the islands by their favorable climate. Missionaries brought the first modern health services, and early in the twentieth century the well-known Queen's Hospital and School of Nursing were opened, as was the Palama settlement, formed originally by nurses to combat tuberculosis. Both are in Honolulu, the modern capital city. In 1959 there were twenty-three such schools in the islands, one of them at the University of Hawaii. Their students include a wide variety of racial stocks, oriental and occidental, and all kinds of racial mixtures. A distinguishing characteristic of the Hawaiian people is the remarkable lack of racial prejudice and discrimination. English is the dominant language, and the system of nursing follows very closely that of the continental United States. The Hawaiian Nurses Association is a member of the American Nurses Association, and the status of nursing in general is similar to that on the mainland.

PUERTO RICO

Puerto Rico, which remained under the government of the United States after the Spanish-American War, has a different history. The first efforts to establish a modern school of nursing began in 1904, at San Juan, under the auspices of the Presbyterian Mission. In 1916 another school was organized at St. Luke's Memorial Hospital. Most of the pioneer Puerto Rican nurses were trained in these two schools under such experienced nurses from the United States as Amy Pope and Ellen Hicks. Encouraged and supported by them, some of their graduates began to tackle the bad nursing situation in the island's public hospitals. It took tremendous stamina to stand up against the combined pressure of family mores, social disapproval, corrupt politics, and stiff medical and often religious opposition. Rosa Gonzales, one of these pioneers, tells the story of their struggles in her pamphlet *Unknown Facts.*[7]

Modern nursing is now well established in Puerto Rico. Hospital and public health services are expanding. Several nursing schools, both public and voluntary, are on the accredited list of the National League for Nursing. They include the pioneer schools referred to above, which had a great influence on nursing on the island. The School of Tropical Medicine, affiliated with the University of Puerto Rico, also has a nursing department under the direction of a well-qualified public health nurse, Célia Guzman. Another school of nursing under Catholic Sisters is established at St. Mary's University in Ponce. The hospitals under the Veterans Administration are attempting to raise nursing standards under the guidance of trained Puerto Rican nurses. These nurses, especially in the larger cities, are well organized, one group being a constituent of the American Nurses Association and the other a unit of

[7] Tr. from the Spanish by Mrs. Grace DeW. Lugo Viña with R. Gonzales, San Juan: Imprenta "Venezuela," Cristo 6, 1929.

the National League for Nursing. An important advancement in organization was the creation in 1930 of the Board of Nurse Examiners, which controls the education and licensure of nurses on the island.

AMERICAN VIRGIN ISLANDS

In the American Virgin Islands, formerly Danish, nursing has been influenced by the Sisters of the Danish Lutheran Church who were sent to the islands to care for the sick. When the United States assumed control, nurses were trained for a time by the government. In 1952 the civilian government took over, and the United States Public Health Service and the Children's Bureau worked closely with local health departments to improve the care of children. Midwives practice in the homes, but at the present time the trend is toward hospital care of maternity patients. In 1954 the Virgin Islands Nurses Association was admitted as a constituent of the American Nurses Association. The islands have a nurse practice act which helps to maintain better standards of care.

INTERNATIONAL RELATIONS AND ACTIVITIES

American nurses started early to enter into closer relations with nurses of other parts of the world, not only in the International Council of Nurses, but in the contacts of nurses of different countries during the two World Wars and by increased travel, service, and study. Missionary, Red Cross, and later United Nations and other agencies contributed to this wider understanding and cooperation, as did study scholarships and fellowships from the Rockefeller, Kellogg, and other foundations and the nurse exchange plan developed by the International Council of Nurses. (These are discussed more fully in Chapter 20). The temporary removal of the International Council of Nurses' headquarters to the United States during World War II and the holding in 1947 of its first postwar congress in this country did much to stimulate the interest of American nurses in international nursing affairs.

In the United States, as in Great Britain, the new nursing movement found many conditions favorable to its development and also some formidable obstacles that tended to obstruct or delay progress. Some of the barriers were the size and newness of the country, the mixed elements in its population, and its politics. Nevertheless, leaders soon appeared who succeeded in introducing the new ideas which spread rapidly, aided by the growing prosperity of the country, by advances in medical and public health services, and by the women's movement. Though the young vocation met many of the same problems and went through much the same stages as it did in Britain, many variations can be seen in the nursing systems of the two countries and in the steps taken to put the work on a sound educational, legal, economic, and ethical basis. An important point is the constant interchange of ideas and the close cooperation of nurses of these countries which have continued for nearly a century and have done much to lay the foundations for international cooperation among nurses of the world.

SELECTED BIBLIOGRAPHY

Alger, George W. "Lillian D. Wald," *Am. Jo. Nurs.*, March 1960, 354-357.
American Association of Industrial Nurses' Journal. New York: Am. Assn. of Ind. Nurses. Published monthly.
American Journal of Nursing. New York: Am. Jo. Nurs. Co. Published monthly.
American Nurses Association. *An American Challenge.* New York: ANA. N. d.
———. *History of the ANA Professional Counseling and Placement Service, Inc.* New York: ANA, 1951. Mimeographed.
———. Publications. New York: ANA. On Intergroup Relations Program, Professional Counseling and Placement Service, Research and Statistics Unit, Economic Security Unit, Industrial Nurses' Section, Public Health Nurses' Section, Legislation, Headquarters, Membership, Constitution and By-laws, The Older Nurse, State Boards, Executive Secretaries, Studies of Nursing

Functions, Registries, State Approved Schools of Nursing, Ethical Code, Public Relations, American Nurses Foundation, and others.

Bixler, Genevieve K., and Leo W. Simmons. *The Regional Project in Graduate Education and Research in Nursing.* Atlanta: Southern Reg. Ed. Bd., 1960.

Breckinridge, Mary. *Wide Neighborhoods: A Study of the Frontier Nursing Service.* New York: Harper, 1952.

Brown, Esther Lucile. *Nursing for the Future.* New York: Russell Sage Foundation, 1948.

Burgess, May Ayres. *Nurses, Patients and Pocketbooks.* New York: NLNE, 1928.

———. *Nursing Schools Today and Tomorrow.* New York: NLNE, 1934.

Committee on the Function of Nursing. *A Program for the Nursing Profession,* New York: Macmillan, 1948.

Committee on Nursing and Nursing Education in the United States. *Nursing and Nursing Education in the United States.* New York: Macmillan, 1923.

Cowan, M. Cordelia (Ed.). *The Yearbook of Modern Nursing.* New York: Putnam's, 1959.

DeWitt, Katharine. "The Journal's First Fifty Years," *Am. Jo. Nurs.,* October 1950, 590-597.

Duffus, R. L. *Lillian Wald: Neighbor and Crusader.* New York, Macmillan, 1938.

Faddis, Margene O. *The History of the Frances Payne Bolton School of Nursing.* Cleveland: Alumnae Assn., 1948.

Goostray, Stella. "A Time to Every Purpose," *Am. Jo. Nurs.,* July 1952, 818-820.

———. "Mary Adelaide Nutting," *Am. Jo. Nurs.,* November 1958, 15-24.

Gowan, Sister M. Olivia, and Sister M. Maurice Sheehy. "Contributions of Religious Communities to the Development of Nursing Education," *Tr. Nurse and Hosp. Rev.,* April 1938, 404-409; June 1938, 652-655, 700.

Gray, James. *Education for Nursing: A History of the University of Minnesota School.* Minneapolis: University of Minnesota Press, 1960.

Gruening, Ernest. "Alaska Proudly Joins the Union," *Nat. Geog. Mag.,* July 1959, 143-185.

Hampton, Isabel A., and Others. *Nursing of the Sick 1893.* New York: McGraw-Hill, 1949. Pp. 1-12.

Haupt, Alma C. "The Metropolitan Nursing Story," *Quart. Bull. for Met. Nurses,* November 1951, 143-185.

Hawaii. Territorial Commission on Nursing Education and Nursing Service. *The Nurse of Tomorrow.* Honolulu, T. H., 1952.

Hughes, Everett C., Helen MacGill Hughes, and Irwin Deutcher. *Twenty Thousand Nurses Tell Their Story.* Philadelphia: Lippincott, 1958.

International Council of Nurses. *National Reports. 1933,* 8-9; *1947,* 9-15; *1949,* 6-12; *1957,* 101-104; *1961,* 98-100.

Johns, Ethel, and Blanche Pfefferkorn. *The Johns Hopkins Hospital School of Nursing, 1889-1949.* Baltimore: Johns Hopkins University Press, 1954.

Koch, Harriet Berger. *Militant Angel.* New York: Macmillan, 1951.

Lee, Eleanor. *History of the School of Nursing of the Presbyterian Hospital in New York, 1892-1942.* New York: Columbia-Presbyterian Hosp., 1942.

Lewis, Edith Patton. "Mary M. Roberts, Spokesman for Nursing. *Am. Jo. Nurs.,* March 1959, 336-345.

McManus, R. Louise. "Nursing Research—Its Evolution," *Am. Jo. Nurs.,* April 1961, 76-79.

Montag, Mildred L. *Community College Education for Nursing.* New York: McGraw-Hill, 1959.

Moore, Louise. *Practical Nursing Training Comes of Age.* Washington: Govt. Print. Off., 1954. U. S. Off. of Ed. Voc. Ed. Div., Misc. No. 3468.

Munson, Helen W., and Katharine Stevens. *The Story of the National League of Nursing Education.* Philadelphia: Saunders, 1934.

My Oath. Fiftieth Anniversary Publication of the Mills School of Nursing. New York: Bellevue Hospital, 1937.

National Association of Graduate Colored Nurses. *Four Decades of Service.* New York: Nat. Assn. of Colored Grad. Nurses, n. d.

National League for Nursing. Publications. New York: The League. On Accrediting, Administration, Clinical Teaching, Collegiate Education, Curriculum, Finance, Head Nursing, Nursing School Libraries, Nursing Education, Nursing Service, Standards, Teaching, University Schools, Public Health Nursing. Publications of the League Exchange, and others.

National League of Nursing Education. *The Curriculum for Schools of Nursing.* New York: The League, 1927.

———. *A Curriculum Guide for Schools of Nursing.* New York: The League, 1937.

———. *Standard Curriculum for Schools of Nursing.* New York: The League, 1917.

National Organization for Public Health Nursing. *Manual of Public Health Nursing.* New York: Macmillan, 3rd ed., 1939.

———. *Public Health Nursing Curriculum Guide.* New York: NOPHN, 1954.

———. *Survey of Public Health Nursing.* New York: Commonwealth Fund, 1934.

Nelson, Josephine (Ed.). *New Horizons in Nursing.* New York: Macmillan, 1950.

Newell, Hope. *The History of the National Nursing Council.* New York: NOPHN, 1951.

Nursing Outlook. New York: Am. Jo. Nurs. Co., Published monthly.

Nursing Research. New York: Am. Jo. Nurs. Co. Published quarterly.

Nutting, M. Adelaide. *A Sound Economic Basis for Schools of Nursing.* Putnam's, 1926.

———, and Lavinia L. Dock. *A History of Nursing.* New York: Putnam's, 1907-1912. 4 vols. Vol. III, Ch. II; Vol. IV, Ch. IV.

Practical Nursing. New York: Nat. Assn. for Prac. Nurse Ed. Published monthly.

Reissman, Leonard, and John H. Rohrer (Eds.). *Change and Dilemma in the Nursing Profession: Studies of Nursing Service in a Large General Hospital.* New York: Putnam's, 1957.

Robb, Isabel Hampton. *Educational Standards for Nurses, with Other Addresses on Nursing Subjects.* Cleveland: Koeckert, 1907.

Roth, Anna. *Thirty-Five Years of the Massachusetts State Nurses Association.* Boston: The Assn., 1938.

Schaffter, Dorothy. *What Comes of Training Women for War.* Washington: Am. Coun. on Ed., 1948. Part Three.

Serbin, Oscar N., Jr. *Paying for Medical Care in the United States.* New York: Columbia University Press, 1953.

Shoemaker, Sister M. Theophane. *History of Nurse-Midwifery in the United States.* Washington: Catholic University of America Press, 1947.

Stewart, Isabel Maitland. *The Education of Nurses.* New York: Macmillan, 1943. Ch. III-IV.

———. "Elizabeth Chamberlain Burgess," *Am. Jo. Nurs.,* August 1958, 1101-1105.

"Isabel M. Stewart Recalls the Early Years," *Am. Jo. Nurs.,* October 1960, 1426-1430.

The Story of Nurses House. Babylon, N. Y.: Nurses House, 1954.

Teachers College, Columbia University. *Twenty-five Years of Nursing Education in Teachers College, 1899-1925.* New York: Columbia University Press, 1926.

Thatcher, Virginia S. *History of Anesthesia.* Philadelphia: Lippincott, 1952. Ch. 3, Part III.

Thoms, Adah B. (Comp.) *Pathfinders A History of the Progress of Colored Graduate Nurses.* New York: Kay Printing House, 1929.

The Tradition and Destiny of the U. S. Army Nurse Corps. N. d.

Twenty Years of Nurse Midwifery. New York: Maternity Center Assn., 1955.

The U. S. Cadet Nurse Corps and Other Federal Nurse Training Programs. Washington: Govt. Print. Off., 1950.

U. S. Office of Education. *Practical Nursing: An Analysis of the Practical Nurse Occupation with Suggestions for the Organization of Training Programs.* Washington: Off. of Ed., 1947.

United States Public Health Service. Publications. Washington: Govt. Print. Off. On Cost of Collegiate Programs in Nursing, Public Health Service, Federal Grants, Clinical Resources, State Nursing Surveys, Nursing Activities in Patient Units, Head Nursing Activities, Nursing Aides in Hospitals, Veterans Administration Nursing, Federal Government Nursing Services, and others.

Vreeland, Ellwynne M. "Fifty Years of Nursing in the Federal Government Nursing Services," *Am. Jo. Nurs.,* October 1950, 626-631.

Wald, Lillian D. *The House on Henry Street.* New York: Holt, 1924.

Werminghaus, Esther A. *Annie W. Goodrich: Her Journey to Yale.* New York: Macmillan, 1950.

West, Margaret, and Christy Hawkins. *Nursing Schools at the Midcentury.* New York: Nat. Comm. for Improvement of Nurs. Serv., 1950.

White, Walter. *How Far the Promised Land?* New York: Viking, 1955.

Yamanura, Douglas S. *Functions and Role Concepts of Nursing Service Personnel.* Honolulu: University of Hawaii, 1956. Mimeographed.

Yost, Edna. *American Women of Nursing.* Philadelphia: Lippincott, 1947.

Zeis, Dolores M., and Edna Porter. "Public Health Nursing in the 49th State," *Am. Jo. Nurs.,* October 1958, 1376-1379.

CHAPTER 12

Canada

THOUGH entirely self governing, Canada retains close ties with Great Britain and the United States, from which it is separated by a 4000-mile boundary extending from the Pacific to the Atlantic. Nine of its provinces lie on or close to this border; the tenth, Newfoundland and part of the Labrador coast, stretch out into the Atlantic Ocean farther north. Between this strip of provinces and the Arctic Ocean are the Yukon and Northwest Territories which, though rich in mineral wealth, fish, furs, and timber, are sparsely settled and not as well developed politically. While Canada's land space is larger than that of the United States, its population is only about one tenth that of its neighbor, the great majority living within two or three hundred miles of the international boundary. Added to descendants of native Eskimos and Indians and of the two nations, France and Britain, who settled first in Quebec, Ontario, and the Maritime Provinces, are large numbers of more recent arrivals from Europe, Asia, the United States and other parts of the world.

The province of Quebec, which is predominantly French speaking, has retained many of the laws and customs as well as

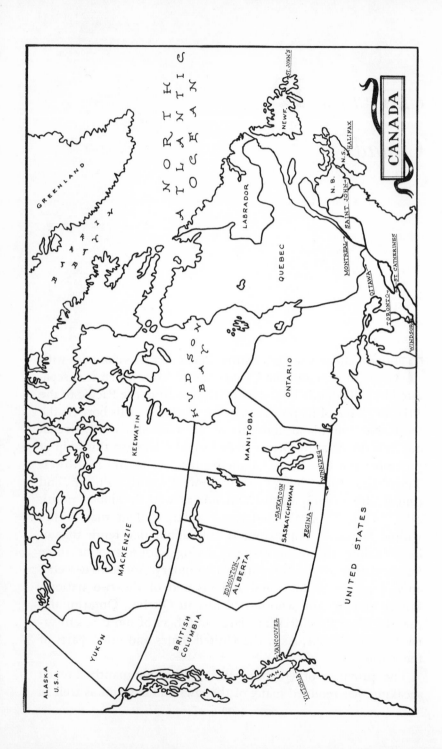

the religion of Old France. The predominant language, laws, and political institutions of the rest of the country are British in origin. Canada's task of building a close-knit, independent, and prosperous nation has been especially difficult because of these geographic, climatic, ethnic, and cultural conditions and the fact that the United States had reached independence earlier and had become a wealthy industrial nation. Since around 1900, however, many factors have contributed to the rapid growth, and maturity of this country. Among these are such organizations as the League of Nations, the United Nations, and the British Commonwealth, in all of which Canada has played an influential role. It is also an important link between the Old World and the New. All of these forces and others such as air travel and world wars have been instrumental in the development of Canadian nursing and help to account for the great strides made in this period.

MODERN NURSING SCHOOLS AND LEADERS [1]

The beginnings of modern nursing in Canada as well as its earlier historical background have been outlined in Chapter 8. From this it will be noted that the two North American countries started their first Nightingale schools at about the same time. Though Dr. Theophilus Mack of the small General and Marine Hospital, St. Catharines, Ontario, was the first to propose a plan for the training of nurses in Canada (1864), he did not send Miss Money over to London to study the new system until 1873. On her return with two trained nurses and two probationers from Guy's Hospital, a separate home was established near the hospital, and this became the headquarters of the first school of nursing in Canada. Chiefly because of its small size and location in a small town, it was soon overshadowed by the larger hospital schools that developed in leading cities. The first of these at the Toronto General Hospital was opened in 1881

[1] A more complete account of the history of Canadian nursing will be found in *Three Centuries of Canadian Nursing* by J. M. Gibbon and M. S. Matheson, to whom we are indebted for a number of facts about this period.

under Mary Agnes Snively, an ex-teacher who had gone to Bellevue Hospital, New York, for training and was considered one of its leading graduates. In 1890 Norah Livingston, an American-born daughter of British parents and graduate of the New York Hospital School, succeeded after many others had failed in introducing a modern school at the Montreal General Hospital. These two held their positions for many years and because of their ability as administrators and trainers and their resolute, indomitable spirit have been honored as the chief leaders of the modern nursing movement in Canada.

Before 1900, twenty hospital schools had been established in towns and cities along the transcontinental railroad linking Montreal in the east with Victoria in the west. The Winnipeg General Hospital School, founded in 1887, was the first west of the Great Lakes. The first Roman Catholic sisters to open such a school were the Grey Nuns in Ottawa (1898), after which more were opened in Ontario and in other provinces. Canadian schools had little or no difficulty in attracting good applicants. Indeed, for many years the supply exceeded the demand, and schools across the border, which were multiplying more rapidly, attracted many Canadian candidates. Most of them found good positions there and remained. This flow continued until World War I, when the demands of the armed forces left many vacancies at home. Later, as the nursing field in Canada widened and as American citizenship became a requirement for registration in many states, the number of applicants from Canada declined. There has always been a close relationship, however, between nurses of the two countries and much borrowing back and forth of each other's ideas as well as personnel. British nurses also found positions in the new country and took an active part in the up-building of the young profession in Canada as they did in other parts of the world, including the United States.

FIELDS OF NURSING SERVICE

At first private nursing was the chief opening for graduate nurses in both countries, apart from a few paid positions in hospitals. The organization in 1898 of a national plan similar to the Queen Victoria Jubilee Institute for Nurses in Britain led to a wide extension of district nursing under the Victorian Order of Nurses for Canada introduced by Lady Ishbel Aberdeen, wife of the then Governor General. Though at first opposed by prominent medical men who feared lay leadership in such health programs, it had strong financial and moral support from the Canadian public, and soon local and provincial branches began to open throughout the country. Later, cottage hospitals as well as the service of visiting nurses and nurse midwives were developed in the more remote areas. Charlotte MacLeod, a Canadian graduate of the Waltham Training School in Waltham, Massachusetts, who was the first superintendent of the VON, brought with her a group of nurses from that school to initiate the program.

In addition to this nationwide plan, which had no parallel in the United States, a few local district nursing associations developed in Canada. Before 1900 at least one nurse, Louisa Clark, was employed by a hospital (the Winnipeg General) to follow up dispensary patients in their homes and the Margaret Scott Nursing mission was organized as a visiting nurse service in the same city. Boards of Health soon began to employ nurses for home visits and school nursing was started in her native Toronto by Lina Rogers (Struthers) who had initiated a similar service in New York City. Among federal nursing services the oldest, other than military, was the Indian, which later included Eskimo groups and provided both hospital and visiting nursing.

Military nursing began in 1887 when a few volunteer trained nurses served in the Riel Rebellion in western Canada. A similar group joined the Queen Alexandra Imperial Military Nursing Service of Britain during the South African War (1899). Shortly after that the Canadian Government established its own corps of Army Nursing Sisters, giving them (unsolicited) the relative rank of junior officers. (The title "Sister" for secular nurses was used in Canada only in the armed services).

During World Wars I and II many Canadian nurses served with their own troops at home and overseas and made an excellent record. In addition, they greatly expanded their professional experience by contacts with British nurses and with those from the various overseas dominions and the United States. Special recognition should be given to Elizabeth L. Smellie, a Canadian graduate of the Johns Hopkins Hospital School of Nursing who served in both wars and was for many years Chief Superintendent of the Victorian Order of Nurses. She was the first nurse to receive the rank of Colonel when Matron-in-Chief in the Royal Canadian Army Medical Corps and many honors came to her also for her distinguished service in the VON. These were in recognition not only of her administrative ability and leadership but of her many gifts of personality and character which helped to win support for her work among all classes and made her a national figure.

NURSES' ORGANIZATIONS, ORGANS, AND LEADERS

As noted in Chapter 11, nurses of Canada had joined with those of the United States to form the American Society of Superintendents of Training Schools for Nurses (1893) and the larger Nurses Associated Alumnae of the United States and Canada (1896). Leading nurses of both countries were active in these groups and helped to support the first collegiate program for graduate nurses (at Teachers College, Columbia University, New York), opened in 1899. This program in which two Canadians, Isabel Hampton Robb and Adelaide Nutting, took a leading part and of which Miss Nutting in 1907 became the first director (with the rank of professor), continued to attract many nurses from Canada as well as from the United States and other parts of the world. The influence of both leaders extended far beyond the borders of any one country through their writings as well as their inspiring personalities.

Though there were may regrets over the severing of ties between the nurses of the United States and Canada, this separation became necessary in order to carry forward the plans of the International Council of Nurses, which was organized on a provisional basis in 1899. Mary Agnes Snively, who was its first treasurer and active in its formation, retired when the decision was made to admit only national nurses associations as members, and under her leadership Canada began to form its own national group composed of alumnae and provincial associations. This became the fourth member of the ICN in 1909. By 1922 nursing laws had been secured in all the provinces, and in 1930 the Canadian Nurses Association became a federation of provincial associations, each with its own secretary and headquarters and complete autonomy in dealing with its own problems.

The national headquarters and staff, with the CNA executive committee and an enlarged and progressive professional journal, provided a clearing house and a coordinating center for all matters concerned with Canadian nursing. Special mention should be made of Jean Wilson, for twenty years the efficient and influential executive secretary of the CNA for much of this accomplishment. During most of this time she also edited the *Canadian Nurse* which had evolved from a small alumnae quarterly to a national journal. In 1932 Ethel Johns, a gifted writer with an exceptionally wide nursing experience, became the full-time editor of this publication and made it one of the world's outstanding nursing journals. Under her successor, Margaret Kerr, it continued to develop and is now a bilingual publication with English and French editions.

ADVANCES IN NURSING SERVICE AND EDUCATION

World War I, which lasted in Canada as in Britain from 1914 to 1918, was a period of strain and ferment that led to many changes in both countries. Public health work, which had been developing before the war, now began to expand rapidly. The Canadian Red Cross, which before the war had concentrated chiefly on disaster nursing, turned more toward preventive and public health work and began to offer scholarships for nurses and subsidies for the development of postgraduate courses. A number of Canadian nurses before 1920 had taken such courses in colleges and universities in the United States. That year two outstanding Canadian universities, McGill and Toronto, began to offer one-year programs for graduate nurses, the first under the leadership of Flora Madelaine Shaw and the second under Kathleen Russell. In 1919 the first five-year program in Canada which led to a university degree was offered under the joint auspices of the University of British Columbia and the Vancouver Hospital School of Nursing of which Ethel Johns was then director. This degree was in nursing and applied science and was open to qualified applicants to the school of nursing, which continued to offer the three-year diploma program. In 1925 the Toronto University School added to its postgraduate nursing programs Canada's first basic course for nurses which was not under hospital control. This was made possible by substantial aid from the Rockefeller Foundation and was under the leadership of Miss Russell. It attracted many foreign as well as Canadian students.

Since 1920 several other Canadian universities have developed either basic or postgraduate programs or both. The first School of Public Health Nursing for French-speaking students was opened at the University of Montreal in 1925. It affiliated a little later with l'Institut Marguerite d'Youville and developed degree and diploma courses in nursing education and hospital administration for French-speaking religious sisters and lay nurses. In response to a request from the Roman Catholic sisterhoods, including the cloistered orders, a papal dispensation was received which allowed nursing sisters to attend lectures and classes in· approved institutions with the permission of their mother superiors. This did much to aid in the improvement of hospitals and schools of nursing in Quebec Province and other French-speaking sections of Canada.

Such influences were greatly strengthened by the Congress of the International Council of Nurses, which met in Montreal in 1929. Under the able leadership of Jean Gunn, then president of the Canadian Nurses Association, and Mabel Hersey, chairman of the Congress committee, all groups joined in plans for welcoming and entertaining the guests, who included a number of religious sisters from the old lands as well as many from the new. The cloistered sisters of Hôtel Dieu received a special dispensation to attend some of the meetings, and the lovely statue of Jeanne Mance in the public square beamed in benediction on the many visitors who brought flowers in her honor.

EARLIER SURVEYS AND STUDIES ON NURSING IN CANADA

During the 1920's the shortage of applicants in schools of nursing had become serious and was giving much concern to medical and hospital as well as nursing organizations. In 1929, through the initiative of the Canadian Nurses Association, a committee, in which the Canadian Medical Association joined, decided to undertake a nationwide study of nursing education in Canada. It was conducted by Dr. George M. Weir, a well-known educator and sociologist, who, after conferences with many groups, questionnaire studies, and visits to schools of nursing, published his *Survey of Nursing Education in Canada* in 1932. As in similar studies of that period in the United States and Britain, many serious weaknesses were found in the existing system of hospital schools, and important reforms were recommended with the endorsement of the committee. One which the author was allowed to include without such endorsement was that schools of nursing should be incorporated into the general educational system of the country and supported by the government. The Weir Report was an important milestone in Canadian nursing and was widely read and quoted in other countries.

The picture of low nurse supply was changed during the depression in the '30's when many were unemployed because neither hospitals nor patients could afford such service. A number of the smaller and weaker hospitals closed their doors at that time, but no radical changes in the system were made. The survey, however, had an important influence on public opinion and led to other studies, such as *The Proposed Curriculum for Schools of Nursing in Canada,* which appeared in 1936. This was sponsored by the Canadian Nurses Association and conducted by a special committee whose chairman was Marion Lindeberg, Director of the Department of Nursing Education at McGill

University. *The Curriculum* and a later *Supplement,* were valuable guides to national and provincial groups interested in building a broader and sounder foundation for the emerging profession of nursing in Canada.

WORLD WAR II AND POSTWAR DEVELOPMENTS

When this war broke out, Canada was one of the first to join the Allies, and its nurses were soon serving in its armed forces, the Red Cross, and similar organizations. The recruitment of nursing sisters for the Army Corps was at no time a serious problem, for there was always a long list of applicants, but the gaps left at home had to be filled. Laws were passed to prevent nurses from accepting positions outside the country without permission. Nursing schools were expanded, funds were secured from the government to help with educational and service programs, studies were made to determine the demand and the resources available, and quotas were set up for the different services. After the war many nurses who had been in active service took advantage of the offer of government stipends for advanced study, and a number dropped out for health and other reasons. The shortage continued to be acute, especially in hospitals which were then increasing in number and size and demanding much larger nursing staffs.

In 1926, in response to a request of the Department of National Health and Welfare on behalf of its Interdepartmental Committee on Professionally Trained Persons, the Canadian Nurses Association presented its *Report on Nursing Service.* This combined available statistical and other data on supply and demand and their implications with a clear statement of the larger issues and trends in nursing. The increasing difficulty of recruitment and the large number of drop-outs were noted, as were the need to limit wastage, conserve nurse power, and correct inherent defects in the whole system. This report was accompanied by a formal request by the CNA that the Dominion Government make a complete survey of the nursing situation as a basis for future estimates of nursing needs.

Another study in 1950 that provided valuable data on the supply of nurses was made for the Committee on Public Health Practice in Canada by Dr. J. H. Baillie, a leader in the health field, and Lyle Creelman, a widely experienced, well-prepared public health nurse who became internationally known for her work in the World Health Organization. This showed that, though there were marked variations in the standards of different provinces and of city and rural districts, in no part of Canada was the accepted minimum for essential health personnel met. For example, instead of the estimated minimum of one public health nurse for every 2000 to 2500 of the population, the average for Canada was one to 5200, and of the nurses employed only 38 per cent had special public health preparation.

The war experience had brought about much closer collaboration between organized nurses and official departments of health and welfare and had led to a greater public appreciation of the country's dependence on this professional group. The idea of public support for nursing service and education was growing. The general population was deeply interested in national plans for health and medical care, and, though few Canadians were ready to go as far as Britain had gone in adopting a tax-supported system of health insurance for the whole population, several provinces (especially those in the West) were promoting health subsidies of various kinds and voluntary health insurance plans were making rapid progress. While practical nurses, nursing aides, and similar nonprofessional workers were employed in increasing numbers, this did not relieve the pressure for more registered nurses and especially for student nurses, who still carried the heaviest part of the nursing load in hospitals. Members of the Canadian Nurses Association were greatly concerned about the whole situation. Although they aided in recruitment campaigns to secure more applicants for nursing schools, they also continued their efforts to improve such schools, hoping in this way to attract not only more students but a larger number with higher educational qualifications. It will be noted that nursing problems here were much like those in Great Britain and the U.S.A.

RECENT EXPERIMENTS AND STUDIES

At the meeting of the Association in 1945 a resolution was adopted, approving a demonstration to determine whether a professional nurse might be prepared adequately in less than three years. This led in 1948 to the establishment of the Metropolitan Demonstration Training School for Nurses at Windsor, Ontario, which was supported by a grant of $40,000 a year for four years by the Canadian Red Cross Society and directed by Nettie D. Fidler, member of the nursing faculty of the University of Toronto. The chief objectives were to establish nursing schools as educational institutions—separate entities in their own right—and to demonstrate that a skilled clinical nurse could be prepared in less than three years if schools were given control of the students' time. The *Report of the Evaluation of the Metropolitan School of Nursing, Windsor, Ontario* (1952) by Dr. A. R. Lord, a well-known educator, concludes with the statement that "nurses can be trained at least as satisfactorily in two years as in three and under better conditions, but the training must be paid for in money instead of in services." The stubborn financial and other issues involved in the conversion of schools from service agencies to educational entities are revealed in the story of this school. Though it was discontinued after the four years were up, it had made a distinctive contribution to nursing education and its results were widely studied in Canada and elsewhere.

Another experiment along similar lines was started in 1950 at the Atkinson School of Nursing at the Toronto Western Hospital under Gladys J. Sharpe, who directed both the school and nursing service. Its purpose was to find a solution for the hospital's problem of attracting good applicants to its school and to test the belief of its sponsors that this could be accomplished by making the training more attractive and giving it more of a professional status. To carry out the new plan, the school was given the necessary administrative and financial independence to compress the basic course into two years. A third year of internship was added, which freed students from classroom as-

signments and offered varied experience which added substantially to their professional competence and at the same time
helped to stabilize the hospital's nursing service. The results
were evaluated by another eminent educator, Dr. W. Stewart
Wallace of Toronto University, whose *Report on the Experiment in Nursing Education at the Atkinson School of Nursing,
Toronto Western Hospital from 1950 to 1955* leaves no doubt
about the success of the experiment. Its influence is seen in the
new Nightingale School opened in Toronto in 1960 under
Blanche Duncanson who came from the Atkinson School and
follows its general plan. Students must meet university entrance
standards and their fees are paid by the Ontario government.
Though independent of any hospital, this school arranges for
clinical experience in several. Its students must also meet provincial registration requirements.

Although these and other studies, experiments, and plans did
not solve the problem of providing a more adequate system of
education in nursing that would produce the number and kinds
of nurses Canada needed, they did arouse a good deal of public
interest in the question and led to a greater sense of responsibility on the part of the government, the people, and the nursing profession. Physicians and educators also were becoming
more concerned with these issues.

MOVEMENT FOR ACCREDITATION OF SCHOOLS
OF NURSING

This began as a project of the Catholic Hospital Council of
Canada and owes much to the leadership of Sister Denise
Lefebvre of l'Institut Marguerite D'Youville of Montreal, who
was also an active member of the Canadian Nurses Association.
In 1955 she was made chairman of a special committee of the
CNA to plan a pilot project that would study and recommend
ways and means of evaluating and accrediting schools of nursing
in Canada and of determining their readiness for such a program. Under the leadership of Helen A. Mussallem, a pilot
study in twenty-five schools was successfully completed, and in

1960 further plans were made to work with schools in interpreting the accreditation plan. Though the principles have been accepted in general the plan has not been put into effect at this date.

PROGRESS TOWARD OTHER PROFESSIONAL GOALS

While they put much emphasis on the improvement of schools of nursing on both basic and postgraduate levels, Canadian nurses did not overlook the fields of service in which their members were engaged and the need to keep abreast of changing demands. They recognized that nurse assistants and aides were needed and provided for their training and certification. They also gave attention to public relations and publicity and secured good support and cooperation from the public as well as from educational, medical, hospital, governmental, and other responsible groups whose understanding and support were essential to nursing progress. Studies had been made of the ethical, economic, legal, and social problems of their members and of human relations, salaries, pensions, and personnel policies in general. The pros and cons of collective bargaining had been considered and some experiments made, but though most of the provinces have passed laws which give professional associations the right to function as bargaining agents the majority of nurses so far seem to prefer other methods of negotiation.

Canadian nurses have taken an important share also in the work of the International Council of Nurses and the Florence Nightingale International Foundation and have been active in Red Cross service at home and abroad. They have shown much interest in the World Health Organization, in which Dr. Brock Chisholm, a Canadian physician, was the first Medical Director and Lyle Creelman, after several years service as a public health nursing administrator, was in 1954 appointed Chief Nurse Consultant in WHO, with headquarters in Geneva. During the difficult war and postwar years student and graduate nurses contributed generously to the support of nursing schools and other projects in the devastated countries, and from the early days on many nurse missionaries as well as other Canadian nurses have volunteered for service in foreign lands.

Looking back over the modern period and considering the handicaps under which the young profession of nursing had to work in this vast northern country with its immense frontiers, one is impressed by the combination of such pioneer work with the progressive studies and programs undertaken by organized Canadian nurses. Many of those who were engaged in these studies were themselves taking advanced programs to prepare for such work, and several had received higher degrees. It should be noted that they have had exceptionally good support from the allied professions, the foundations interested in health, the Red Cross, the government, and the Canadian people who in general have retained a high regard for this profession.

SELECTED BIBLIOGRAPHY

Canada. National Health and Welfare Department. *Study of the Functions and Activities of Head Nurses in a General Hospital, Planned and Conducted by . . . at the Request of the Canadian Nurses Association, and with the Cooperation of the Ottawa Civic Hospital.* Ottawa: The Dept., 1954.

The Canadian Nurse. Montreal: Can. Nurses Assn. Published monthly.

Canadian Nurses Association. *Information on Nurses and Nursing in Canada.* Montreal: CNA, 1953.

——. *A Proposed Curriculum for Schools of Nursing in Canada.* Montreal: CNA, 1946.

——. *A Supplement to a Proposed Curriculum for Schools of Nursing in Canada.* Montreal: CNA, 1946.

Emory, Florence H. M. *Public Health Nursing in Canada; Principles and Practice.* New York: Macmillan, 1945.

[——]. "Structure Study Committee," *Can. Nurse,* September 1950, 745-746.

Gerard, Sister Catharine. "Our Golden Jubilee," *Can. Nurse,* September 1959, 783-786.

Gibbon, John Murray. *Victorian Order of Nurses for Canada, The 50th Anniversary 1897-1947.* Montreal: VON, 1947.

International Council of Nurses. *National Reports. 1933,* 10-12; *1947,* 16-18; *1949,* 14-19; *1957,* 14-19; *1961,* 4-17.

Livingstone, M. Christine. "The History, Aims, and Programme of the Victorian Order of Nurses for Canada," *Int. Nurs. Rev.*, October 1956, 42-47.

Lord, A. R. *Report of the Evaluation of the Metropolitan School of Nursing, Windsor, Ontario.* Montreal: CNA, 1952.

Martin, Paul. "Nursing and Canada's National Health Program," *Can. Nurse,* October 1954, 781-785.

Merrick, Elliott. *Northern Nurse.* New York: Scribner's, 1942.

[Mussallem, Helen K.] *Spotlight on Nursing Education—The Report of the Pilot Project for the Evaluation of Schools of Nursing in Canada.* Winnipeg: CNA, 1961.

Nutting, M. Adelaide, and Lavinia L. Dock. *A History of Nursing.* New York: Putnam's, 1907-1912. 4 Vols. Vol. IV, Ch. IV.

Schmitt, Louise M. *Report of the Status of Basic Nursing Education Programs in Saskatchewan.* Saskatoon, Sask.: [Saskatchewan Reg. Nurses Assn.], 1957.

Walker, Mildred I. "Communications and the Structure Study of the CNA," *Can. Nurse.*, March 1954, 181-183.

Wallace, W. Stewart. *Report on the Experiment in Nursing Education of the Atkinson School of Nursing. The Toronto Western Hospital 1950-1955.* Toronto: University of Toronto Press, n. d.

Weir, C. M. *Survey of Nursing Education in Canada.* Toronto: University of Toronto Press, 1932.

Wilson, Lola. *Cost Study of Basic Nursing Education Programs in Saskatchewan.* [Saskatoon, Sask.]: Saskatchewan Reg. Nurs. Assn., 1958.

——. *The Story of the First Three Years.* Regina, Sask.: Saskatchewan Reg. Nurs. Assn., 1957.

CHAPTER 13

Australasia

Situated on the opposite side of the globe are two English-speaking democracies, New Zealand and Australia, which though about a thousand miles apart and differing in size and in various national characteristics, have much in common. As members of the British Commonwealth of Nations and of the United Nations, they also have responsibilities for administration of East New Guinea and Papua and many of the smaller islands in the South Pacific Ocean. The progressive spirit of their people and the strategic position of these two countries give them, in spite of their relatively small populations, a wide influence in world affairs. This is especially true in regard to social and health services.

AUSTRALIA

Northwest of New Zealand and directly south of Indonesia lies Australia, the largest island and smallest continent in the world. Though covering about the same area as the United States, much of the interior is arid and uninhabitable except by

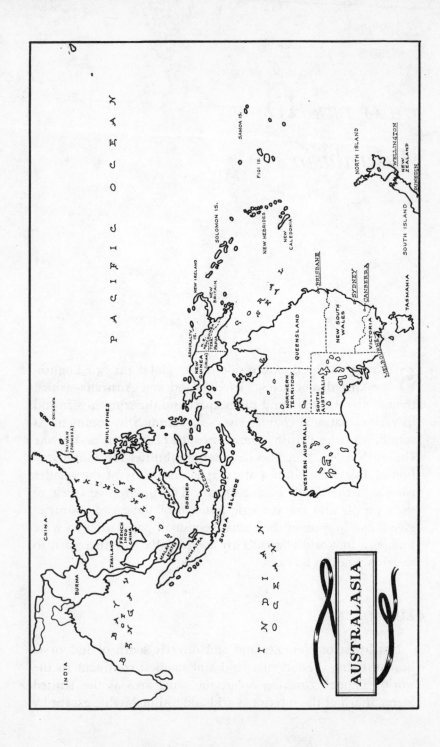

AUSTRALASIA

PACIFIC OCEAN

INDIAN OCEAN

BAY OF BENGAL

INDIA
BURMA
CHINA
THAILAND
FRENCH INDO CHINA
MALAY STATES
SUMATRA
BORNEO
JAVA
CELEBES
SUNDA ISLANDS
PHILIPPINES
TAIWAN (FORMOSA)
OKINAWA

SOLOMON IS.
NEW IRELAND
NEW BRITAIN
ADMIRALTY IS.
N.E. NEW GUINEA (AUST.)
PAPUA
NEW GUINEA (DUTCH)

NEW HEBRIDES
NEW CALEDONIA
FIGI IS.
SAMOA IS.

WESTERN AUSTRALIA
NORTHERN TERRITORY
SOUTH AUSTRALIA
QUEENSLAND
NEW SOUTH WALES
VICTORIA
BRISBANE
SYDNEY
CANBERRA
MELBOURNE
TASMANIA

NORTH ISLAND
SOUTH ISLAND
NEW ZEALAND
WELLINGTON
DUNEDIN

the native aborigines gradually dying out. Of a population of about ten million, the great majority live in an area within 500 miles of the south and east coasts behind which is the "outback" and bush country, where a few hardy settlers carry on farming, sheep raising, or mining. With the growth of air travel much has been done in recent years to open up other areas to new settlers. Although most of those who came earlier are of British stock, later arrivals were of varied origins, chiefly European. Australia's six states, including Tasmania, are organized on a federal plan similar to that of the United States. A sense of national unity was slow to develop, largely because of the lack of a strong central government, early rivalries among the states, and the hardships of travel.

Economic conditions are generally good; indeed, Australia is often called "the working man's paradise." With strong labor and socialist backing, the governments of these states have been among the first to pass laws providing for old-age pensions, maternity allowances, child endowments, invalid and widow's pensions, and free or inexpensive hospital, medical, and nursing services. Though the people of the two British Commonwealth countries in the South Pacific have much the same viewpoint on such matters and in general have kept close to the mother country, they differ a good deal in their systems of government and in their national characteristics. The Australians are generally considered to be more like the western Americans while the New Zealanders resemble the British and many are of Scottish origin.

NURSING SCHOOLS AND SERVICES

Australia was apparently the first to get direct aid from Miss Nightingale in establishing the new system of nursing. In 1867, at the request of Sir Henry Parkes, Colonial Secretary, a superintendent, Lucy Osborn, and five nurses were sent from the Nightingale School to start a training school at Sydney Infirmary. Later groups from this and other British schools and their Australian graduates went from one hospital to another, organizing training schools in the main cities along the coast and on the island of Tasmania. Some medical opposition was met at the start, but this soon subsided, and since then the relations between these two groups have been exceptionally cordial and cooperative. All kinds of hospitals, large and small, general and special, began to develop training schools, whose lady superintendents held the chief positions of influence and leadership in local nursing groups.

Apart from such positions, private nursing was the main field for earlier graduates who usually lived together in nurses' clubs or cooperatives. Beginning in 1885, district nursing associations were organized in most of the cities, and nurses themselves developed hourly nursing to supplement district and private nurse services. Bush nursing, started in the State of Victoria to supply nurses for the more isolated areas, was supported and aided in its organization by the Countess of Dudley, wife of a Governor General. The original idea was to extend the scheme to the whole country, as had the Queen's Nurses of Britain and the Victorian Order of Nurses in Canada, but this plan did not materialize. The Australian Inland Mission was another voluntary organization that provided nursing service for the hinterland and the nearby Pacific islands. These services attracted the hardier and more adventurous nurses whose pioneering spirit is illustrated in many thrilling stories. A noted example is Sister Elizabeth Kenney, widely known for her "polio" work, whose isolation in a doctorless district led her to discover and promote a new method of treatment that made her world famous. In recent years the much publicized service of flying doctors has tended to strengthen these nursing outposts. Ambulance planes and a system of pedal wireless stations now make it possible for settlers in such remote areas to get free medical advice and, when necessary, the service of doctors and nurses who are specially trained for this work.

Health teaching by district nurses developed with increasing emphasis on maternal and child health. State-supported mothercraft and baby health centers are widely distributed, and the sisters in charge (most of them nurse midwives) advise on feeding problems and prescribe diets in accordance with standard medical practice. Sometimes a mobile center is set up in a railway car which goes to small outlying stations on a regular schedule and is switched to a side line for clinics. School nursing, tuberculosis nursing, and other specialized programs also emphasize health teaching, which is combined with bedside care and health-center work. Australia provides similar services for East New Guinea, Papua and other nearby islands where health conditions are backward, and many nurses have gone into these areas to teach native workers. Military nursing, which started during the Boer War, followed much the same plan as that in other British countries. Australian nurses served with distinction in many parts of the world during World Wars I and II, and some of them have been active in the World Health Organization and in other agencies of the United Nations. Susan Haines of Tasmania is especially well known for her distinguished career in international nursing.

NURSING ORGANIZATIONS AND REGISTRATION

Here, as in many countries, hospitals developed sporadically and with few controls, and there were wide variations in size as well as in the type and quality of medical and nursing services. A few leading nurse superintendents who recognized the danger met with some interested physicians in a conference in Sydney in 1892 to consider the formation of an association similar to the British Nurses' Association formed in Britain, but no agreement was reached, chiefly, it was said, because they could not decide how to define the term "trained nurse." In 1894 Miss Milne of Tasmania, an active exponent of state registration, also urged organization but with no results. In 1899, at a meeting in Sydney attended by nurse and medical delegates, an association was formed with its headquarters in that city. Though at first named for the State of New South Wales, it was soon expanded and called the Australasian Trained Nurses' Association, its main object being to develop a system of nurse registration for the whole country. The *Australasian Nursing Journal,* which was started in 1903 as its official organ, became one of the world's oldest professional nursing magazines. Soon after, the rival state of Victoria developed the Royal Victorian Trained

Nurses' Association with its own magazine (*Una*) and its head-quarters in Melbourne. These state associations concentrated at first on registration laws to protect the public and their own nurse members. (Physicians and other supporters were accepted as members of these associations.) Queensland was the first (1912) to pass such a law, and by 1928 all the other states had similar laws. Efforts to put nurse registration under federal rather than state control continued but with no success. In 1946, however, public health functions were transferred to the Central Government, and a nurse, Miss Peterson, was appointed Director General of Nursing for the Commonwealth. It was hoped that this would lead to a closer coordination of nursing standards and would raise the educational level of all Australian schools of nursing.

During most of this time Australian nurses did not have membership in the International Council of Nurses, though Susan McGahey of Australia had served one year as president of the ICN before 1904. After that date national membership ceased to be granted on an individual basis and was open only to national organizations which had as officers and voting members only fully trained nurses. It was not until after World War I that the state associations in Australia decided to form such a national organization—the Australian Nursing Federation—with a federal council to manage its affairs. Its first meeting was held in 1924 in Sydney, where its headquarters were located. E. P. Evans was Honorary Secretary until 1919. In 1937 this organization was admitted to the International Council of Nurses. A permanent secretary, L. Mavis Avery, was appointed secretary-general in 1951 and permission was given in 1955 to add the word "Royal" to its title.

Before this a national branch of the Florence Nightingale International Foundation had been organized in Australia, and Red Cross groups as well as nurses were active in raising scholarships which admitted several Australian nurses for a year or more of study in the International Course in London. There they met and compared notes with nurses in general and also acquired better preparation in various branches of nursing. Those who served abroad during the war years also helped to stimulate many of the changes that came later in Australian nursing.

SOME RECENT DEVELOPMENTS

In Australia, as elsewhere, the education and service of nurses, including their economic status, were directly affected by post-war changes in national health services. Under the Labor Government the trend was definitely toward the adoption of a "free medicine" scheme similar to that of Great Britain and New Zealand, but owing chiefly to medical opposition and the election of a new government this scheme was voted out, and a new plan which has attracted wide and favorable attention was adopted in 1950. Its main object was to bring the cost of first-rate medical service within the means of the entire population by the active cooperation of federal and state governments, insurance companies, organized medical and hospital groups, and representatives of the people. Under this plan the great majority of Australians are insured in voluntary agencies for most health services, the government providing for those who are unable to meet such costs.

Though the new scheme was introduced gradually, there was some difficulty in meeting the demand for nurses brought about by this measure and by the greatly increased immigration after the war. The marked expansion of hospital and other health services led to an increase in nurse education facilities on both basic and more advanced levels. Leading nurses realized that standards should be raised to attract larger numbers of well-qualified applicants. Though the better known schools in the larger centers had introduced preliminary courses and other modern improvements, there were still many in the more remote areas that had done little to modernize their programs and entrance requirements. There was also a great need for more well-prepared nurse administrators, sister tutors, and other specialists.

At a conference of the Florence Nightingale Memorial Committee of Australia in 1946 it was decided to form an Australian College of Nursing with headquarters in Melbourne. This institution is similar in many ways to the Royal College of Nursing in Britain. Its members are called fellows, and one of its main projects is the Australian Postgraduate School of Nursing, which opened its doors in 1950. Its regular courses range from four months to a year, and short refresher courses are offered, all of which are open to nurses of Australia and to those from other countries who qualify. Sydney also has a New South Wales College of Nursing connected with the University of Sydney and the Royal Prince Albert Hospital, partly supported by grants from the Federal Department of Education. Tuition is free in both centers and in other postgraduate courses which prepare nurses for maternity and child-welfare work. These courses attract nurses from neighboring countries in Asia and the South Pacific as well as from Australia. Substantial increases are reported in the numbers of fully prepared general nurses and also in those who have taken their training in psychiatric, children's, maternity, and other specialized institutions.

In their economic status Australian nurses have kept abreast of other groups of workers in their own country and seem to consider their incomes, hours, and retirement and other benefits satisfactory. They have secured these results largely by joining trained nurses guilds or hospital workers unions and by using the official machinery for collective bargaining. Such negotiations are now compulsory for all groups except those whose incomes are in the higher brackets. Every three years representatives of nurses meet with those of employers in the industrial relations courts provided for this purpose. Agreements are reviewed and adjustments made which are binding for the next period. The forty-hour week and yearly vacations of about four weeks are accepted nationally.

Contacts between Australian nurses and those of other countries have been increasing steadily, and many more nurses from Australia are visiting and studying in Canada, the United States, and Britain. The Congress of the International Council of Nurses, which met in Melbourne in 1961, furthered this exchange of ideas and increased the interest of nurses of other countries in Australia and New Zealand. The president of the Royal Australian Nursing Federation at the time of writing is

Gladys Schott. Other outstanding nurses who are well known in international circles are G. N. Burbidge and Ethel Gray, all three leaders in their own country and active in local, national, and international nursing affairs.

NEW ZEALAND [1]

This country is composed of two main islands, North and South, which cover about the same area as Great Britain and North Ireland and have a population of about two million. Colonized shortly before 1850 by British settlers and becoming a self-governing dominion in 1907, New Zealand developed rapidly and, in spite of its small size, has won for itself an enviable reputation among the nations for the good health of its people and its generally high standard of living. Though the British settlers retained a strong attachment to their motherland, they were determined to chart their own political course and to avoid the extremes of wealth and poverty from which the old land suffered. They have evolved an economic system that tends to equalize wealth and opportunity for all their people, including the native Maoris who occupy a position of social, educational, and political equality and to whom all careers are open. Although they are encouraged to keep their own language and distinctive culture alive and tend to prefer life among their own people, many have qualified for professional and other occupations, including nursing.

This country prides itself on being a kind of experimental laboratory in which new political, social, economic, and health plans have been demonstrated, often before they have been tried elsewhere. The fact that the area is small and the government highly centralized helps to make such experimentation possible. The New Zealand Government, for example, was the first to give women the vote (1893). Enlightened public health policies resulted in the lowest infant death rate in the world and a generally high health standard for the entire population, which is predominantly rural. It will be noted also that many activities

[1] For a more detailed account, see Mary I. Lambie, *Historical Development of Nursing in New Zealand 1840-1950* (Wellington: Dept. of Health, 1951).

elsewhere sponsored by voluntary agencies are here performed
by the state.

INITIAL STEPS IN NURSING, AND EARLY LEADERS

The first New Zealand hospitals were developed in a hap-
hazard way and were much like those of the pre-Nightingale
period in Britain. In 1882 a progressive British physician, Dr.
Grabham, was appointed Government Inspector of Hospitals.
Having himself seen the effect of the Nightingale revolution at
home, he started at once to introduce the new system. British
trained nurses were sent for, placed in three of the larger
hospitals, and, with Dr. Grabham's backing, systematic nurse
training was started with a few selected recruits. Realizing that
physical and other conditions must be improved to attract the
right kind of young women, Dr. Grabham suggested that an
eight-hour day and three-shift plan be tried out in the Wellington Hospital. This experiment was apparently the first of its
kind in any hospital. By 1889 schools had been organized in
three of the chief cities, Wellington, Auckland, and Christ-
church, and their trained nurses were soon introducing the new
system into other parts of New Zealand. As in Britain, the
matrons (also called lady superintendents) held a strong position
and became the nursing leaders in the larger centers. Since these
were few and far apart, there was little contact at first between
local groups.

Dr. Macgregor, who succeeded Dr. Grabham, also stood for
progressive policies in nursing and hospital work. In 1895 he
appointed as assistant inspector of hospitals, Mrs. Grace Neill,
said to be the first woman to occupy such a position in any
country. This highly competent Scottish nurse had broad experience not only in her own field and country but in Australia where for a time she had been a factory inspector. Gifted
with strong personality and character, she soon gained much
influence in both hospitals and schools of nursing. With
the authorization of the government, she gave special attention
to the moral and physical conditions of women workers in hospitals as well as to nurse training. Visiting Britain in 1899, she

was invited to represent New Zealand at the London meeting at which the International Council of Nurses was organized and at which state registration was discussed and endorsed by the new organization. On her return, she proposed such a measure to Dr. Macgregor, who approved it and secured permission from the New Zealand Government to prepare a law, which was passed in 1901. This was the first complete act of the kind, though in 1891 South Africa had taken the first step toward state registration of nurses by putting a clause in its Medical Act and thus giving the Medical Board authority to administer it. This power in New Zealand was invested in the Department of Hospitals, in which the nurse inspector had much influence. Later, in 1906, private hospitals were put under the Act and their schools were inspected and registered if satisfactory. Though some matrons at first feared that these schools would lose their individuality and they themselves their authority under the new system, this fear subsided as the benefits were recognized.

A Midwives' Act, which followed in 1904, not only registered midwives but created several state-aided schools to train them. Such schools came under the direct supervision of Mrs. Neill and of her successor, Hester Maclean, who was appointed in 1906. Nursing and midwifery were thus closely related in New Zealand and progressed together, many nurses qualifying for registration in both fields. Miss Maclean, who was Australian born and trained, had gone to Britain for special preparation in district nursing and midwifery and was therefore well equipped to help direct the new national program for maternal and child health which opened the year she arrived. She also had many gifts of mind and character which strengthened her influence and made her the outstanding nursing leader in this country for many years.

EXPANSION OF NURSING SERVICES, VOLUNTARY
AND GOVERNMENTAL

The year 1906 saw the beginning of a nationwide voluntary organization which was to have a great influence on child health in this and other countries. Its leader was Dr. Truby King, internationally famed for his experiments in infant feeding and his gift for popularizing and promoting his program of child care. To sponsor this program, the Royal New Zealand Society for the Health of Women and Children was formed (commonly called the Plunket Society after its Patroness, Lady Plunket, wife of the Governor General then in office). The society developed local branches in all parts of the country, through which funds were raised for the work of its large staff of nurses and midwives and for the support of six or more Mothercraft Centers. These were called "Karitane" after the home of Dr. Truby King in Dunedin, where the first center was started in 1907 to teach mothers the care and feeding of their babies, to prepare baby nurses (in a one-year course), and to give trained nurses and midwives short postgraduate courses in child care. Stimulated by this voluntary preventive and educational program, the government in 1907 passed the Child Welfare Act which marked the beginning of a broader concept of its responsibility for the national health and welfare. The Plunket organization remained a separate entity and continued to raise funds and to develop infant welfare centers in urban areas, while the public district nurses who served in rural communities carried on similar activities. In recent years voluntary and official agencies were more closely coordinated and their standards became almost the same.

Another important step was taken in 1909 when a law was passed giving the Health Department authority to provide district hospitals for the remote "backblock" areas or, where such aid was impractical, to pay private or district nurses, as required, for home care. To further such services in the Maori settlements, some of the native girls were prepared as nurses and did so well that soon they were serving in many other districts also. In 1912 a law was passed providing for medical inspection for school children, and district nurses then combined school nursing with their family health services. Industrial nursing (called occupational health) was longer in developing, but it is now included in the general nursing program. Private nursing was never a major branch and has steadily declined in importance, for relatively few nurses now are employed in that field. Hourly nurses are used when needed to supplement district nurses' services.

Military nursing at the start of World War I was represented by a very small group attached to the British Queen Alexandra's Service. At the urgent request of the New Zealand Trained Nurses' Association, the government offered to supply nursing service for its own fighting men and released Hester Maclean to organize and direct this nursing unit of the New Zealand Army. Five hundred or more nurses from this small country served on the European front and in the South Pacific and made an excellent record, gaining at the same time a wider concept of their profession in their contacts with nurses of other countries and in their varied experience not only in Europe but in the Fijis, Samoas, and other neighboring tropical islands. Later, when New Zealand was given a mandate for several of these Pacific islands, its plan of nursing and health work was established there and put on a permanent basis. During and after World War II the World Health Organization and other international groups working on similar problems employed many New Zealand nurses for such positions, and some Asian and other countries sent their nurses to New Zealand for special training.

It is interesting to note that one of the chief leaders in promoting modern health work among the natives of the South Pacific Islands is a Maori physician, Sir Mani Pomare, whose Knighthood was received from the British Crown. With the aid of the Rockefeller Foundation he has trained men attendants to assist physicians in the prevention and treatment of hookworm, leprosy and other chronic diseases in this area.

REORGANIZATION OF NURSING AND HEALTH SERVICES

Following World War I and the influenza epidemic in which the medical and health resources of New Zealand had been stretched to the utmost, a Royal Commission of Enquiry was appointed. Among its recommendations was one urging the reorganization of the Health Department and its merging with the Department of Hospitals. At this time nursing was made a distinct division under its own head with increased autonomy and a larger staff. During the depression of the '30's, when unemployment was serious and the Labor Party came into power, the country moved definitely toward a comprehensive national health insurance plan which took shape in the Social Security Act of 1938. This provided medical and health care, preventive and curative, for the entire population, the total cost, including the education of personnel, being paid for by direct taxation and other public funds. Though at first opposed by some medical and other influential groups, the plan had strong popular support and was carried out with comparatively little friction or confusion. This was partly because it was introduced gradually over a period of years, beginning with the maternity and infancy services which had long been partly supported by public funds. Toward the last came the dental service, which provided free treatment for school children and much reduced rates for adults. District nursing also was generally extended at this time.

The need for nursing personnel was met by various means, among which were an active recruitment campaign and extension of existing categories to include nursing aides (similar to assistant nurses in Britain), dental nurses, and other special groups. Such workers were prepared as a rule in one to two years. The minimum age limit for registered nurses was reduced to twenty-one years, and though some schools voluntarily raised their educational requirements for admission to college matriculation standing the minimum remained, as in Britain, at school leaving, around the age of fifteen. A few college graduates have entered in recent years.

In spite of increasing pressures, nursing continued to be the most popular occupation open to women. Its economic status has kept pace with that of other occupations, such as teaching, and there has been little competition from other health and social specialties. Drop-outs and turn-overs have remained relatively low, and morale has been well maintained. A forty-hour week (approved when the new law was passed) was delayed for some years chiefly because of the shortage of domestic staffs in hospitals. However, hours have never exceeded forty-four a week, with one full day off. This and other delays and adjustments were accepted in good spirit. During this period the number of men nurses was increased, especially in mental hospitals, where the training was eighteen months. In the Pacific islands most native nurses, both men and women, were given initial training similar to that of aides, and those who were qualified for more advanced work were then admitted to regular nursing schools with a time allowance for previous work. As general education improved and other requirements were met, such applicants were admitted directly to programs leading to registration.

Nurse Education and Registration

A comparsion of the major developments in nursing in New Zealand with those in other countries so far studied reveals several differences in the sequence of steps and in the way new policies were initiated. For example, in New Zealand public hospitals were under legal control before nursing schools began, and state registration of nurses preceded the national organization of nurses by eight years. The initial steps were taken by government officers, and the administration of nurse registration was centered in the Department of Hospitals from 1901, when the act was passed, until 1925, when it was revised. Only then were organized nurses and similar medical and hospital groups represented on the registration board. In 1906 private hospitals and sanitaria were put under government inspection and regulation. Since most of these establishments were very small and had limited clinical and financial resources, few met the requirements set for training hospitals. Later a plan for affiliation with larger hospital centers was tried without much success. Largely because of these policies, nursing schools in New Zealand are relatively uniform with few far above or below the prescribed requirements.

There has also been a tendency from the early days to keep the standards close to those of Britain, thus favoring the exchange of nurses between New Zealand and the mother country. This tie was strengthened during World War I when many New Zealand nurses not only served in Britain but often remained for added study or experience. The prestige so gained led other nurses to follow their example, with the result that a large proportion are partly British trained. New Zealand also attracted many nurses from the old land, among them a number of sister tutors who helped to introduce the preliminary course and the block system of theory and practice. After state registration laws were passed in the British Isles (the first in 1919), a plan for reciprocal registration was arranged between the two countries. Regulations and requirements, though not identical, were quite similar. These influences were further strengthened by the wide use of nursing textbooks, journals, and other nursing literature from Britain.

During and after World War I contacts were made with Canada and the United States. Before Hester Maclean's retirement in 1923, her assistant (and successor), Jessie Bicknell, was sent abroad for a year of travel and study. On her return she proposed that a five-year basic nursing program (with specialization in the last year) be developed in Otago University to prepare better educated applicants for higher posts in nursing schools and services. This plan was actively supported by the nurses' association and adopted. Janet Moore was then sent to London to prepare to direct programs in hospital administration and teaching, and Mary Lambie went to Canada and the United States to prepare for a similar position in district and public health nursing. Difficulties arose later over the financing of the Otago program, and in 1927, after two years' trial, it was discontinued, and a one-year postgraduate diploma program was set up to accommodate sixty students a year. This was located in Wellington and was administered by a committee representing the Victoria University College, the New Zealand Department of Health, and the Wellington Hospital, all of which contributed to its eight-month courses in teaching, hospital administration, and public health nursing. With the exception of a few who paid their own fees, all students received bursaries covering full expenses, most of which came from the government but some from individual hospitals and voluntary agencies.

The Plunket Society and some other large agencies of a similar type set up independent service courses which were usually shorter. To keep general staffs up-to-date, brief summer refresher courses, chiefly in clinical and technical subjects, were given in such educational centers. The New Zealand Registered Nurses Association, at the time of writing, was negotiating with the University of New Zealand to establish a special school at which graduate nurses might take advanced courses in administration of nursing services, research, and nursing education. This project had the support of the Department of Health of the New Zealand Government.

The Nurses Act of New Zealand has been revised from time to time to adapt it to changing conditions. When first passed, it recognized only one category of registered nurses—the graduates of three-year courses. The Act as now revised provides for the recognition of baby, maternity, psychiatric, dental, and other special types of nurses and for nursing aides. Maternity nurses and midwives may practice with or without full general nursing preparation. As in Britain, the general nursing program did not include maternity nursing, but in 1937 when the Nurses and Midwives Act was passed this provision was covered. Many nurses then took an extra half year of preparation to qualify for the midwives' certificate.

Though the basic program had a "preventive bias," the chief emphasis was on bedside nursing, and in general the course was stronger in practice than in theory. The postgraduate program for nurses established in Wellington in 1928 and financed by the government offered courses in administration, public health nursing, and medical social work. Postcertificate courses in clinical nursing (usually of six months' duration) are held throughout the country.

Organized Nurses and Their Work

Although nurses in New Zealand have much influence and control in their own positions, they seem to expect the nurses in government posts to take the lead in national nursing activities that elsewhere are initiated by voluntary groups. For example, the first steps toward a national organization were taken in 1908 when Miss Maclean called together representative nurses from the whole country and presented the idea of a national organization. Out of this conference came the New Zealand Trained Nurses' Association which elected a hospital matron, Mrs. Kendall, as its first president and Miss Maclean's assistant, Jessie Bicknell, as secretary. In addition to fully trained nurses, active members included midwives, maternity nurses, and some physicians. An important adjunct to the NZTNA was the small journal *Kai Tiaki* (Maori for watcher or guardian), which Miss Maclean edited and published from 1908 to 1922 when it was bought by the association. She then continued as volunteer editor until her death, when a paid editor-secretary was appointed. When the new association applied for membership in the International Council of Nurses and found that it could not qualify unless all its voting members were fully trained nurses, the group decided to give physician members a special consultant status and others, who did not meet full requirements, associate membership. With these changes the association was admitted in 1912.

Though the ICN did not function actively during the war and immediate postwar years, many New Zealand nurses who served abroad became aware of international nursing trends and especially of the part that voluntary nurses' organizations were taking in the registration battles in Britain. No doubt this helped to bring about the passage in 1925 of a new nurses' and midwives' act in their own country which transferred responsibility for administration of registration to a General Nursing Council on which the Nurses Association was well represented. This Council had broad powers and was able to initiate a number of needed improvements in nurse and midwife training which reflected a growing concern for standards and a greater awareness of registration trends in other countries.

The renamed New Zealand Registered Nurses Association at this time began to give more attention to the economic and ethical problems of nurses. Some of the members were conscious of the conflict between their Nightingale traditions and ethical teachings and the principles of trade unionism held by the majority of New Zealand citizens. In 1908 labor sympathizers in the government pushed through a law requiring an eight-hour, three-shift, six-day-week plan for all hospital employees. The newly organized nurses persuaded them to make some adjustments for staff nurses, but nurses in training were put on the straight eight-hour day. This was another "first" that met some criticism from nurses in other countries largely because of the arbitrary way in which it was interpreted by labor groups who knew nothing of hospital or nursing requirements.

During the '30's and '40's, when the economic and health structure of New Zealand was undergoing progressive socialization, the chief attention of nurses in all branches of service and education was given to meeting the growing demand for service and trying to work out a nationwide salary scale to be used as a basis for negotiations between the Nurses Association and employers. At first such negotiations were voluntary, but in 1936 a law was passed making it compulsory for all occupational groups to set up arbitration machinery. The Registered Nurses Association then secured the right to represent its members (including midwives and student nurses) in such negotiations. This was the first nonunion association of nurses to participate actively in collective bargaining. A succession of problems connected with this and similar laws that followed took much of the association's attention for years and gave its members a wide experience in such matters.

During recent decades the New Zealand Registered Nurses Association has grown rapidly and more than forty branches have been organized in different parts of the country. In addition to a matrons' section, it has two others devoted to public health and nursing education. It also has an affiliated student nurses association, formed of individual councils representing the different schools and having its own funds and activities. This group was especially active in raising Florence Nightingale scholarships for study abroad. During the '40's New Zealand nurses doubled their yearly funds for such scholarships and awarded four or more for nurses in war-devastated countries who came to New Zealand for study. The association then had only about 4500 graduate and 3000 student-nurse members. This interest no doubt was partly because one of their leading New Zealand nurses, Mary Lambie, was then president of the Florence Nightingale International Foundation.

This capable and dynamic director of the government's nursing division was later closely associated with the World Health Organization, which employed New Zealand nurses in many difficult posts. The association cooperated also with the Red Cross and the Order of St. John in the training and supervision of voluntary aides and active service with sea, land, and air forces in the European and Pacific areas and in the Middle East, where the nurses from this little island are well and favorably known. Among those who held important posts was Mrs. Fieldhouse (formerly Miss Reid), for some time chief nurse in the Far East region of the World Health Organization. She was also active in strengthening the educational structure of nursing in New Zealand in an effort to prepare nurses for their increasing responsibilities as leaders. Since the great majority of nurses in this country seem to prefer to work with patients and families in rural and other communities to executive, teaching, and other positions, it was evident that efforts were needed to attract and develop a larger proportion of broadly educated nurses for such positions and also for research in the field of nursing.

The record of modern nursing in these two English-speaking countries in the South Pacific reflects the strong influence of British attitudes and patterns in nursing and the basic characteristics of pioneers in a new environment. They did not have in their population the wide variety of national influences represented in the United States and Canada, and apparently there were fewer ex-teachers among their founders or nurses who in general were acutely aware of the educational needs and problems of the new vocation. New Zealand was exceptionally fortunate in its government officers, both medical and nursing, and chiefly because of their foresight avoided many of the nursing problems that caused so much trouble in the homeland as well as in America. One notes, however, that leadership in such matters has been left chiefly to nurses in government positions. Australia also was late in developing strong professional leadership partly because of its vast area and scattered population. Nurses in both countries are now recognizing the need of a larger proportion of qualified leaders and are working on this and other problems that directly affect their professional status and effectiveness.

SELECTED BIBLIOGRAPHY

Bridge, E. Ruth. "The Control of Nursing in New Zealand," *Int. Nurs. Bull.* Vol. VI, no. 3 (1950), 10-12.

"Bush Nursing Across a Continent," E. Francis, "The Beginnings of Bush Nursing in Victoria," 30-32; K. H. Barnes, "A Silver Chain in Western Australia," 32-33; E. J. Whicker, "In the Out Back of New South Wales," 34-35; Doris Noller, "Horseback to Helicopter in Tasmania," 36-39; Janet Scott, "In the Gulf of Carpentaria," 39. *Int. Nurs. Rev.*, April 1958, 30-39.

Davis, R. A. "Public Health Nursing amongst the Maori People in New Zealand," *Int. Nurs. Rev.*, October 1956, 21-25.

International Council of Nurses. *National Reports. 1947*, 30-32, 64-65; *1949*, 38-42, 84-87; *1957*, 36, 72-74; *1961*, 3-5, 62-63.

Lambie, Mary I. *Historical Development of Nursing in New Zealand 1840-1950.* Wellington: Dept. of Health, 1951. Pamphlet.

"New Zealand Reflects," *Int. Nurs. Rev.*, October 1959, 14-16.

"Nursing Programmes in New Zealand," *Int. Nurs. Rev.*, March/April 1961, 14-17.

Nursing in South Australia First Hundred Years 1837-1937. Adelaide: Vardon, 1938.

Nutting, M. Adelaide, and Lavinia L. Dock. *A History of Nursing*. New York: Putnam's, 1907-1912. 4 vols. Vol. IV, Ch. IV.

Pidgeon, E. C. "Pioneer Nursing in Australia," *Int. Nurs. Rev.*, October 1956, 38-42.

Salter, Kathleen. "School Dental Nursing in New Zealand," *Int. Nurs. Rev.*, Feb., 1960, pp. 62-67.

CHAPTER 14

Northern Europe

THOUGH relatively small in area and population and moder-
ately endowed with material resources, the five northern
European countries here considered—Sweden, Norway, Denmark, Iceland, and Finland—have won an important place
among the nations for the sturdy character and intelligence of
their people and their political, social, and cultural achievements. The first four of these countries are Scandinavian in
race, language, and culture, and though their people speak
different dialects they seem to find little difficulty in understanding each other. The Finns have a different ethnic origin
and language but were influenced greatly by the Swedes who
ruled Finland for six centuries before 1809. After about a century of Russian rule, Finland in 1919 became an independent
republic. The people of all five countries are predominantly
Lutheran in religion and social democratic in their political
systems. Though strongly individualistic in their personal
affairs, they have shown a marked ability for social cooperation,
the results of which are seen in their successful promotion of the
cooperative movement in business and trade and their leadership in such causes as woman's suffrage, world peace, adult edu-

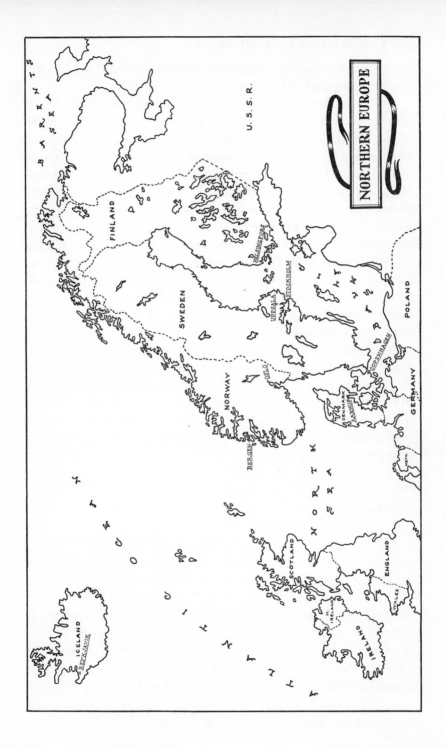

cation, public housing, and health insurance, as well as in medicine, nursing and public health.

Up until about 1840 hospital and nursing work in these northern countries was backward as it had been in other parts of the world. The first impulse toward reform came from the Kaiserswerth Deaconess movement. Introduced by the Lutheran Church and stimulated by a religious revival, this work attracted attention among serious-minded women, a number of whom entered Deaconess Training Institutes in Germany or at home, where they were prepared for teaching, nursing, and other religious and charitable vocations. Attention was then drawn toward Britain by Miss Nightingale's work in the Crimea and her nursing reforms at home and in other parts of the world. Soon after, the Red Cross, with its patriotic appeal for volunteers, found a ready response here as in other European countries. For some time these differing concepts of nursing and nurse training led to some confusion and conflict. Then, too, many physicians in these northern countries had studied in Germany or France, where medical chiefs had complete control over the selection and training of all personnel in their departments. This continued to be a controversial issue long after the Nightingale system had been introduced in a few continental schools.

SWEDEN [1]

Queen Sophia, a deeply religious, social-minded German princess, inspired and directed the first stage of the new movement in Sweden, and her influence is still strongly felt through the nursing school Sophiahemmet (Sophia Home), maintained in her memory by the Swedish Royal Family and other loyal friends. The queen's interest in this work was shown first in the founding in Stockholm in 1851 of a Lutheran (Kaiserswerth) Deaconess Institute, of which she became friend and patron. She was active also in developing a plan for Red Cross nursing after

[1] The chief reference here is Elisabet Dillner's *Eight Decades*, an English summary of her longer *History of Nursing in Sweden*.

1864, when the Geneva Convention was signed and Sweden started to organize a Red Cross Society to carry on such work. A letter from one of Queen Sophia's ladies-in-waiting to Florence Nightingale then brought an invitation to send a Swedish pupil to the London school for training, and Emmy Rappe, a member of an aristocratic family, was selected and sent in 1866 as a protégé of the Swedish Red Cross Society. She spent six months as a lady probationer at St. Thomas's Hospital, returning to Sweden in 1867 to start a six months' course in the surgical ward of a new hospital at Uppsala, a university center. Miss Rappe was made head nurse over a single ward in which during the next decade she trained sixty to seventy nurses in surgical nursing. This experiment under the Red Cross apparently had little or no influence on conditions in the hospital as a whole, which remained backward. The Queen then decided to open in 1884 a small nurses' home in Stockholm where serious-minded, intelligent women from good families could receive instruction based on religious principles and where some liberal education could be included with nursing instruction. Through the interest of a prominent physician, practical experience was secured in a nearby hospital where moral and physical conditions were more satisfactory, even though the old system of nursing remained unchanged.

Queen Sophia next visited London incognito to observe the Nightingale system and was so impressed that her family and friends raised a fund to purchase a large property in Stockholm on which they built the spacious Sophiahemmet referred to earlier. Alfheld Ehrenberg, a Swedish nurse who had been a lady probationer in London and Liverpool, was the first lady superintendent and Queen Sophia herself was president of the board. Attached to the school was a small private hospital over which it had direct control. Here nurses were able to demonstrate and practice a higher quality of nursing and to gain experience in the handling of private patients as well as in general management and teaching. Most of their practical experience, however, was still in the wards of other hospitals where the older system prevailed and in which untrained attendants did most of the nursing. Efforts to introduce the English plan met with no success, and Miss Ehrenberg, who considered any other plan unworkable, resigned.

She was followed by a new superintendent who was a teacher, not a nurse, and the school continued under such direction until 1947 when Gerda Magnusson became the first nurse superintendent. This pattern of an independent school conducted by a recognized educator and staff and relatively free from the demands of outside hospitals for routine service became the approved pattern in Sweden. It had some definite advantages, including freedom to select good candidates, to give them sound systematic instruction, which was quite broad in scope, and to have them live under good home influences much as they would in a deaconess motherhouse. In 1893 this school appointed the first full-time nurse teacher on record, Sally Peterson. It also inaugurated the first block system with alternating periods of theory and practice. The practice consisted chiefly of more responsible technical and administrative functions, since most of the actual nursing and housekeeping duties were still performed by paid ward helpers. Gradually the old-time head nurses were replaced by those who had completed their training in this and other schools.

Another distinctive feature of the Sophiahemmet was the Sophia Sisterhood, which reflected the influence of the deaconess motherhouse pattern. Eligible students might apply for membership in the sisterhood after their first year at the school. They had to be willing to accept any position to which the superintendent assigned them (usually institutional or district nursing or mission work) and to live on a nominal salary with a pension to care for them in illness and old age. The Sophiahemmet also had its own chapel and resident chaplain as well as a home for its aged and ailing sisters. The continued patronage of the Royal Family of Sweden undoubtedly did much to strengthen the school's prestige and to give powerful support to its graduates in the reforms they undertook later. Another school which also had powerful backing from influential social and political groups was that of the Swedish Red Cross, established in 1891. It was more secular and military in character but attracted superior applicants, usually from the middle or upper classes.

The graduates of these schools filled most of the important positions in Swedish nursing and were sometimes sent to other countries such as Norway, which remained under the Swedish Crown until 1905.

PROBLEMS AND DEVELOPMENT IN NURSING EDUCATION
AND SERVICE

Around the turn of the century the number of public hospitals was increasing rapidly. Most of these were under the control of county councils with some under city councils or belonging to deaconess or other private associations. Untrained helpers still did most of the domestic and bedside nursing work in nearly all Swedish hospitals. With the advances in medical and surgical work, when medical staffs in public institutions were often overloaded with new technical procedures, some doctors began to select and train young women of better intelligence to assist them in their work. Thus began a number of so-called hospital nursing schools, the training in which varied in length from three months to seven years. There was no uniformity of content, even from ward to ward of the same hospital, and no agreement on what the terms "nurse and nursing" meant. Leading Sophia Sisters and others who were in touch with conditions in Britain and elsewhere became so outspoken in their criticism that in 1919 the government started an investigation that lasted four years. Of the six appointees on the commission, two were physicians and three nurses, one of the latter being secretary. No agreement was reached on the functions of nurses, and the law that was passed shortly after defined such persons only as those who had passed through a complete training of at least two years in a state-recognized school. This law, however, made it illegal for hospitals to start schools without state permission and authorized the appointment of a lady inspector of nurses to be attached to the State Department of Health.

For more than twenty years this position was held by an able resolute Sophia sister, Kerstin Nordendahl, through whose efforts (with strong Royal Family and government support) the number and standards of nursing schools in Sweden were strictly regulated. Gradually, all of these schools became independent of hospitals in administration and financing, the nursing school and nursing service each having its own director, staff, and budget. The Swedish Medical Board in 1922 issued a uniform plan of instruction which was revised from time to time, the course being lengthened to at least three years, excluding probation. This board also decided on the maximum number of student nurses to be admitted each year and how they were to be rationed among the schools. These and other regulations were made chiefly on the recommendation of the state inspector. The fact that by this time women in Sweden had the vote, that Swedish nurses had in 1910 organized a national association, and that its president, Berta Wellin, an able and eloquent Sophia sister, was one of the first women members of the Riksdag (parliament) undoubtedly helped to strengthen the position of the state inspector in her exceptionally difficult task.

NURSING ORGANIZATIONS AND SERVICES

In its earlier years most of the activities of the Swedish Nurses Association had to do with the development of postgraduate courses to prepare nurses for more important positions in hospitals, schools, and municipalities. The first six-month course for matrons and teachers was established in 1917. Shortly after, some state aid was secured for it, but the association continued to contribute to its maintenance and otherwise to support its work. In 1920 the State College of Public Health Nursing was developed as a government institution under the direction of the state inspector. Only public health nurses who had taken this six-month course were appointed to positions. Though it required some time to prepare nurses for all the municipalities in Sweden, the standards established were uniform throughout the country, and these nurses did much to meet the health needs of the rural communities in which most of the Swedish people live.

The next step was to broaden the narrow basis of clinical experience provided by nursing schools and to develop postgraduate courses in such branches as mental, pediatric, maternity, and contagious disease nursing. Though midwifery and nursing are quite separate in Sweden, many public health nurses, especially in isolated areas, have qualified and practiced in both professions. Compared with conditions in many countries, where specialties such as X-ray and laboratory work were being turned over to non-nurse technicians, there were still many Swedish nurses who held such posts and who helped to provide post-graduate courses in these areas. Other nurses continued to fill positions that elsewhere were held chiefly by trained social workers. Some graduates of the deaconess schools also qualified as parish nurses. Private nursing has been a minor branch in this country, the chief reason being that a large proportion of sick patients are cared for in hospitals, where under the voluntary health insurance system, individual costs have been relatively small. Hospital positions open to trained nurses were chiefly those of nurse administrators, teachers, head nurses and assistant nurses in the wards.

The Economic Revolution

Although the number of schools was relatively small (since 1920 never until recently above thirty) and the supply of trained nurses was strictly controlled, this did not lead, as one might expect, to higher salaries and better economic conditions for nurses. Most of the older generation of Swedish nurses, who were influenced strongly by deaconess ideals and traditions, refused to consider the growing protest of the younger generation against their low economic status, the old-fashioned regulations which barred them from many forms of recreation open to other girls of their own age, and in some cases their sober outdoor uniforms and the title "sister" with its religious connotations. A few, especially in the depression, had begun to join trade unions in the hope of bettering their lot.

Among the more outspoken of the young modernists was Gerda Hojer, an independent-minded graduate of the Red Cross School who took a course in the London School of Economics with the purpose of finding out what could be done to improve these conditions. After her return she was elected, and served three years, first as executive secretary of the Swedish Nurses Association, then as president. During that time she helped its members to work out a plan in cooperation with a federation (formed by the medical and other professions) in which she represented nursing. This group sought to improve the economic status of professional workers in public service who, in general, earned lower salaries than many industrial workers. As a result of their efforts, the government was persuaded to pass laws between 1936 and 1940 which gave the professions the right to bargain independently for their members provided they represented fifty per cent of the practitioners in their field. Though not the first nursing group to take such action, the Swedish Nurses Association, which had joined the International Council of Nurses in 1929, attracted considerable attention among nurses of other countries because of its bold and persistent efforts.

Earlier, in 1920, the Northern Nurses Union had been formed as a regional group composed of the nurses' associations of the five countries here discussed. It met every two years to consider common problems and to compare notes on other matters of mutual interest. This organization undoubtedly had a strong influence on nursing developments in all its member countries and was the first of several regional groups later formed by countries belonging to the International Council of Nurses.

Some Postwar Developments

Neutral Sweden suffered much less than its neighbors during World War II, but its nurses carried many extra responsibilities and gave generous aid to their colleagues in other countries. By 1945 the shortage of nurses had become so acute that a state commission composed of physicians, nurses, and other groups was appointed to study the situation. Its first report revealed some disturbing facts and recommended long-needed changes in the education of nurses and auxiliary personnel. Although the number of nurses had increased fivefold in the preceding four decades, auxiliaries had increased tenfold. Sweden, compared with other countries having modern health services, had a strikingly low number of fully qualified nurses, midwives and nursing helpers for its population. Most of the helpers were still trained on the job and had little or no organized instruction. There were then only twenty-four state-approved schools of nursing, of which seven were private and the others supported by the provinces.

The commission recommended a substantial strengthening of the basic training for hospital helpers and stipulated that all students entering nursing schools must begin by taking this course. Those who wanted to go further but did not have regular high school education (often lacking in rural districts) were urged to attend people's high schools for basic science and general education. The subsequent course in nursing schools was to be shortened to two years and nine months and was to contain more intensive theoretical and practical instruction. A period of six months, or longer if needed for such branches as operating-room and laboratory work, was allowed for specialization. Midwifery training was to be based on at least two years of the nursing course as soon as this could be arranged. Among many other suggestions was the establishment of a State School of Nursing to serve as a demonstration and experimental unit for the entire country. Provision was made for free training for all nurses; state scholarships for the theoretical blocks and student service in hospitals covering room and board. More recent developments have included studies of several aspects of nursing education, such as requirements for entrance to basic schools, standards of education for both basic and postbasic students, preparation for psychiatric nursing, and the use of nursing personnel in hospital nursing services.

In 1948 Gerda Hojer, then president not only of the Swedish Nurses Association but also of the International Council of Nurses, had been elected member of the Riksdag, and in 1949 Sweden was host to the nurses of the world when the ICN met in Stockholm. Many wondered how a small association of about 10,000 nurses was able to handle such a large gathering, with all the side trips and extras provided. However, the population as a whole, from the Royal Family down, offered their help.

Associations of nurses in the neighboring countries also arranged conferences before and after the Stockholm meeting, thus giving the visitors a chance to get a comparative picture of nursing in the entire northern area. Guests who attended were impressed not only by the efficiency and courtesy of these dignified, upstanding northern nurses but by the differences that existed in their nursing systems and the lively but friendly debates among them on these and other questions. Such close relations were furthered by the exchange system arranged by the Northern Nurses Union in which hundreds of their nurses were given an opportunity to live and work for a year or more in a neighboring country.

DENMARK

Before 1850 nursing conditions in Denmark, as elsewhere were backward. A small Danish Deaconess Institute had been started in 1836, but neither this nor the Red Cross movement that came later had much influence in bringing about reforms. The first effort to improve these conditions began in a new municipal hospital in Copenhagen through the efforts of a progressive director of hospitals, Dr. C. E. Fenger. Working with him to develop better nursing services was an able young woman, Henny Schulz, who was to become a leader in the new nursing movement. In 1883 she went to London to study the Nightingale system at St. Thomas's Hospital and was soon convinced that a similar scheme should be developed in her own country. It was not until 1897, however, that the first training school for nurses in Denmark was organized at the Municipal Hospital. Shortly after a London-trained Danish nurse started a preliminary course at the State Hospital in Copenhagen. This did much to give beginners in nursing a more uniform preparation, but since the hospital had no general superintendent of nurses the students who completed the course were routed through the various hospital departments, in each of which the medical chief and his personally chosen head nurse decided how and what they should be taught.

In the next two decades several other schools were opened

in Copenhagen and in a few outside centers. These varied greatly in their organization and standards. In 1913 Charlotte Munck, a well-educated Danish nurse who had been trained under Anna Maxwell at the Presbyterian Hospital, New York, was appointed superintendent of nurses at the beautiful new Bispebjerg Hospital in Copenhagen. She accepted on condition that she be given complete charge of the nursing service of the hospital as well as of the school of nursing and that she select her own nursing staff. Her success in this famous institution did much to spread the ideas for which she stood, and she soon became a widely respected and beloved leader in the national nursing organization and in the movement as a whole.

PROFESSIONAL ORGANIZATION AND EFFORTS
TOWARD STANDARDIZATION

Leading Danish nurses were in touch with the new trends toward professional organization and registration in Britain and America in the 1890's, and they, too, recognized the need to bring about greater uniformity in the preparation of nurses. A Danish suffragist, Mrs. Charlotte Norrie, who had had a brief training in nursing, was present at the 1899 meeting in London when the International Council of Nurses was launched. The Danish Council of Nurses was formed the same year and she was elected president. Later, however, when the decision was made to work for a systematic three-year program of theory and practice and to make this a requirement for membership, she resigned and Mrs. Tscherning (the former Henny Schulz) was then elected. This was a fulltime paid position which included the work of executive secretary, management of the Council's[2] headquarters, and editorship of its journal, *Tidskrift for Sygeplejersker,* which first appeared in 1901. Under Mrs. Tscherning's able and courageous leadership for nearly thirty years, the Council became a powerful force in bringing about reforms in nursing schools and services.

Though the Council members believed in state registration,

[2] This and the following references relate to the Danish Council of Nurses unless otherwise specified (pp. 287-291).

they wanted to be sure that the three-year standard was in force in most schools before asking for a law. Their first step was to require all members of the Council to wear its official badge on duty, indicating that they were fully qualified nurses. In 1913 the members proceeded to study hospitals that were conducting schools of nursing, and this led to their division into two groups. The first had the necessary facilities for a full three-year program but the second could provide only one or two years of training. The Council also fostered the extension of preclinical education by encouraging the establishment of preliminary schools in the larger centers. To help the country districts, it turned to the local folk high schools for which this country is famous. In 1927 one of these schools (Testrup) was transformed into a nursing high school which offered a combined preclinical and adult education program to prospective nurse students who had passed the ninth grade.

In 1933 the first nurse registration law was passed, and the approval of schools and the control and supervision of nursing education became the responsibility of the National Health Service. At this time all health services came under a compulsory health insurance plan.

Some Developments in Nursing Service and Postgraduate Education

The main opportunities for trained nurses at first were in hospitals, but soon district nursing was begun in both rural and urban communities, which, with the advancement of public health, called for more of a preventive and teaching emphasis. There was little demand here for private nurses, since most of the sick were cared for by hospital or district nurses under the new health insurance plan. Trained midwives in Denmark had for more than a century held an excellent professional position and attended nearly all normal births; thus the nurse-midwife did not develop here as in Britain and in some of its dominions. Most nurses, however, had training in the care of maternity patients. Relatively strong emphasis was given to mental nursing in the general training program. The Danish Council, which conducted its own private nurse exchange or registry, helped its members to secure added training in psychiatric, maternity, and communicable-disease nursing. When an over-supply of nurses developed, the council found employment for some of its nurses in other countries where they became well and favorably known for their nursing skill and general competence.

On the initiative of the National Health Service a postgraduate school of nursing education was established in 1938 at the University of Aarhus. This was made possible by generous donations from the Rockefeller Foundation and the Danish Life Insurance Companies. Such funds covered expenses for the first few years, after which the state assumed financial responsibility. The immediate purpose was to prepare public health nurses to serve in municipalities under the new health act in reducing infant mortality and morbidity. The training, however, was broadened to qualify such nurses for service in schools, industry, and tuberculosis dispensaries as well as in infant welfare. Soon other courses were offered to prepare administrators in nursing services and schools and teachers for schools of nursing. The Danish Council of Nurses provided some scholarships for students and took an active interest in the school. Ellen Broe, who in 1951 became Director of Studies of the Florence Nightingale International Foundation, was one of the teaching group that established this center of postgraduate nursing education. Many Danish nurses have studied abroad and have shared in such international projects as those of the World Health Organization. In recent years studies have been made on the curricula of schools of nursing in order to integrate public health nursing content into the basic curriculum. The State Registration Act of 1956 reflects these and other educational advances.

SOME ECONOMIC AND PROFESSIONAL DEVELOPMENTS

The Danish Council of Nurses, in addition to all its other activities, has undertaken some major business and professional enterprises. It has owned and managed convalescent and recreational homes for its members, handled relief and scholarship funds, arranged for pensions, and published not only a journal but textbooks for nurses. With the aid of the city, which gave the land (a city block), it built the large Nurses House in Copenhagen, which provides, in addition to its spacious administrative offices, apartments and rooms for members and guests at a minimum rate. Maria Madsen, for many years the Chief Officer of the Council, was largely responsible for the planning of these various services and activities.

In the late '30's when economic conditions became quite acute the Council realized that something must be done to improve hours, salaries, and other conditions of service. Failing to make much impression on the executive officers of state and local institutions and agencies, this body secured permission to function as a bargaining agency and proceeded to appoint its negotiators and to set up its policies and proposed salary schedules. Contrary to predictions, its cause got good support from the public. Council members showed not only professional solidarity in this campaign but exceptional dignity, self-discipline, and social responsibility. Though many of them placed their provisional resignations in the hands of the negotiators to be used at their discretion if other arguments failed, due consideration was given to the safety of patients and to the upholding of professional principles.

During the German occupation of their country in World War II, Danish nurses like other citizens showed their discipline, unity, and stamina in spite of many dangers, impositions, and restrictions. One of their distinguished nurses Eli Magnussen, Director of Nursing Education in the government, was imprisoned during the war. Later she served as chief nurse consultant in the East Mediterranean area of the World Health Organization, where she made an important contribution to international nursing.

Immediately after the war the head of the National Health Service in Denmark appointed a committee to study the nursing situation. Sitting on this committee were five members of the Danish Council of Nurses and two from the National Health Service. Three government reports recorded the results of its work. The first two, based on a job analysis made by engineers, dealt with the lack of nurses, nursing functions in general hospitals and in mental institutions, and plans for improving service in both. The third dealt with the education of nurses in a survey of recent trends and the quantitative and qualitative need for nurses in the future. It also recommended a mandatory bill for registered nurses, which was put into effect. Maja Foget, Director of Nursing Studies of the Nursing Division of the National Health Department of Denmark, included in this report a chapter on the development of nursing education in that country which has been very helpful in the preparation of this summary on Danish nursing.

NORWAY

Norway and Sweden were united under the same Crown until 1905, and their nursing systems up to that time were of much the same pattern. The Deaconess Institute (established in 1868) took the first steps toward modern nursing under Cathinka Guldberg, who was trained in Kaiserswerth and was the first nursing sister in Norway. In 1894 the Norwegian Red Cross opened a training school under two Sophia sisters, and shortly after another one-year school was set up by the Norwegian Women's Public Health Association. Later this group took on the care of war wounded and showed an intensely social and patriotic spirit as well as a strong belief in women's capacities for social action. This is a notable example of a voluntary organization of women citizens who pioneered in a program of health and nursing education for an entire country. Branches soon developed all over Norway, and, as the work grew, nurse training schools were opened by them with the object of employing their graduates chiefly in community health work under the Association.

In 1900 the first direct contact with Britain was made by two nurses from Bergen, who after a period of hospital experience returned to develop the British plan of training in two municipal hospitals of Bergen and Oslo. Independent and hospital-affiliated schools continued to develop side by side, and in 1961 there were twenty-nine basic and two post-basic schools in Norway. There were then about 3000 students in these schools and about 9000 graduate nurses for a population of more than three million.

PROFESSIONAL DEVELOPMENT

Norwegian nurses began in 1912 to unite in the Norwegian Nurses Association in order to safeguard their profession and its rights as well as to free it from many unauthorized persons who were working as nurses without training. They were also determined from the start to establish higher and more uniform standards in their schools and set the three-year course as their goal. The chief leader in this movement was a determined, intelligent, and capable nurse, Sister Bergliot Larsson, who had gone to Edinburgh, Scotland, in 1909 for special training in fever nursing, intending at that time to go into the mission field. She was urged to return to a position in Norway and soon threw herself with all her missionary zeal and strong feminist bent into the work of nursing organization. This resulted in the founding of the Norwegian Nurses Association, of which she was the first president. As in most other Scandinavian countries, this was a fulltime paid position. The Association joined the International Council of Nurses in 1922, and its journal, *Sykepleien* ("Sick Nursing"), was started the same year. State registration was a primary object; but since the three-year standard was opposed by the organized medical profession the Norwegian Nurses Association, like the Danish Council, started by admitting to membership only graduates of three-year schools approved by the association. This plan continued until 1949, when a three-year-law was finally passed.

Beginning in 1925 the Nurses Association also conducted one-year postgraduate courses for nurses preparing for institutional and public health work and other special branches. This school, directed for many years by Sister Bergliot, was closed during World War II, and the attractive headquarters of the Nurses Association in Oslo was taken over by the Army of Occupation along with the funds of the association. The president, Sister

Bertha Helgestad, fortunately escaped to Sweden before she was arrested for opposing these and other plans. A woman "commissar" was put in charge, but the nurses kept up a shadow organization until peace was restored. They then got possession of their building, though not of all their funds and properties. Many nurses, in addition to their regular work, served in the underground and showed exceptional courage and stamina during these hazardous years. Some went with their army to Britain where they were in active military service. The year after the war's end, a congress was held in Oslo of the reunited Norwegian nurses, their colleagues of the Northern Nurses Union, and guests from other countries belonging to the International Council of Nurses. To the 2400 nurses who attended and to the people generally who rejoiced with them, this was a deeply moving and unforgettable experience which showed the spiritual kinship as well as the professional strength and solidarity of the northern nurses and the great respect and affection in which they were held by the population at large.

There was much to be done to help restore nursing schools and services in Norway, especially in the devastated northern area. Plans were made to put the new registration law into operation and to strengthen the curriculum of nursing schools. Norwegian nurses also took an active interest in the program of hospital rebuilding and expansion and were represented on building committees which repaired the war damage and put up new hospitals. In 1947 the state established a new post-graduate school for public health nurses which provides free tuition and maintenance for fifty selected students each year and offers a comprehensive modern program. The other post-graduate courses also have received state support and increased facilities.

Norway, which had long had a form of health insurance, partly voluntary and partly compulsory, began after the war to lean more strongly toward the compulsory system. Its national health service is much like that of Britain, with whose people the Norwegians have close ties. The general status of nursing in both state and private services is similar to that of other northern countries. Norwegian nurses have developed plans for negotiating economic questions with state and other employers. The eight-hour law for both student and graduate nurses has been in force since 1937. This country seems to have no serious shortage of good applicants to nursing schools nor any special difficulty in finding nurses to fill even the isolated posts on the rugged Norwegian coast or in the remote rural settlements. Norwegian nurses have been studying nurse placement and the use of auxiliary nursing personnel in hospitals. From these and other indications it would seem that they are moving in much the same direction as nurses in other northern countries.

FINLAND

This plucky little country to the far north has been a battleground for centuries between East and West. Since 1919, when it became an independent republic, it has gone through many crises that threatened its freedom and integrity, but the sturdy spirit of its people has never failed, even when after World War II a rich part of its territory was lost to Russia and its population was then resettled at the cost of the Finnish state. With the highest literacy rate in the world and a record of having been the third country to give women the vote, it was also one of the first to give this group an important place in economic and political life and to allow them equal opportunities for education and for independent careers.

BEGINNINGS OF MODERN NURSING

The first step toward a modern system in Finland was taken by a few deaconesses in 1867. Through them, a friendly surgeon, Dr. F. Saltzman, became interested in opening a wider path for educated women in nursing. He started a six-month course for secular nurses in the Surgical Hospital at Helsingfors (1889) and secured as matron a well-qualified nurse, Anna Broms, who had taken training in Sweden and Edinburgh on a state scholarship. Like too many of the first leaders, she died early, a victim of overwork, but her followers carried on, and by 1892 the nursing course had been rounded out and lengthened to one year. Then in 1904 Baroness Sophie Mannerheim, a tall, handsome, well-educated member of a distinguished family, who had been trained in the Nightingale School in London, was appointed matron.

Madame Mannerheim (as she preferred to be called) became an outstanding leader of nursing in her own country and later as President of the International Council of Nurses was known and admired by a wider circle. To her is often attributed the "go-ahead" spirit of the Finnish nurses, their ambition to travel and study in other countries, and their success in putting their work at home on the highest possible basis.

PROFESSIONAL ORGANIZATIONS OF NURSES

The Nurses Association of Finland, organized in 1898, was one of the earliest and the most active and ambitious in its undertakings. It not only initiated and managed the new Central Preliminary School and Home opened in Helsingfors (1906) but started district nursing (1912) and promoted school nursing. Ellen Nylander, the first director of the Central School, was sent to the London Hospital to study its preliminary school and later to New York, where she attended lectures in Hospital Economics at Teachers College. Madame Mannerheim, president of the Nurses Association of Finland, attended the International Council of Nurses meeting in Paris (1907), and two years later her group joined the ICN. After World War I she was elected president of this world body and invited the first postwar congress to meet in Finland (1925). What this meant to a small country that had just secured its independence and had gone through a distressing civil war can scarcely be imagined. The congress, which had not met in full session since the eventful meeting in Cologne in 1912, was a remarkable success, and the nurses and people of Finland made a deep impression on those who came from all parts of the world to reestablish the bonds of friendship and to rebuild their international organization.

Differences in language and often in viewpoints between the

Finnish-speaking and Swedish-speaking peoples of Finland (the latter now a minority) led to the formation of a second national nurses association called the National League of Trained Nurses of Finland whose president for many years has been Kyllikki Pohjala. She has also edited its official magazine, *Sairaanhoita-jalehti* (meaning "Journal of Nursing"). Miss Pohjala has been a member of the Finnish Parliament for many years and has served as a delegate to the United Nations. The two organizations later joined in a federation called the National Council of Nurses of Finland through which both were represented in the International Council of Nurses. They have also united in support of many national projects. The National League has been active in organizing local and provincial branches and in keeping these in touch with each other and with national nursing affairs.

The Nurses Association of Finland, which now has a smaller membership (chiefly from around Helsinki), has had a strong influence in promoting progressive educational and public health nursing programs in this country. Its journal, *Epione,* started in 1908 is named for the Greek wife of Asklepios, god of medicine. One of its outstanding leaders is Venny Snellman, who in 1924 introduced public health nursing in Finland under the auspices of the Mannerheim League and in 1931, when its work was transferred to the government, became head of the new National Division of Nursing. She has been widely recognized in international as well as national nursing circles. Her associate, Tynne Luoma, who succeeded her as head of the division, was its first director of public health nursing. The chief medical officers in the state Department of Health have given excellent support to the recommendations of their nurse associates, and the Parliament even in times of national stringency has recognized the vital contribution of nurses to the national health and morale.

RECENT EDUCATIONAL AND OTHER DEVELOPMENTS

For many years the chief controversial issue between physicians and nurses in Finland was the three-year course. In the earlier days two classes of nurses were prepared, the first taking three years or more and the second from one and one half to two years. After a long battle, state registration was secured in 1929 with a three-year minimum requirement and provision for the inspection of schools. Gradually the shorter programs were eliminated, four central preliminary schools were organized in different sections of the country, and short postgraduate programs for head nurses and public health nurses were provided, all with government support. When larger numbers of qualified educational personnel were available, all the schools (fourteen) were able to give the complete program. Of these, ten were owned and supported by the state, one by a municipality, and three by deaconess organizations. Since World War II, a fine new state school, the Helsinki College of Nursing, which has both basic and postgraduate programs, has been opened in a large modern building. This experimental school helps to develop and try out new plans for the country as a whole and to prepare educational and other specialists for the more responsible positions. The Rockefeller Foundation has given liberal grants to its work and to other nursing and health projects and has awarded many nursing fellowships for study, chiefly in Canada and the United States. Because of the influence of these countries on Finnish nursing, neighboring nurses often called this country "little America of the North."

During the war years of the forties, when Finland was isolated and the nurse shortage was acute, pressure became stronger for a cut in the basic program. Two committees were appointed by the government to consider this question, one composed of nurses and the other of physicians. Meeting as a rule in the early morning before their day's work began, the nurses were the first to present a plan. This was a modified form of the one outlined in the Goldmark Report of 1923 (U. S. A.) In addition to the introduction of a group of attendants or aides, they proposed a twenty-eight month basic curriculum for nurses with an eight-month postbasic option to be selected from such special branches as mental nursing, midwifery, and public health nursing (in some cases the last two combined with a few months added). After graduation and registration and with satisfactory experience, the nurse might take an advanced course in administration or teaching. Though this compromise did not satisfy the other committee, it was accepted as a basis for experimentation. The law as amended in 1957 requires two and one half years for the basic program.

Meanwhile the demand for nurses continued to increase, the estimated need being 1000 graduates each year. The country has a ratio of one nurse to 3000 people, every health district having at least one public health nurse. Though Finland has not gone so far as the rest of northern Europe in adopting socialized medicine, a large proportion of its people is insured through voluntary group plans. All district nursing services and most hospitals are tax supported, as are nearly all schools of nursing. These schools are independent of hospitals and have their own nurse directors, staffs, and budgets. Although the College of Nursing in Helsinki is not affiliated with a university, its educational status is on approximately the same academic level, and its imposing building is a part of the fine new medical center which is one of the architectural sights of this beautiful modern city.

Another unique unit in this group in which nurses have an active interest is the Children's Castle, which grew out of a small institution founded by Sophie Mannerheim for the care of neglected children. This is now housed in a new building for which funds have been raised chiefly by children and their friends. Its work covers a wide variety of nursing, medical, educational, and research activities, all focusing on the study and improvement of child health and welfare. Many other examples could be given of the originality, initiative, and indomitable spirit of the Finnish people. Regardless of their war losses, their insecure position on the Soviet border, and their austere conditions of life, these strong-fibered and courageous northerners go right on caring for their people up to the Arctic Circle and beyond and also planning and building for the future. In the far north where the migrant Laplanders often mix with their own people they have helped to provide needed health services for both groups, also to build rest homes for travelers to this beautiful and picturesque region.

ICELAND

This little island in the North Atlantic, with its scattered population of less than a half million, though self-governing, was under the Danish Crown until 1941 when it became independent. In 1933 its first and only school of nursing was established at the capital at Reykjavik by state law, and in the same year a nurse practice act was passed which automatically registers all graduates of that school. Icelandic nurses go abroad in fairly large numbers to take postgraduate courses.

The Icelandic Nurses Association, founded in 1919, joined the Northern Nurses Union in 1922 and the International Council of Nurses in 1933. Its capable first president, Mrs. Sigridur Thorvaldsen, did much to bring its scattered members (about 260) together, to plan meetings in Reykjavik and in some outlying districts, and to edit its small quarterly the *Icelandic Nursing Review*. Most nurses are employed in the hospitals or in antituberculosis, infant and maternal welfare, and similar programs under the Health Department of Iceland. Public health and social problems have been complicated by the large numbers of foreign troops who were stationed in that country during and after World War II. Though native intelligence is relatively high in Iceland, isolation from other lands has hampered progress in many ways. Air travel has now brought its people much closer to both Europe and North America, and the hope is that these contacts will lead to a freer exchange of nursing and medical personnel and to better opportunities for the professional development of nursing.

Like the English-speaking group of nations, these northern countries possessed many cultural, economic, religious, and political assets that provided a favorable soil and climate for the growth of modern nursing during the last century. Among their peoples were many who responded to the call for nursing service reform, including some outstanding leaders who were recognized and respected in many countries other than their own. They met many of the same obstacles that were encountered by nurses in the English-speaking countries, and although they were willing to learn from others they also had the courage and initiative to experiment along new lines.

SELECTED BIBLIOGRAPHY

Ahla, Mervi. "College of Nursing Helsinki Finland," *Int. Nurs. Rev.*, January 1957, 7-11.

Arnadottir, Thorbjorg. "Nursing in Iceland," *Am. Jo. Nurs.*, April 1950, 22.

Bone, Agnes I. C. "Nurse Training in Denmark," *Nurs. Times*, December 17, 1954, 1407-1408.

Darnell, L. M. "Nursing Schools and Hospitals, in Scandinavia and Finland," *Nurs. Times*, March 3, 1951, 211-217.

Davies, M. "Report on a Visit to Scandinavia during July and August, 1949," *Int. Nurs. Rev.*, Summer 1950, 9-15.

Goff, Hazel Avis. "Report of a Study of Public Health Nursing in Europe," *Int. Coun. Nurses Congress Rep.*, 1933, 156-161.

Hallsten-Kallia, Armé. "International Influences on Nursing in Finland," *Am. Jo. Nurs.*, March 1946, 154-156.

International Council of Nurses. *National Reports. 1933*, 13-15, 16-17, 28-29, 41-42, 49-50; *1947*, 19-23, 24-26, 40-41, 54-57, 62-63; *1949*, 20-24, 25-29, 47-50, 73-76, 80-83; *1957*, 26-29, 30-32, 45-47, 78-80, 90-92; *1961*, 18-20, 22-26, 34-35, 66-67, 77-79.

Madsen, Maria. "The Danish Council of Nurses Through Fifty Years," *Int. Nurs. Bull.*, Autumn and Winter, 1949, 5-8.

Magnussen, Eli. "The Danish Way," *Am. Jo. Nurs.*, August 1960, 1126-1129.

Moriarty, Honora R. *Educating the Nurse in Norway.* Oslo: Akademisk Forlag, 1954.

Nordendahl, Kerstin. "Nursing in Sweden," *Am. Jo. Nurs.*, November 1948, 694-696.

Nutting, M. Adelaide, and Lavinia L. Dock. *A History of Nursing.* New York: Putnam's, 1907-1912. 4 vols. Vol. III, Ch. III.

Reimann, Christianne. "First and Second Nursing Congress of Northern Countries of Europe," *Int. Nurs. Bull.*, January 1924, 25-27.

Schroeder, Ellen Margarette. "Nursing in Denmark," *Am. Jo. Nurs.*, April 1937, 255-260.

[Schwartzenberg, Anna]. "Editorial," *Int. Nurs. Rev.*, July 1946 [1-8].

Spilling, Regnhild, and Gustav Vig. "Public Health Nursing in Norway," *Int. Nurs. Rev.*, May 1957, 37-41.

[Swedish Nurses Association]. *Survey of Advanced Education of Nurses in the Northern Countries Autumn 1952.* [Stockholm]: Swedish Nurs. Assn., 1956.

World Health Organization. *Seminar on Team Work in Nursing Services.* Geneva: WHO, 1955.

CHAPTER 15

Central and Southern Europe

W<small>E</small> <small>NOW</small> turn to the countries where, under the fostering
care of the Church, organized nursing had its origin in
the early centuries of the Christian era. Part I traced the development of several kinds of religious nursing groups, first the
deaconesses, then the monastic and military orders, and following them some of a more democratic and secular organization
such as the Catholic Sisters of Charity and the Lutheran Kaiserswerth Deaconesses. The religious orders with their motherhouses were stronger in this part of Europe than in the north
and had deeper roots. The servant-nurse system which was often
associated with the older hospital orders later became dominant
in municipal and military hospitals. As the trade union movement spread, this group of secular hospital workers consolidated
their position and political influence, making reform extremely
difficult. Other conditions that helped to hold back the new
ideas in nursing that were developing across the Channel from
the 1860's on were the walls of prejudice created by long-standing political, religious, and racial feuds involving Britain and
such powerful continental rivals as Germany and France. The
last two, representing the Teutonic and the Latin races, differed

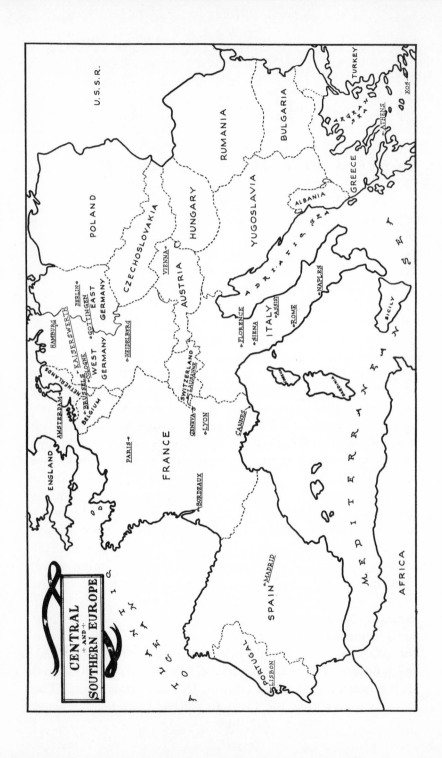

in their national origins, cultures, and racial characteristics as did those of Slavic and other European peoples. Nevertheless, there were many similarities in their nursing systems in modern as in older times.

GERMANY

Germany was a comparatively late arrival among the great powers, but by 1850 it was a strong military nation and a leader in industrial, educational, and other fields. Although it was advanced in many ways, its government and institutions were organized on authoritarian and class lines, and men of the ruling caste who were in all key positions exercised autocratic power. Even in the family women had little opportunity to develop initiative or independence, and in the religious motherhouses priests and pastors held chief authority which extended into the hospitals in which the sisters were employed and often led to controversies between the religious and secular authorities over moral and other questions. Miss Nightingale, who was in close touch with the situation in German secular hospitals, was outspoken in her criticism of the prevailing system and insisted that the whole nursing service should be put under a capable woman matron or superintendent with authority to select, train, and discipline both staff and pupil nurses. Such a plan was unthinkable to most German physicians and hospital administrators of this period, but there were a few notable exceptions. For example, in 1869, a famous German medical leader Rudolf Virchow, in a talk to a women's organization, urged them to help in developing nursing on a strictly secular and humanitarian basis. He advised them to organize schools in all large hospitals, to encourage educated women of high character to enter them for training, and to prepare such nurses for responsible positions in both men's and women's wards.

After 1864, when the German Red Cross was organized, it began to recruit some volunteers from socially prominent families and to give them a brief course in first aid. With the sudden outbreak of the Franco-Prussian War in 1870, military hospitals were soon overflowing. Appalled by the general confusion and loss of life, the Empress Frederick, daughter of Queen Victoria and mother of Kaiser Wilhelm, with her husband's and mother's approval, consulted Miss Nightingale who sent Florence Lees, one of her expert nurses, to give advice and help. The notable success of this able nurse-administrator in reorganizing nursing services led the Empress, on the advice of Miss Nightingale, to interest herself in a plan to prepare young women of good social standing for nursing service on a broad community basis.

With the help of influential German women, the Victoria House, named after the Empress, was established in Berlin in the early '80's. It was similar in many ways to the Sophia Home in Stockholm, opened at about the same time. Both incorporated some elements of the German motherhouse system, and in both nurses in training could apply for membership in a secular sisterhood whose members remained under the head of the school, received a small allowance, and were available for appointment wherever they were needed. Louise Führmann, the first director, who was prepared in London, succeeded after some delay in setting up a connection with a suitable hospital where nursing experience could be secured under the direction of trained head nurses. A similar plan was developed in Erica House, which was connected with the large Eppendorf Hospital in Hamburg and supported by a private association of that city.

The German Red Cross later followed much the same system in reorganizing its nurse training and service on a national basis. It built a number of Red Cross hospitals as well as motherhouses, though in some cases it contracted with large public hospitals to supply their nursing services. These motherhouses which attracted nurses from the better families, gave the Red Cross sisters a dignified and influential position. Though under the control of their *Oberins,* or heads, they had much more freedom than the sisters in religious motherhouses and could join in social and cultural activities, handle their own economic affairs, and even terminate their contracts and seek other positions without incurring the stigma attached to the religious sister who left her motherhouse. Many of these sisters, however, contracted with the Red Cross to remain on its staff for life and were thus assured of care in illness and old age.

The popularity of the secular motherhouses and the growing rigidity and strictness of the deaconess system led the Lutheran Church to develop a new kind of organization, the *Diakonie Verein*. These groups attracted better educated applicants and prepared them for the more responsible posts, chiefly in teaching nursing and social work. Members lived together but were allowed much greater individual freedom than was possible under the deaconesses. Competition for recruits soon became acute, and these organizations also competed for contracts with hospitals and other agencies that employed nurses. It was not unusual to have several groups of sisters belonging to different motherhouses employed in the same institution, each being assigned to its own wards or wings and having little or no contact with the others and no coordination at the top.

THE PROFESSIONAL MOVEMENT IN GERMANY

Toward the end of the nineteenth century both religious and secular motherhouses began to find serious difficulties in supporting their members through life, and this led to an exodus of nurses who sought greater economic security as well as more freedom. These free or "wild" sisters, as they were sometimes called, then began to compete in the open market with the domestic or practical nurses. They were severely criticized by religious and other groups but were fortunate in finding an able sympathetic friend and leader in Sister Agnes Karll. She herself had left her Red Cross Motherhouse, believing that the whole system was economically unsound, since it could not produce and support enough nurses for the needs of a powerful and growing nation. Sister Agnes also held that it tended to isolate nurses from each other and to produce too many immature "shut-in" personalities. Endowed with statesmanlike vision, keen intellectual powers, and a boundless love of humanity, she was also an unusually able organizer. Coming to the nurses' help at the same time with sympathy and support were prominent members of the new woman's movement, then becoming active in Germany, and looking on sympathetically but still unknown to the German nurses were the nursing leaders in other countries who in 1899 had begun to organize internationally.

Many bitter and distressing articles written by nurses and sisters had appeared in print, and Sister Agnes Karll had concluded that, unheard of as it was in Germany at that time, nurses must unite outside the motherhouses to remedy these conditions. She consulted some of the suffrage leaders and was invited by them to one of their annual meetings, where it was agreed that "the only practical remedy for all abuses is self-organization." At that historic meeting the entire nursing situation was discussed, and the feminists promised their moral support to the nurses in their efforts to organize themselves professionally. The majority of nurses, however, opposed this step, the matron of a large Red Cross hospital expressing the typical conservative view that "nursing uncontrolled by motherhouses, is impossible." Nevertheless, in 1903 the German Nurses Association was founded. In 1906 it started its journal, *Unterm Lazarus Kreutz,* a militant organ ably edited by Sister Agnes Karll. The next year was to see the International Council of Women meeting in Berlin and with it the International Council of Nurses. At this congress the German association entered the international bond and found a warm welcome from other pioneers, most of whom had been going through a similar struggle, though none more dramatic and stirring.

The German nurses, who had so difficult a step to take in organization, carried registration through in a surprisingly short time and with comparatively little opposition. Legal regulation was in harmony with German ideas, and the disorder in nursing standards had become notorious. For example, there had been practicing nurses who could claim "examination by a physician" after a few weeks' lecture course. In 1905 the Federal Council accepted the draft of an Act regulating the practice of nursing for the German Empire, and in 1907 it went into effect in Prussia under the Minister of Education. Though elementary, it put an end to irresponsible short courses and encouraged more thorough training. In Germany as a whole, however, persons with the required hospital experience who passed the state examination could still be registered whether or not they had entered a school and received regular training. The medical men who signed such certificates approving the holder's competence had the final decision in such cases.

Small as it was, the German Nurses Association did much progressive, constructive work. It produced the evidence which led to a careful study and publication of the facts about the serious health conditions among religious and secular nurses due to pathological fatigue and the high mortality in these groups from tuberculosis, cardiac conditions, mental breakdowns, and suicide. Public agitation finally brought governmental intervention and some improvement in hours and working conditions. A learned scientific report, *Overstrain among Nurses,* presented by a German physician, Dr. Hecker, at the Cologne Congress of the International Council of Nurses in 1912, made a deep impression on those who attended and led many to push for better health conditions for nurses in their own countries. The congress with its impressive setting and striking pageants was an artistic as well as a professional success and attracted large groups of nurses from Germany and other countries. This marked the highest peak of the professional nursing movement in Germany.

PERIOD OF DISORGANIZATION AND REGIMENTATION

During the war of 1914-1918 many shortcuts and compromises were made in nurse training and service. Conditions were more chaotic in the postwar period when political disorder and disastrous inflation led to a serious crisis in hospitals and health services. Many free-lance nurses were unemployed, and those who clung to the motherhouses for shelter and some degree of security often received only subsistence. At this time the state welfare program was greatly expanded to care for the growing numbers of dependents, especially the war orphans and foundlings. Workers in this field were called *Fuersorgerinnen* (from the word *Fuersorge,* meaning to care). They were part nurse and part social worker and had a year or more of training in a school of social work and about the same in a hospital. Many nurses and young people interested in nursing took up this work. District or public health nursing, as developed in Britain and America, had little place in Germany or in other countries of central Europe and the line between nursing and social work was almost indistinguishable. This was true also of nursing and housework, the care of healthy children, certain kinds of police and prison reform duties, and medical technology. The preparation of nurses reflected this lack of a clear definition of what constitutes nursing. The death of Sister Agnes Karll shortly after the war was a serious blow to the professional movement in German nursing, and though her followers kept the German Nurses Association alive through the difficult period that followed no real progress was made.

Under the Hitler regime, which began in 1933, a new Nazi nursing sisterhood, popularly called the "Brown Sisters" was organized and attracted many of the Führer's devoted followers. Then in 1937 all nurses' organizations were absorbed into the totalitarian state, which became the chief employer for all kinds of health and welfare services. Nurses who did not belong to one of the four large motherhouse groups (the Roman Catholic, Deaconess, Red Cross, and Nazi sisterhoods) were required to join a miscellaneous fifth group, the Association of Independent Sisters and Attendants, which included those in Sister Agnes Karll's Association. The only concession made was that women nurses were classed with other women workers, whereas men nurses were under the control of an industrial union. All were regimented under political leaders and worked under their orders. Political orthodoxy became a dominant factor in obtaining and holding positions, and those who did not conform often lost their posts. Although more uniform standards of preparation were framed into a new nursing law that covered the whole country, the minimum standard was low, and all schools, including those of the Red Cross, were under the direction of men physicians. The former matrons became their assistants. Only eighteen months' training was required at first (later two years), and for a good part of this time the trainee might serve as a mother's helper in a private home. Instruction was to cover 200 hours and was based on one specified text book.

POSTWAR REORGANIZATION

Some optimists hoped that the enforced union of the different nursing groups at this time might lead to a more permanent self-governing national organization, but after the Nazis' defeat the former motherhouse groups withdrew into their own closed circles and most of the free sisters were too disorganized and disillusioned to take much interest in uniting. This was difficult in any case because of the division of Germany into four zones under British, French, American, and Russian control. A few followers of Sister Agnes Karll revived the German Nurses Association under the name Agnes Karll Verband. This group also began to discuss plans for a general reorganization of nursing, and with the encouragement and help of leading nurses of the Western occupation forces some conferences were arranged. In 1948 the German Nurses Federation was formed to include the Agnes Karll group and nurses from the Red Cross and *Diakonie* Societies, but the religious motherhouse groups as well as a number who had joined trade unions remained outside. With the help referred to, the federation succeeded in building the nucleus of a professional group that began to assume some responsibility for nursing leadership in the new Germany. The membership of professional nurses (1958) was 21,000. Legislation for nurses then varied with the locality, but some new laws intended to raise nursing standards were passed.

The federation was admitted to the International Council of Nurses in 1949 at the Stockholm Congress, and German nurses were welcomed back to the international circle which their early leaders had helped to form. The federation's president was Erna von Abendroth, a well-educated German nurse with a doctor's degree in economics, who was director of the Werner Schule, formerly located near Berlin and now connected with the University of Göttingen. This school, developed earlier by the German Red Cross, offered courses for graduate nurses who were preparing for positions of leadership in teaching and administration. In the early '50's a modern collegiate school of nursing was opened at the University of Heidelberg with the assistance of the Rockefeller Foundation. It had a well-qualified faculty, most of whom had been sent to Canada or the United States for special preparation and its director was Oberin von Lersner. This first independent nursing school in Germany, had some difficulty in securing support from many German nurses who considered it too modern. It admitted well-educated girls and provided a broad and sound basic program on a university level as well as postgraduate programs in nursing education and public health nursing. The plan was to develop leaders to further the progress of modern nursing in Germany. Recent reports from West Germany indicate other gains in basic education, such as better selection of students, longer preliminary periods, payment of tuition, and longer programs in some schools.

As to the future of modern nursing in this country, much depends on the strengthening of its democratic forces and on the success of nurses in gaining greater freedom and more individual responsibility. An encouraging sign of wider interest in education was the formation in 1953 of the German Committee of the Florence Nightingale International Foundation. Its first project was a study of Florence Nightingale and her ideas concerning nursing and the raising of funds for scholarships to enable some German nurses to study abroad. How far the motherhouse pattern can be integrated into the new structure is still a vital question. Without some modification of the powerful position of the heads of the various motherhouses and the national motherhouse organizations there would seem to be little chance for professional nurses to achieve either unity or independence. A significant development in this direction was the passage in 1957 of a new Nursing Law which provided for the education and practice of nursing on a national basis.

Little is known of the nursing situation in Eastern Germany, but indications point to much the same kind of reorganization that has gone on in the other countries of eastern Europe under the communist system, discussed in Chapter 16.

AUSTRIA

The Austrians, though closely related to the Germans in language and culture, are less homogeneous in their racial components and more cosmopolitan in their outlook and interests. They also are considered more easygoing and lighthearted than their strenuous and efficient neighbors. Though there is little difference in the general patterns of nursing in the two countries, Austria has more Roman Catholic nursing sisters and fewer deaconesses. The majority of religious sisters, as well as of Red Cross nurses and hospital attendants until quite recent times have had comparatively little systematic training.

The first modern school of nursing in Austria was the Rudolfinerhaus in Vienna, founded in 1902 through the interest of the famous Viennese surgeon Theodor Bilroth. Like the Sophia Home in Stockholm and the Victoria House in Berlin, it had some of the characteristics of a secular motherhouse and of the Nightingale School in London. Like them, it attracted a superior group of applicants who received their practical experience in a private hospital, one of the few built especially for use as a nursing school adjunct. The fact that this institution has apparently retained its prestige through all the ups and downs of the past years is a tribute to its founders. Most of the large public hospitals in Austria at the time of its founding were staffed by nurses who had little but practical training. In 1914 a nurse registration law was passed, but since it did not require a systematic course of training its effect on national standards was not very great.

After World War I, when Austria suffered from a serious food shortage and high mortality rate, especially among the large number of war orphans and illegitimate children, American public health nurses headed by Alma Haupt and Hortense Hilbert were sent over under the Commonwealth Fund to help organize a public health nursing service in Vienna. They found some willing and intelligent helpers who cooperated actively in the services established. Most of these services were of the *Fuersorgerinnen* type with a combined training of elementary nursing and social work which was then considered the best preparation for work of this kind. Some of these later rounded out their nursing training in Britain and America.

One important postwar development was the famous *Kinderclinic* built up with the aid of foreign friends by the renowned child specialist Professor von Pirquet and his able nurse assistant Hedwig Birkner. This became a widely known teaching and demonstration center that attracted doctors and nurses from Austria and other countries. Dr. Julius Tandler, Director of the Department of Health in Vienna also gave staunch support to modern plans which emphasized health teaching and prevention as a part of the nurses' preparation.

PROFESSIONAL AND EDUCATIONAL DEVELOPMENTS

In 1933 a small group of nurses, including some who had studied or worked in other countries, formed the Trained Nurses Association of Austria which joined the International Council of Nurses in 1935. Fredericka Zehtner, Superintendent of Nurses at the Rudolfinerhaus, was especially active in promoting this organization. A few years later when Austria was absorbed by Nazi Germany, the group was dissolved. After the collapse of Germany, Austria regained its identity as a separate nation but not for some time its full freedom and economic stability. In 1947 the League of Red Cross Societies sent one of its field representatives, Lilli Petschnigg, to Austria to help rehabilitate as far as possible the nurses and nursing services of the Red Cross and other groups. By remaining there for more than a year and working first with one group then with another she was able to bring nurses together in conferences and study groups. In 1948 it was decided to reorganize the Trained Nurses Association, with Oberin Marie Strobl of the Rudolfspital as president. Its members were required to meet the minimum state qualifications specified in the new nursing law of 1949 (two years' systematic training), irrespective of their political, religious, racial, or social status or motherhouse affiliations. In the following year the Association had 2000 members and a national magazine under the name *Die Krankenschwester,* the nurses of each province being responsible in turn for one monthly issue. Committees were appointed to study nursing conditions and to make plans for the future.

Recent reports indicate that active nurses are about evenly divided between religious and lay groups. The motherhouse system predominated in both groups and such houses received more applications than they could accept. Since the majority of Austrian nuns then had no formal training as nurses, schools were set up especially for them. Other schools were opened by the Red Cross and by the provinces, many at first on a rather insecure economic and educational basis. The Red Cross schools qualify nurses for state diplomas and also prepare nursing aides. Their motherhouses, in addition to supplying nurses for civilian hospitals, enter into contracts with the military to provide a certain proportion of their personnel for service in time of war. Plans have been made to offer postgraduate courses to those who are to hold administrative posts in civil and military institutions and to send some nurses abroad on scholarships or through exchanges with other countries.

Faced with serious conditions and forces tending to discourage and disorganize nurses and to keep them separated into many different groups, the Trained Nurses Association of Austria has shown remarkable initiative, courage, and leadership. It has not only united the scattered groups of nurses but has taken steps to improve their educational and economic status and to meet the nursing needs of the country at a time of great hardship and uncertainty. The contribution of the League of Red Cross Societies as well as of the Austrian Red Cross was an important factor in the success of this undertaking.

SWITZERLAND

Protected by its high mountains and by its policy of neutrality, this small country has managed to keep out of European wars and to maintain its independence for centuries. It is composed of three main sections, which were originally parts of Germany, France, and Italy. The inhabitants of these sections have retained the language and many of the characteristics and customs of these respective countries. Since the German section is much the largest, the influence of Germany has been greater, especially in such matters as health and education. Switzerland is further divided into twenty-two cantons, or states, which are almost completely autonomous, some of them being situated in remote valleys where people have little contact with the outside world. This has made it difficult to bring about anything like uniformity in institutions, customs, and laws. The latter are written and enforced almost entirely by the individual cantons. Actually the Federal Government of this republic has little power except with respect to military defense and external affairs. This helps to explain the long delay in giving Swiss women the vote as well as some of the peculiar features of the nursing system and the difficulties met by Swiss nurses in achieving control of their preparation and standards.

EARLY NURSING SCHOOLS

All the traditional systems of nursing found in the rest of Europe were represented here in 1850 and still can be found in some parts of the country. The first attempt to modernize nursing was made in 1859 in Lausanne, when Count and Countess de Gasparin founded and endowed the Normal Evangelical School for Free nurses (usually called *La Source*). Their purpose was to demonstrate that secular nurses without vows could give service as good as that of nuns or deaconesses. Though Miss Nightingale's plan for nurse training had been announced before this and had influenced it, the Nightingale School in London did not actually open until a year later. Like it, *La Source* accepted only applicants of good character and family background and required them to live in a training home under a woman head. One important difference was that here the system of training was put under a medical man who not only directed the teaching but, with the cooperation of some of his colleagues, provided nursing practice and supervision in the homes of their patients. Shortly after the start a small children's ward was set up in the nurses' home under a nurse who taught the students before they were sent out to care for private patients. Later the school was put under the Swiss Red Cross, and though its graduates took increasing responsibility for teaching and supervision in both homes and hospitals the director continued until 1952 to be either a physician or a clergyman.[1]

Another pioneer school, the *Bon Secours,* was founded in Geneva in 1905 by a social-minded woman physician, Dr. Champandal, to provide a visiting nurse service for babies of poor families. The first students were daughters of her friends who became interested in her work. These girls paid fees, lived in a common home, and were trained for community service, much of their experience being in homes and small clinics, where they worked directly under physicians. At the founder's death, the school became the property of the Association of the Old Students (Alumnae), the only nursing school known to operate under such a group.

These two schools, both supported by private individuals or agencies, had little contact with each other or with the larger public hospitals, where for centuries nursing had been carried on by deaconesses or Roman Catholic sisters or by paid workers, both men and women. Though the employees in the Swiss hospitals were in general of a better class than the servant-nurses in neighboring countries at that time, no national or cantonal standards for nurses existed until the Swiss Red Cross was entrusted by the Federal Government with the task of securing quotas of nursing personnel from the various cantons to serve with the national army in case of mobilization. A Red Cross Commission of prominent citizens, all men, then set up a few qualifications and gave its Red Cross diploma to those they considered eligible. The same diploma was given to nurses prepared by schools and to others certified only by hospital physicians. One general textbook which might or might not be supplemented by a few medical lectures was the basis for the brief examination prescribed. Though the schools received a nominal sum proportionate to the numbers of nurses they were able to provide for the national service, there was no inspection

---

[1] As noted in Chapter 11 Dr. Alfred Worcester followed the general *La Source* plan in setting up the Waltham School in Massachusetts in 1885.

of such schools and no effort was made to improve or unify their standards. Indeed, the Swiss Red Cross apparently gave more attention to the preparation of voluntary aides than to the education of well-qualified nurses.

BEGINNINGS OF PROFESSIONAL ORGANIZATION

In 1910 the Swiss Red Cross Committee on its own initiative formed an Association of Red Cross nurses, with physicians as officers. The chief purpose of this group was to prepare for war or other national emergencies. Apparently, the Swiss trained nurses did not become aware of the international professional movement until around 1925 when the office of the International Council of Nurses was set up in Geneva. Finding that membership in the Red Cross Association did not admit them to the International Council of Nurses, a few leading nurses decided to organize the National Association of Nurses of Registered Training Schools, which set up its own requirements and list of schools whose graduates might apply. This association, under its president, Miss Hofmann, joined the ICN in 1937 and was just beginning to function actively when World War II broke out.

With the mobilization of the army and the nurse reserves, the marked inequality of standards and the lack of unity in Swiss nursing became more apparent. The need for greater uniformity in the training of nurses led to a union of the two groups in the Swiss Trained Nurses Association. For a short period membership was open to members of both the organizations mentioned with the understanding that from then on all trained nurses in Switzerland would be prepared in duly approved schools of nursing. The *Bulletin des Gardes Malades,* which had started in 1906 under a medical editor, was taken over as the organ of the new association and edited by a nurse. Membership in the ICN was extended to the new association in place of the original member. (The name was later changed to the Swiss Association of Graduate Nurses, which is composed of several different groups.)

One of the primary objects of the Trained Nurses Association was to secure for organized nurses a more responsible role in determining the educational and professional standards of nursing in Switzerland. As a first step toward that goal, an agreement was reached with the Swiss Red Cross whereby a Red Cross Nursing Committee was constituted, with equal representation from the Red Cross and the Nurses Association. Under the able leadership of its first president, Monika Wuest, the association made great strides toward its long held object of becoming the official spokesman for the nursing profession in Switzerland. Concurrently, an important step was taken by the Red Cross to award the Red Cross diploma only to fully qualified graduates of approved schools of nursing. Organized nurses then began to work for regular inspection of schools and better educational programs. By 1946 there were 20 schools with 1200 students, and much had been done to bring about more uniform standards. Though no federal nursing law has been passed in Switzerland, there is now an intercantonal covenant approved by the Federal Government, and directors of public health ratify nurses' diplomas as being valid in all cantons.

An important development in 1950 was the founding by the Swiss Red Cross of a postgraduate school, its purpose being to prepare nurses for the more responsible positions in Swiss nursing. This was located in Zurich, and its first director was Monika Wuest. Another step forward was the reorganization of the *Bon Secours* School in Geneva. With the aid of its own graduates, the Rockefeller Foundation, and other friends, this old school established close relations with the University of Geneva as well as with the state authorities in education and health and developed a broadened clinical program which emphasized public health nursing throughout. Marjorie Duvillard, a well-educated alumna who had been nursing consultant in South America for three years, returned in 1948 to direct this school, which is an outstanding example of the more recent trends in nursing education. Another Swiss nurse who did a great deal to forward all these projects was Yvonne Hentsch, who has held for many years an important position as head of the Nursing Division of the League of Red Cross Societies, with headquarters in

Geneva. More details of the work of the League are given in Chapter 20.

THE NETHERLANDS

This is one of the Low Countries, lying between Germany and France, which are close neighbors also of Britain and of the Scandinavian countries. Holland and Belgium, at one time united, have faced many disasters from war and natural calamities. Although they have been influenced by their neighbors, especially by Germany, France, and Britain, they have developed a distinct individuality of their own. This is apparent in their nursing history, which presents many examples of the stubborn fighting spirit and independent attitude of their people.

In the middle of the nineteenth century the nursing situation in Holland was much like that in other parts of Europe. No reforms were undertaken, apparently, until 1874 when a group of liberal-minded philanthropists formed the White Cross Association of North Holland. One of the committees had for its object the training of women nurses of good character and education outside religious motherhouses. In 1879 these men, on the advice of a pioneer feminist who was trying to find suitable fields of work for educated women, sent a few candidates for experience and training to an Amsterdam hospital. As in other places where the reformers had no control over the physical and moral conditions within the hospital, this experiment failed. In the early '90's a new attempt was made by Miss Reynvaan, a distinguished lady of high birth and humanitarian ideals. Impressed by the example of Miss Nightingale, she took the post of matron in the Wilhelmina Hospital in Amsterdam, and with the support of a progressive superintendent cleaned up some of the worst conditions. Most hospitals, however, refused to make the changes needed to attract a better class of women nurses and to give them proper status and training. The liberals continued their efforts, and to meet their criticism the more conservative hospital and medical groups formed in 1892 the Association for

Sick Nursing (known as the *Bond*). Matrons and some practicing nurses were allowed to join but had little voice or influence in shaping its policies.

Organization Under Nurse Leadership

When the Matron's Council in Britain was planning for the organization meeting of the International Council of Nurses in 1899, Miss Reynvaan and another nurse from Holland were invited. The year following a self-governing society of nurses called *Nosokomis* (the Greek word for nurse) was formed in that country with the support of leading feminists and of a few sympathetic physicians. Mrs. Aletrina, the first president, like Mrs. Fenwick, was married to a physician who championed the nurses' cause and gave valuable help in launching the association and editing its journal (also called *Nosokomis*). The Aletrinas attracted the interest of another well-educated and gifted nurse, J. C. Van Lanschot Hubrecht, who took on the work of secretary. In 1909, as president, she led *Nosokomis* into the International Council of Nurses and became an active member of the small group of "dynamos" that piloted the international nursing movement in its early days. A special feature of *Nosokomis* was that it excluded hospital matrons because its leaders considered this group too closely identified with the *Bond* to give active support in their fight against long hours, poor teaching, and overwork.

Though small in size, *Nosokomis* accomplished much because of its militant spirit, direct aims, and persistent efforts. In addition to its attacks on bad economic conditions, it developed its own system of examinations, translated and published textbooks, circulated a professional library, conducted courses for graduate nurses, and urged that nursing schools be put under the Minister of Education. In 1907 the government was finally induced to consider the registration question, and the *Bond* then took the lead in opposing the movement using many of the same arguments that the British Hospitals Association was then using in its antiregistration campaign. A registration law was finally passed in 1921, and the progressives, though not satisfied with all its details, accepted it as a fair beginning. They then showed a magnanimous spirit in deciding to replace *Nosokomis* by a larger and more inclusive organization of registered nurses called the National Association of Nurses of the Netherlands.

The International Council of Nurses accepted the new association on condition that only nurses with full general training would be active voting members. This meant that a large proportion of nurses whose preparation was entirely in mental hospitals could join only as associate members. Gradually, however, many of them qualified in other clinical fields and the majority of schools broadened their programs. As in Sweden, the ratio of untrained or partly trained to registered nurses was high in Holland. Although the majority of the registered nurses were employed in hospitals or in private nursing, a few began to branch out into public health work, chiefly in specialized tuberculosis, school, and infant-welfare programs. Others took up different forms of social and health work, including programs for delinquent girls and women which led some to qualify also as policewomen.

Until quite recently the government had sent many nurses to the Netherlands Indies where they helped to establish hospital and health work and to train Indonesian nurses. With the loss of the colonies, most of these nurses returned home and had to be readjusted to life and work in Holland. Before 1947 nurses from the Netherlands took postgraduate courses in Great Britain, United States, and elsewhere and led in developing new educational and service programs. In that year graduate courses of one to two years were developed at home, through the efforts of the National Nurses Association of the Netherlands, in preparation for more advanced positions in executive, teaching, and public health work.

It was evident that this organization had inherited the vigorous pioneering spirit of *Nosokomis,* though the high aims of that group were not all realized. During the hard and dangerous war years it had to suspend its activities and to conform to the new order of the Nazi invaders. Since that period, it has concerned itself chiefly with problems of reconstruction, the nurse shortage, and its contributing causes, which were largely economic. Strengthened by their new rights as citizens, nurses appealed to the government and were advised to join other nurses' groups, including the unions, in their efforts to secure better hours, salaries, and general working conditions. A federation of professional and nonprofessional nurses' organizations was formed, with Miss Menalda, then president of the National Nurses Association, as its head. The appointment of a leading nurse to the Ministry of Health to give special attention to these and other important matters and the interest of a sympathetic Minister of Health greatly improved the prospects for effective action on long-standing economic and educational problems. Among other changes, the Ministry prepared a new national law governing the practice of nurses which also provided for improvements in the scheme of nurse education.

BELGIUM

Whereas the people of the Netherlands are relatively homogeneous in race and culture and predominantly Protestant in religion, the Belgians belong to two distinct ethnic groups and are bilingual. The French-speaking Walloons are closely related to the Latin peoples in culture and religion, and the Flemish-speaking to the Dutch and Germanic. Though often incompatible, these two groups in Belgium have shown a high degree of loyalty to their country and ability to work together in times of need.

From 1850 to 1900 nursing conditions were definitely backward, though a few attempts had been made by interested physicians to give lectures to the uneducated hospital attendants and even to introduce matrons into some of the public hospitals. The modern movement was started in 1907, when Dr. Depage, a prominent and progressive Brussels physician, whose wife was also deeply interested in nursing, decided to establish the Belgian School of Certified Nurses on English lines and applied to the London Hospital for a trained matron to head it. Edith Cavell, who was to become internationally renowned for her tragic fate and noble example in World War I, was the nurse sent, and the school was later named for her and for Marie Depage who perished in the Titanic disaster. In the ten years that Miss Cavell gave to nursing in Belgium, she met much opposition, chiefly because of her foreign origin, her strict English discipline, and the long four-year hospital training required in her school. However, with the support of Dr. Depage and a group of medical and hospital friends who stood with him, the school continued its work.

In 1908 their opponents succeeded in securing a royal decree creating an official nurse certificate which was to be given to anyone with or without practical training or experience who passed a government examination. Dr. Depage and his friends immediately organized a Federation of Training Schools for Nurses, which consisted of a few hospitals whose boards were willing to open their wards for nurse training under certain stipulated conditions. The federation then began, with Miss Cavell's aid, to lay down a suitable program of combined practice and theory and to help the hospitals to organize the new system. Most of these hospitals were run by nuns, who then started to prepare themselves for their new responsibilities. Shortly after (1913), the federation secured another royal decree requiring at least one year of hospital training for nurses and giving higher recognition to those with two or three years more.

The new plan was just getting started when Belgium was invaded and World War I began. Many daughters of leading Belgian families volunteered for service in military and civil hospitals, the Belgian Queen and some of her ladies-in-waiting setting an example. Contact with the trained nurses who came from several countries to help led some of these volunteers to round out their preparation for the state examination and to become professional nurses. One of these, Countess D'Ursell, later took postgraduate work in New York and became one of the leaders in Belgian nursing.

A major influence in her own and other schools continued to be Edith Cavell's example and her last letter to her Belgian nurses urging them to carry on the work they had started together and giving them her motherly blessing before she went out to face the firing squad. This letter included the widely quoted message, "I realize that patriotism is not enough. I must have no hatred or bitterness toward anyone." Her own country honored her with a statue in London, one of the four then commemorating famous women, of whom two were nurses (the other, Florence Nightingale), and two were queens (Anne and Victoria).

PROFESSIONAL ORGANIZATION AND RECENT DEVELOPMENTS

Belgian nurses showed their initiative and professional spirit when they began to organize as a self-governing group first in Brussels (1918) and four years later in the country as a whole. The National Federation of Belgian Nurses joined the International Council of Nurses in the same year, and in 1933 the Federation and the French nurses' association were joint hostesses to the ICN congress, which met for half the week in Paris and the other half in Brussels. Their official magazine *L'Infirmière,* and most of their other literature, is published in French and Flemish. The two groups have cooperated well, and the religious sisters in nursing have worked closely with the lay nurses. Like the Beguines of Flanders who helped to initiate the secular orders in the twelfth century, they realized that nursing must be adjusted to the conditions and needs of the times and have taken their full share in the work for professional advancement.

With the aid of educational and public health groups and substantial contributions from the Rockefeller Foundation, a modern school of nursing was established in connection with the University of Brussels and its Medical School and the large Saint Pierre Hospital. This provided both basic and postgraduate programs and was directed for many years by Cècile Mechelynck, an exceptionally dynamic and well-prepared nurse. The Edith Cavell-Marie Depage Institute (successor to the pioneer school) carried on a modern program under Mlle Marie Bihet, one of the school's capable graduates, who was elected president of the ICN in 1953. There is also a well-established normal school at the University of Louvain, where selected nuns and lay nurses are prepared to direct and teach in nursing schools. The Government of Belgium in 1957 gave special recognition to nursing by establishing a Higher Council of Nursing Schools in its Ministry of Public Health and by providing for representation for training school directors and professional organizations.

At that time, by Royal decree, nursing education was integrated into the general structure of public education and nursing was "reclassed" on a higher educational level. By this means the general entrance requirements were raised, the basic program was extended, and additional preparation in certain fields was provided for graduate nurses. These provisions, effective in 1960, gave the schools an opportunity to prepare for the changes. Nursing schools also received government grants on the same basis as other schools. Although in 1956 there were forty-six approved schools with an average of more than 70 students each, Belgium like most other countries suffered from a shortage of nurses. To meet this deficiency, a group of practical nurses was introduced under the title *garde de malade,* and a course covering four months of regular instruction and one year of practical experience in a hospital was established.

In recent years postbasic courses in public health nursing, midwifery, psychiatry, administration, and teaching have been developed. In 1939 the University of Louvain began offering an advanced course of two academic years leading to a degree for nurse instructors, and the University of Brussels, assisted by the Rockefeller Foundation, has offered similar courses. Also, studies have been undertaken in the field of public health nursing.

World War II again disrupted the life of the country, disorganized nursing, and led to serious economic and other problems. The National Federation of Belgian Nurses was suspended, and all nurses were compelled to join the Union of Manual and Intellectual Workers. When they were again free, the various groups of nurses went back to their prewar status. In 1945 a National Congress of Belgian Nurses met in Brussels and the whole nursing situation was freely discussed, especially the relationship between the professional nursing group and the government union, which included nurses and other personnel engaged in health and social work. The union group had helped to raise salaries and improve hours and conditions of work in nursing and to look after the economic and legal rights of its members. Since it did not engage in political activity and was in general sympathy with the ethical and educational objectives of the non-union National Federation of Belgian Nurses, the federation agreed to broaden its membership to include nurse members of the government union in the hope that it would lead to more effective measures for the material and professional security of all nurses in Belgium.

This trend toward a closer relationship between the nurses' associations and the free unions will be noted in some other European countries. It was one of the topics discussed at the conferences in Brussels arranged by the Belgian Federation the following year (1946), when nurses of Holland, France, and Switzerland met with them. The formation of the Western European Group was an outcome of this conference. Like the Northern Nurses Union, it is a regional organization that functions within the general framework of the International Council of Nurses and meets between congresses. Standing for the same principles it is concerned with the same kind of problems as the larger organization and helps to keep the national groups in touch with the ICN. Since the first meeting, the group has been enlarged to include representatives of other ICN member associations in the part of Europe discussed in this chapter.

LUXEMBOURG

This small nation has no complete nursing system of its own. Most of its nurses were trained in surrounding countries, especially in Belgium, with which it is closely related. As in most other Roman Catholic countries, the nuns have an important place in its nursing service. The small National Association of Trained Nurses and Social Workers, after having had affiliate status in the International Council of Nurses for many years, was accepted into full membership in 1953 as the Luxembourg

Nurses Association. There are no schools of nursing in Luxembourg, but a system of registration was established by law in 1935. In 1956 there were more than a hundred nurses on the list. Nursing here functions under the Ministry of Health.

FRANCE

This country was one of the leaders of western European civilization and among the first to begin to question the feudal and authoritarian concepts of the medieval world and to adopt a more democratic and liberal form of government. Yet the struggle between the absolute power of royalty, nobility, and clergy on the one hand, and the rights of the common man on the other continued both before and after the French Revolution which split the country. Since then France has had periodic swings toward radicalism and reaction with recurrent outbreaks of anticlericalism which resulted in the expulsion of many of the older religious orders from public hospitals and educational institutions and their replacement by lay nurses, men and women. Drawn chiefly at first from the proletarian forces, this group had a strong political influence which has persisted into modern times. The Sisters of Charity were unmolested during the Revolution because of their popularity with the common people, and some of the other orders returned later, but the civil authorities remained in control of public hospitals, and in Paris and some other cities the religious orders did not regain their old position. The Church, meanwhile, imposed more rigid regulations on its own sisterhoods, which did not tend to improve the general nursing situation.

First Efforts to Reform Hospital Nursing

Some leading public officials and physicians had made some attempt at reorganization and reform before the Franco-Prussian War (1870) but with very little success. Interest in nursing was then roused by groups of women volunteers who served in military hospitals and later did some work in local communities. The French Red Cross united and absorbed several of these voluntary groups and initiated a brief teaching program which led to a certificate qualifying the holders to become superintendents and sisters in military hospitals in case of war. The course of lectures given to them by physicians was accompanied by some observation in wards and operating rooms and a little practice in dispensaries but no actual experience in the nursing of hospital patients. Indeed, these institutions were considered unsuitable places for ladies, a point of view which lingered on into the twentieth century.

In the '70's Dr. Bourneville, a liberal-minded and sincerely democratic Paris physician, started to organize a regular teaching program for nurses in the public hospitals. He had read about the reforms in English nursing and had visited a London hospital where he saw the Nightingale system in action. Having great faith in formal education, he stressed lectures by physicians and the study of a textbook which he prepared himself. The lectures were given in four centers and were open not only to employees of the Paris hospitals but to outsiders who wished to attend. Nurses' certificates were awarded to those who qualified by attendance and examination. Applicants who could not read or write were given lessons by school teachers, and those who had no hospital experience were allowed the privilege of walking the hospital wards and seeing some nursing demonstrations. Dr. Bourneville, who continued to fight for his scheme, also helped to bring about some improvements in working conditions, hours, wages, and the like. But without a reorganization of nursing administration and firm support from hospital administrators and physicians in cleaning up the bad physical and moral conditions in the hospitals, no appreciable advance was made.

Early Modern Schools

It was not until 1901 that the Nightingale system was introduced in France by Dr. Anna Hamilton, a physician whose dramatic story has been told more fully in *The History of Nurs-*

ing.[2] This nursing reformer was seriously handicapped by the fact that she was half British by birth, a Protestant with feminist leanings, and an outspoken critic of the nursing system in French civil and religious hospitals. Her troubles started when as a medical student she chose the subject of hospital nursing for her final thesis and raised such a controversy in the medical faculty that she nearly lost her degree. The publication of her thesis under the title *Les Gardes-Malades Congrégationistes Mercenaires Professionelle, Amateurs,* brought bitter attacks from religious, lay, and medical circles. The fact that Dr. Hamilton praised the English system and advocated its adoption in France was especially resented. Nevertheless, she was determined to demonstrate its effectiveness and accepted a position as superintendent of a small Protestant hospital in Bordeaux, where she set up a school (later named for Florence Nightingale) under the direction of an English-trained matron, Catharine Elston. This plan had the support of the mayor of Bordeaux, Dr. Lande, a physician who decided to set up a similar school in one of his municipal hospitals. Although these two schools attracted a number of superior applicants, including some of the Roman Catholic faith, and brought about a marked improvement in nursing and hospital work in a few centers, the British system which stressed practical work and strict discipline never became popular in France nor in most other Latin countries.

Such reforms, however, did help to arouse the interest of influential leaders in organizing two private schools of nursing for well-educated French girls. The first, founded in 1900 by a group of teachers and philanthropists, was popularly known as the Rue Amyot and was directed by Mme Alphen Salvador. The second, founded in 1905, was owned and directed by Mlle Leonie Chaptal, member of a distinguished family quite influential in government, church, and social circles. Though more a social worker than a nurse, she became a recognized leader of French nursing and soon identified herself with the professional group then becoming active in the International

[2] By Mary Adelaide Nutting and Lavinia L. Dock (New York: G. P. Putnam's Sons, 1907-1912). Vol. III, Chapter IV.

Council of Nurses. Both schools were located in Paris and had attractive residences and well-organized theoretical programs. Their chief weakness was that they offered very little practical experience or even observation in hospitals and failed to exert much influence on the city institutions where nursing conditions were still backward.

In 1905 the conflict between Church and State again became acute, and an edict was issued which separated religious and secular functions and powers and resulted in the expulsion of many religious orders from hospitals and the departure of large numbers to other countries. The civil authorities of Paris and some leading medical men then began to give serious consideration to the training of secular nurses in their own municipal institutions under the *Assistance Publique* of Paris. In 1907 they announced the opening of the new Salpetrière Hospital in which they planned to establish a nursing college. This notice attracted the attention of Mrs. Fenwick and other leaders in the International Council of Nurses, and a conference was arranged with Mme Salvador and Mlle Chaptal to discuss the possibility of holding an interim meeting of the ICN when the Salpetrière was to be opened. With the help of these ladies, arrangements were made and the Director of *Assistance Publique* was invited to speak at the ICN's opening dinner. In the eloquent speeches (recorded in the *History of the International Council of Nurses*)[3] many highly optimistic statements were made about the new era in French nursing. Subsequent developments indicated, however, that the ideas of the Paris officials had little in common with those of the ICN leaders present. For example, the new school and nurses' residence were put in charge of men, the teaching consisted of a highly theoretical series of medical lectures, and the plans to start the new hospital afresh with better qualified trainees were largely frustrated by the strong hospital workers' union. Apart from a regulation differentiating the position of nurse from that of ward maid, there was little actual change in the nursing system of the public hospitals of Paris at that time or for some years thereafter.

[3] By Margaret Breay and Ethel Gordon Fenwick (London: ICN, 1900).

WORLD WAR I AND BEGINNINGS
OF PROFESSIONAL ORGANIZATION

When war broke out in 1914, France had only about 200 trained nurses, and they were completely outnumbered and out-ranked by Red Cross and other volunteers who occupied most of the top posts in the military nursing services. Nevertheless, the war experience did much to promote modern nursing in France, largely because of the example of thousands of trained nurses from other countries who served in military hospitals and in the care of civilians behind the lines. Among the agencies that did much for civilian nursing was Anne Morgan's American Committee for Devastated France, which established a public health nursing center at Soissons under the direction of Mary Breckinridge, who tells the story of her pioneer work there and elsewhere in her fascinating biography *Wide Neighborhoods*. Another important outcome was the reorganization and expansion of the Rue Amyot School in its new quarters in Montrouge near Paris. This school was staffed with qualified French nurses who were sent to America for special preparation. Jeanne de Johannis, its director, was one of a number of able war volunteers who recognized the lacks in French nursing and decided to round out her training and to remain in this field. Several other schools were started at this time, one at Lille by four graduates of the Nightingale School at Bordeaux, another by the Faculty of Medicine in Paris as a part of its *Puericulture* (child care) department. Later, with the assistance of the Rockefeller Foundation, modern schools were developed in Lyons, where religious sisters and lay nurses were prepared together, and in some other centers.

After the war Mlle Chaptal led a movement for state registration in order to give legal recognition to nurses of good character who had received regular training or had had acceptable experience of five years or more in hospital work. With the support of influential religious and civil authorities, a national decree was passed in 1922 that awarded a state diploma to such nurses. Two years later all applicants were required to pass a state examination and to submit a record showing that they had attended a state-approved school for at least two years. A Central Bureau of Nursing was set up to keep the state register, to inspect schools, and to conduct examinations, and a National Council on Nursing was appointed to advise the Ministry of Hygiene on such matters.

In the following year (1923) the nurses who had received state diplomas formed the National Association of Trained Nurses of France with Mlle Chaptal as president, and in 1925 it joined the International Council of Nurses. This group included nuns (some cloistered) and a few Protestant deaconesses, graduates of Nightingale, Red Cross, and several other types of schools, and many nongraduates with little or no formal preparation but with approved experience. Considering the diverse elements represented, the differing concepts of nursing and the individualistic tendencies of the French people, this was a real achievement. It was soon evident, however, that the new professional group with its higher educational and ethical standards was relatively weak compared with the large trade unions backed by political influence and armed with such weapons as the strike. In sections where unions were strong the professionals found it difficult to compete, especially for positions in state or municipal hospitals or similar public agencies. Greater progress was made in the provincial hospitals where these difficulties were less marked.

The International Council of Nurses Congress of 1933, which met in Paris and Brussels and brought together large groups of nurses from other countries, did much to stimulate interest in professional nursing. The official magazine, *Infirmière Française,* also helped to keep members in touch with each other and with nursing in France. It had been established earlier under the sponsorship of physicians and nurses with Mlle Chaptal and Dr. Albert Calmette (the well-known tuberculosis specialist) as joint editors. These two had collaborated in starting hospital social service work in tuberculosis dispensaries, their plan being similar to that of Dr. Richard Cabot in Boston. Many French nurses took up this type of work, some being employed as social workers in the large city hospitals where they were able to exercise some influence on the nursing situation in a rather indirect way. Others worked in homes and in child welfare and tuberculosis clinics, which were often under private or voluntary agencies.

Nursing Education Patterns—Basic and Advanced

The state-approved "bifurcated" program for nursing schools differed in several ways from the prevailing patterns in countries discussed earlier. The first year's course was the same for all groups, but in the second year two options were presented, one leading to an institutional nursing diploma and the other to a public health and social assistance diploma. Those who could give three years might take a combined program preparing for both major fields. In the beginning the theoretical side of the work received more attention than the practical, but the latter has been steadily strengthened. Hospital positions were few at first, and the majority of students chose the program in public health and social work rather than that in hospital and nursing school work. The situation has been changing, however, especially since 1946, when the National Association of Trained Nurses succeeded in having a law passed to protect the title of state-registered nurses and to give them precedence in filling state positions. It was difficult at first to enforce this law because of the nurse shortage and the fact that some war volunteers were using social prestige or political influence to get paid positions.

Much has happened in recent years to improve these conditions. For example, shortly after the war, the French Red Cross discontinued all its nurses' aide courses except those for the training of auxiliaries in child welfare work for which this organization had an intensive program. It further concentrated on the improvement of its schools of nursing, of which it had at the end of 1952 thirty-five of a total of 142 then existing in France. A first step was to provide various types of refresher and advanced courses for nurses in leading positions. A second, in 1950, was the opening by the French Red Cross of a postgraduate school of nursing in Paris under the leadership of two French nurses who had received scholarships from the American Red Cross for a year's study in the United States to prepare them for this work. The school, which is open to Red Cross and non-Red Cross nurses alike, prepares the students for responsible positions in teaching and administration and its influence on nursing in France is already proving beneficial. Moreover, for the last few years the directors of all the schools of nursing in France have met under the leadership of a special committee to discuss common problems. These meetings have done much to clarify nursing aims and principles and to unify nursing groups. ·

Thus, although the war and postwar years were extremely difficult for French nurses and there have been times of great discouragement over the whole nursing situation, some substantial advances have been made. The loss of several trusted leaders through death or retirement was keenly felt when the nursing group began to face the reconstruction period, but new leaders are coming forward and the whole outlook is more encouraging.

ITALY

Farther south is another Latin country which has made some important contributions to nursing in the past and has had a long struggle to establish modern nursing on a sound basis. In Italy the first direct contact with this movement came in the '90's. Two vivid pictures of the nursing situation at that time are given in *The History of Nursing*.[4] One was by the wife of a well-known physician, Professor Celli, herself a German nurse and a co-worker in her husband's malaria experiments which were carried on in Italian hospitals and clinics. The other was by Amy Turton, a British lady of independent means, residing in Florence, who became deeply concerned about nursing in visits to the sick in public hospitals. Failing to arouse much interest among her Italian friends, Miss Turton decided that her mission in life was to insert the wedge that would eventually open the closed doors of Italian hospitals to a better class of secular nurses, who would bring about the necessary reforms. Though no longer

⁴ Nutting and Dock, *op. cit.*, Vol. IV, Chap. III.

young, she sought training from an Italian professor of medicine who was sympathetic but knew nothing of modern nursing. Then she wrote to Miss Nightingale, who suggested that she apply to the Edinburgh Infirmary, where she spent one year as lady probationer. Returning in 1894 to Italy she finally succeeded in interesting some patrons who helped her to start a small school in Rome. Shortly after, through the interest of a lady-in-waiting to Queen Elena, another opportunity in Naples was offered to her, and she appealed to Grace Baxter, a former resident of Italy, then in training at the Johns Hopkins School in Baltimore, to come over and help her.

Miss Baxter opened a small private school (the Blue Cross) in Naples and made a valiant effort to prepare the few applicants she had recruited from good middle-class families, but the results were not encouraging. Though several of the Blue Cross nurses did finish the training and gave a good account of themselves later, it was impossible to keep the school going. Some of the difficulties were the lack of funds, the fears of anxious parents, the irresponsibility and immaturity of many of the girls, their dislike of hard work, their love affairs, and the lack of sufficient incentive to complete their training. Miss Baxter remained in Italy and made further efforts to interpret modern nursing to Italian women by teaching home nursing classes and by writing and otherwise supporting efforts to establish nursing on a modern basis.

Amy Turton's little school in Rome had similar difficulties, but because of the interest and patronage of Queen Elena and the cooperation of the medical staff of the new Polyclinic Hospital, it was reorganized in 1910 under an English matron, Dorothy Snell, and a staff of twelve British nurses. The Regina Elena, for years the leading school in Italy, had a three-year course and a good practical as well as theoretical program designed especially to prepare nurses for executive positions in schools and hospitals. Though some of its graduates qualified for such positions, this school with its strict English discipline and strong emphasis on practical training had a limited appeal, especially to girls of the social class from which most of them came, who usually married early and had little desire for professional careers.

Shortly after World War I some American Red Cross workers who knew Italy's health needs were able to send over a group of experienced public health nurses under the able leadership of Mary Gardner to introduce this type of nursing in Italy. They found only about 200 trained nurses in the whole country, very few of whom were suitable for such work. Moreover, neither the prominent physicians consulted nor the Italian people saw the need, and the plan was considered too costly and complicated for their country. Although a few demonstration centers were opened under the Italian Red Cross and several Italian nurses were sent to America and Britain to prepare for such work, the net results were disappointing.

In the years following two types of training were developed by the Italian Red Cross, one in hospital schools where students were interns (in residence), the other where they were externs (living at home) and were given only limited practical experience, chiefly in child welfare and tuberculosis clinics and in home visiting. The visiting nurses, called *infermiera voluntaria,* paid for their training and were expected to serve without salary. Both programs were two years in length and shared the same lectures. Those who passed the theoretical test were eligible for admission to a seven-month postgraduate course in public health nursing which became a requirement for those in state positions.

THE PROFESSIONAL MOVEMENT

In 1920 a small group of Italian nurses organized a national association, which in 1922 was admitted to the International Council of Nurses. After it was discovered that many of its members were of the extern group, this decision was reconsidered and a reorganization was advised. The association continued on its original basis until the '30's, when under the Fascist regime it was absorbed in the corporative state. Although it succeeded in having its members classed with professionals and artists rather than with manual workers and trades, this did not prevent serious losses of status and freedom during the years of Fascist rule. After the war (1946) the association was reorganized as a federation of about seventy provincial groups, its new title being the Italian Nurses Association. Since then it has made a strong effort to recover lost ground and within the decade was admitted to active membership in the International Council of Nurses, with about 1000 members. At that time Italy had about 5000 nurses with state diplomas, 10,000 religious sisters, and 60,000 *voluntaria*. Basic schools of nursing of the intern type were mostly small and relatively few compared with the courses for *voluntaria*. Most of the nuns had no formal training, and this was true also of the majority of practical hospital nurses. The trade unions here as in most other parts of Europe support the practical nurse group in demanding the same returns for their services as those with full preparation. In 1954, however, a law was passed which established a National Registration Board for Nurses which places nursing education and practice under the Ministry of Health and Ministry of Education. It is reported that this is having a favorable effect on the quality of nursing service and the status of professional nurses.

Among the hopeful signs was the growing influence of international organizations, such as the World Health Organization, the League of Red Cross Societies, and the International Council of Nurses, all of which supported a clear distinction between the various grades of workers in nursing, irrespective of class lines, and a definite requirement of both practical and theoretical preparation for general nursing practice and more specialized positions. Such ideas were strengthened by the meeting of the Congress of the ICN in Rome in 1957. Reports indicate that large hospitals are gradually replacing practical nurses and auxiliaries with professional nurses. In 1957 the Federation of Colleges, mainly professional, was made the registration authority for nurses in the country as a whole. Attempts to conduct studies to determine the needs of nursing services and schools are meeting with varied responses. It is evident that professional nurses in Italy still have many difficult problems to solve and need all the help they can get from their sisters in other countries.

PORTUGAL

West of Italy lies the Iberian Peninsula, which has been almost completely isolated from the modern nursing movement until very recent years. Most of the hospitals have continued to depend as they have for centuries on the service of untrained religious sisters and servant-nurses, and the sick at home have been cared for chiefly by their relatives and household servants. Portugal began to introduce modern nursing a few years ago when it opened its first school of nursing. The suggestion for this school came from the National Organization for the Prevention of Cancer, located in Lisbon. Hazel Goff, an American nurse who had pioneered in several European countries was asked to help organize it and she remained until it was in operation. Fernanda Alvez-Diniz, who succeeded her, was later appointed by the World Health Organization as Chief Nurse in its European section. The school had a small but competent staff of Portuguese nurses who had received additional training abroad. Its graduates formed a national association, which has an associate representative in the International Council of Nurses. They have begun to organize different types of nursing services in communities as well as in hospitals. The establishment, near Lisbon, of the first rehabilitation center with a British nurse therapist on its staff has opened up another type of service and training. To help raise nursing standards, the Rockefeller Foundation has brought a few young Portuguese women to the United States for preparation in basic nursing as well as a number of graduate nurses for further study. The work of these nurses and the visits of nurse consultants of the Foundation are helping in the solution of some nursing problems. There is some evidence that the government is taking more active measures to reduce malaria, yellow fever, and other preventable diseases, to improve environmental sanitation and water supply, and to expand hospital facilities. Though a National Syndicate of Nurses, which is state controlled, registers all who practice nursing this does not indicate any national standard of fitness.

SPAIN

Farther east, in Spain, only a small beginning has been made to establish nursing on modern lines. The first attempt to train secular nurses here was made by Dr. Rubio, a Spanish physician who founded the Rubio Institute for this purpose in 1896, with a German nurse in charge. His concept of nursing was so different from both the old and new ideas that it could scarcely be called nursing at all. One aim was to make nurses as unattractive as possible by requiring them to wear a hideous uniform. In 1930 plans were laid for a modern school of nursing to be connected with Madrid University, but they were frustrated by the outbreak of the Spanish Civil War and unstable political conditions. The Red Cross has carried on a course for *visitadores,* who do volunteer health work in many communities. A few Spanish girls of the better class have taken training abroad in the hope of returning to introduce modern nursing at home, but so far there have been few positions open and little support for them or their work.

GREECE

We now come to Greece, which, though closely related to the Balkan group by race, religion, and long association as a part of of the old Turkish Empire, managed in 1821 to secure its independence and to develop its own political, social, economic, and religious systems. For centuries it was a stronghold of the eastern section of the Christian Church and of the Greek Orthodox faith, which is still dominant. Unlike the western or Roman branch of the Church it did not develop monastic orders that specialized in nursing and hospital work, but it did encourage charity, hospitality, and the care of the sick.

The first attempt to develop modern nursing in Greece was made by Queen Olga (Russian) who in the '80's started a small private hospital in Athens, the *Evangelismos,* which gave a year's training in nursing under its first matron, Mrs. Mitsaki, a Greek nurse trained in Germany, and later under Mrs. C. Reinhart from Denmark. At about the same time Greece joined the International Red Cross movement, and this stimulated interest in voluntary Red Cross nursing. Meantime, Cleoniki Klonari had gone to the Massachusetts General Hospital in Boston for training in nursing. On her return she had taken charge of the Children's Hospital (founded in Athens by Crown Princess Sophia) and later sent to the United States a number of qualified students to complete a three-year program in nursing.

At the time of World War I, Athina Messolora, an outstanding Greek graduate nurse, recruited and trained many voluntary nurses for first aid work. These volunteers were given the name of "nurse" until the first nurses graduated from the Hellenic Red Cross School, which had been founded in Athens in 1921 and which included in its program practical experience at the Evangelismos Hospital. This school, which has now added courses for graduate nurses, has remained a potent force in nursing in Greece. Another school, founded at about this time (1923), was opened at the American Woman's Hospital at Salonika, under the direction of Dr. Emilie Willms and Dr. Ruth Parmelee.

The graduates of these early schools in 1925 formed a Hellenic National Graduate Nurses Association, which with Miss Klonari as its first president joined the International Council of Nurses in 1929. This step did much to help the status of the professional nurse in Greece. As in Italy, however, amateurs had a better social status than most trained nurses, and the untrained domestic nurses who held most of the hospital positions were less costly. Since there was little demand for private nurses and most of the country outside the larger cities was unsafe for visiting nurse service, the demand for graduate nurses was limited and some went into other fields of work.

After World War I, the Hellenic Red Cross supplied many volunteers as well as trained nurses for nursing service. The need was greatly increased by the arrival in 1923 of a million Greek refugees from Smyrna who had been expelled by the Turks. In this emergency Alice Carr, an American Red Cross nurse who had served in the eastern area during the war, was sent to Greece by the Near East Foundation. Her successful anti-malaria campaign and work with Greek refugees brought her many honors and tributes from those who had seen her work and studied its results. In 1929 recommendations relative to the preparation of health personnel were made as a result of a request from the Greek government to the League of Nations, by Dr. Haven Emerson of Columbia University, Hazel A. Goff, Red Cross representative, and Elizabeth Crowell of the Rockefeller Foundation.

When World War II broke out, followed by civil war in Greece, serious food shortages and a high mortality from epidemic disease developed. During the period of internal strife the United Nations Rehabilitation and Relief Association (UNRRA) had an active unit in Greece, with Olive Baggallay, a well-known British public health nurse, in charge of its nursing program. This group prepared and helped Greek nurses to develop a visiting nurse service in both rural and urban areas. UNRRA and the Economic Cooperation Administration (ECA) also sent several Greek nurses abroad for study. At this time Greek nurses were doing important work in military hospitals, and when peace was restored it was hoped that they would be able to go forward with the support of their own government and people. Nurses from other countries who have worked with them report that they have great capabilities and do well under experienced leaders. With the help of the League of Red Cross Societies, the Near East Foundation, the U. S. Public Health Service, the World Health Organization, the International Council of Nurses, and other international and national agencies interested in such programs, nursing service is being extended and Greek nurses are now being sent abroad for additional preparation. Legal control of nursing is also becoming a reality. In these and other ways the prospects for continued advancement in nursing service and education in Greece seems definitely promising.

This brief review of the situation in central and southern Europe indicates that in spite of its rich cultural, scientific, and humanitarian traditions there are still some serious obstacles to the development of modern nursing. The situation has been complicated by wars and other disrupting experiences and by religious, economic, social, political, and medical traditions and systems that have made changes difficult. Nevertheless, new ideas and leaders have been developing, and definite progress has been made with the support of international agencies interested in nursing and health work.

SELECTED BIBLIOGRAPHY

"A Belgian University Nursing School," *Nurs. Times,* October 6, 1951, 986-990.

Broe, Ellen. "Some Glimpses of Visits to Schools of Nursing in Europe," *Int. Nurs. Bull.,* Summer 1953, 13-17.

Carr, Alice G. *Public Health, Medicine, and Sanitation in Greece.* New York: Near East Foundation, 1942.

Elster, Ruth. "New Nursing Legislation in Germany," *Int. Nurs. Rev.,* April 1960, 53-56.

Enriques, Bice. "Professional Nurses and their Training in Italy." *Int. Nurs. Rev.,* May 1957, 19-21.

Giunti, Marchesa Irene di Targiani. "Notes on the History of Nursing Care with Special Reference to Italy," *Int. Nurs. Rev.,* May 1957, 12-15.

Hooykaas, Sophie H. "Nursing in the Netherlands," *Am. Jo. Nurs.,* November 1946, 760-762.

Hampton, Isabel A., and others. *Nursing of the Sick 1893.* New York: McGraw-Hill, 1949. Pp. 57-60, 73-78, 79-92, 188-191.

International Council of Nurses. *National Reports. 1933,* 1-2, 6-10, 18-21, 25, 34-35, 39-40, 45, 56, 62, 65-66; *1947,* 27, 34-35, 44-45, 67-69; *1949,* 30-32, 43-46, 56-58, 88-91, 92-94; *1957,* 7-9, 10-12, 33-35, 36-37, 42-44, 55-57, 67-68, 69-71, 93-95; *1961,* 6-7, 8-9, 27-28, 29-30, 31-32, 44-45, 59-61, 80-82.

Judson, Helen. *Edith Cavell.* New York: Macmillan, 1941.

Karll, Sister Agnes. "Report on Nursing in Germany During the Year 1923," *Int. Nurs. Bull.,* January 1924, 28-29.

"Le Bon Secours School of Nursing, Geneva," *Nurs. Times,* June 8, 1956, 519-520.

Ledaskis, A. "Nursing Education in Greece: The Present Programme and Future Aims," *Int. Nurs. Rev.,* January 1957, 48-54.

Mechelynck, Cècile. "The University School of Nursing at Brussels," *Am. Jo. Nurs.,* March, 1937, 238-243.

Messolora, Athina. *A Brief History of the Evolution of Nursing in Greece,* Athens: Hellenic National Graduate Nurses Association, 1959.

Nussbaum, Helen. "Health Services in Switzerland," *Int. Nurs. Rev.,* July/August 1961, 20-23.

Nutini, Stephania. "Advanced Nursing Education in Italy," *Nurs. Times,* May 17, 1957, 547-548.

Nutting, M. Adelaide, and Lavinia L. Dock. *A History of Nursing.* New York: Putnam's, 1907-1912. 4 vols. Vol. III, Ch. IV; Vol. IV, Ch. I-IV.

Petschnigg, Lilli. "Nursing in Austria," *Am. Jo. Nurs.,* January 1956, 61-63.

Pietzcher, Dominika. "Theodor Billroth and the Rudolfinerhaus," *Int. Nurs. Rev.,* May 1930, 259-262.

Seltzer, Lorraine. "Nursing and Nursing Education in Germany," *Am. Jo. Nurs.,* December 1945, 993-995.

Sgarra, Antonietta. "Nursing in Italy," *Int. Nurs. Bull.,* Autumn 1952, 1923.

———. "Organization of the Nursing Profession in Italy," *Int. Nurs. Rev.,* April 1955, 48-54.

Sher, Alice A. "A Visit to Austria," *Int. Nurs. Rev.,* April 1959, 80-84.

von Abendroth, Erna, and Maria Therese Strobl. "Nursing in Germany and Austria," *Am. Jo. Nurs.,* November 1950, 728-730.

Werminghaus, Esther A. "These Are Nursing Students in Heidelberg," *Am. Jo. Nurs.,* October 1955, 1201-1206.

CHAPTER **16**

Eastern Europe

THE chief country in this area is Soviet Russia, which covers nearly a sixth of the earth's surface and extends from the Baltic to the Pacific. Along its western border are the former Baltic provinces of Estonia, Latvia, and Lithuania, now absorbed in the Soviet Union, and several other states from Poland to the Greek border, which are more or less under its control. The population of this whole block and that of China are estimated at approximately a third of the human race. The Soviet Union contains citizens of at least sixty different nationalities and about 180 ethnic groups. In addition to the difference in language, religion, and culture, they represent different stages of development, from primitive nomads to highly civilized groups. All now live under the Communist system of government. Before attempting to outline the present system of nursing and its place in the medical and health structure of the Soviet Union, it is important to get a picture of the medical and health system of pre-Communist Russia.

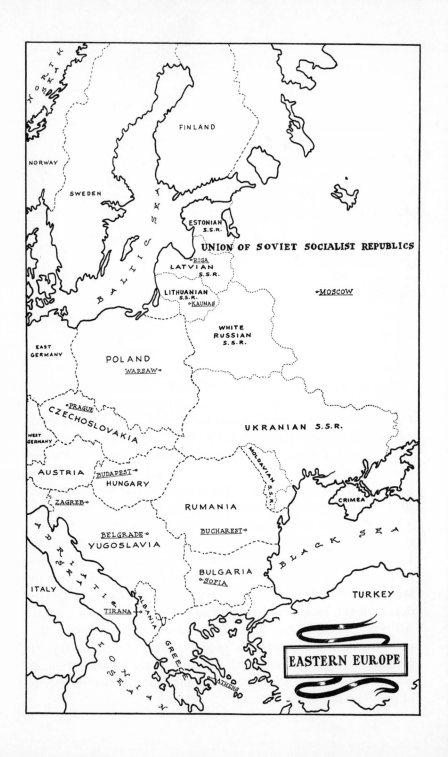

RUSSIA

In his introductory historical summary Dr. Henry Sigerist[1] points out that there were relatively few Russian physicians until 1850 and that most of those employed by the court and aristocracy were imported from European countries. The great majority of the peasant and city workers depended on folk medicine or on the services of local midwives and practical doctors of the barber-surgeon type (the men called *feldshers* and the women, *feldsheritzas*). After 1850 more trained physicians became available, but they were located chiefly in the cities where they were often assisted by midwives and *feldshers* for whose training they were responsible. Medical schools later admitted these two groups for elementary medical courses, and the more promising of such students were often encouraged to take the full medical training.

Nursing in Russian homes of the better class was relegated to family servants, and in hospitals patients were cared for as a rule by ward maids or domestics. Russian and other Orthodox churches of the east did not develop religious nursing sisterhoods, though there were some Sisters of Mercy and a few Russian ladies who served in the Russian Army during the Crimean War in positions similar to that of the Lady Hospitallers of earlier days. They were voluntary workers, usually of upper-class families, and sometimes the widows of army officers. Miss Nightingale noted in her account of nursing in the Crimean War that these lady volunteers had a better status than that of nurses in the old British army hospitals. The Russian word for nurse is *sestra* (sister), first applied to Red Cross nurses and later to trained nurses. The sisters assisted the surgeons with dressings, medicines, and diets and carried some responsibility for ward management but gave little or no bedside care.

In 1864 important medical and health reforms were intro-

[1] Sources used here include Henry E. Sigerist's *Medicine and Health in Soviet Russia* (1933), and *The Report of the United States Public Health Mission to the Union of Soviet Socialist Republics* (1959), supplemented by notes taken by one of the authors on a visit to Soviet Russia in 1933, and more recent reports on the USSR.

duced in Russia under what was called the Zemstvo system, in which the local districts assumed chief responsibility for their own health and charitable services. These services were tax supported and were to be developed on a wide scale, but progress was slow because of the lack of health personnel, the poverty of the people, and the immense areas to be covered. To economize the services of physicians, *feldshers* and midwives manned the larger district centers, where under the general direction of their medical superiors they cared for the less serious medical and surgical conditions and officiated at most of the births, even in the best families. In the 1870's women were beginning to study medicine, and this field rather than nursing attracted most of the better educated Russian women who were interested in health work.

There seems to be no evidence that the Nightingale system ever got a start in Russia, though some Finnish nurses who were so trained were brought in to staff at least one of the de luxe private hospitals in St. Petersburg. A few German deaconesses were employed in a similar way before 1914. According to Dr. Sigerist, the number of two-year nursing schools then was about 100, and there were 18,000 trained nurses in the entire country. From what can be learned of these schools, they were on a lower level than the courses for midwives and *feldshers* and their educational programs consisted of medical lectures with very little practical supervision or training in nursing or ward management. These lacks were reflected in the conditions of most Russian hospitals, which in cleanliness, sanitation, order, efficiency, discipline, and personal care of the sick were much below those in Britain, Scandinavia, and other countries where the Nightingale revolution by that time had brought many reforms.

REORGANIZATION UNDER THE SOVIETS

When the Bolshevik revolution of 1917 occurred, the country was threatened by a serious typhus epidemic, which spread rapidly and forced the new Communist Government to take immediate action in reinforcing and extending its medical and sanitary personnel. The Zemstvo structure was taken over with little change, but the organization and training of medical personnel followed the same general pattern as that adopted for workers in industry and other essential services. Under the dictatorship of the proletariat, the class structure was turned upside down, with workers on top and aristocrats and bourgeoisie at the bottom. Preference in educational opportunities, appointments, and the like was given at first to the proletariat, though this was modified later. Men and women were declared equal, as were professional and manual workers, and all were required to take an active share in the defense and necessary work of the country. Compulsory education, with heavy emphasis on science, was introduced. A system of secular ethics was evolved which called for almost complete subordination of the individual to the authority of the state and the welfare of the country as defined by the new leaders. The antireligious campaign, which was started ostensibly to combat superstition, discriminated against those who continued to follow the older religious faiths. Such changes as these were enforced not only by law but by a system of indoctrination and discipline that began in the cradle and was continued through the schools, youth organizations, trade unions, and other agencies, official and nonofficial.

An important feature of the Soviet system was the adoption of a nationwide scheme based on a detailed analysis of needs and resources and covering all the major services and occupations, including medical and health work. The results of such studies were embodied in five-year plans which were broken down into one-year quotas for every industry and every section of the country. At the start the military services and heavy industries took precedence over everything else, and most of the better educated men were drafted for top positions as officers and engineers. Women in large numbers were assigned to the medical and health services, the proportion of women physicians being as high as seventy-five to eighty per cent. Individuals had very little choice of fields of work or location, such matters being determined largely by the quotas of workers required.

In the medical and health field, as in all major industries, personnel were classified into three categories—lower, middle, and higher—nurses being in the middle medical category along with midwives and *feldshers*. This three-rung vocational ladder of unskilled and skilled labor, semiprofessional and professional groups had its counterpart in an educational plan that provided preparation at each level. This was designed to promote easy transfer and promotion from one stage to the next. Workers were considered eligible for such advancement provided they qualified by additional preparation (which could be secured at little or no extra cost) and had a good record for political orthodoxy and generally approved conduct. Often pressure was exerted to fill the higher level positions, and in times of stress, as in World War II, nurses might be advanced to medical positions without much if any additional preparation. According to recent official reports, a third of the medical women in Russia had first taken nurses' training and many had been midwives or *feldsheritzas*. It is also reported that among all applicants to medical schools nurses are preferred. This helps to explain what seems to be a lack of leaders in the nursing field.

A supplementary part of the medical and health structure was under the Red Cross (called Red Crescent in Moslem areas). This organization, which was purged of its former aristocratic associations, encouraged patriotic service, especially in times of war and national disaster. Until recently, when it was put under the central medical authority, it conducted its own rest homes, hospitals, and sanatoria, and its flying ambulances were staffed by nurses trained for parachute jumping. During World War II millions of citizens took Red Cross courses and helped in sanitary and ambulance brigades on the battlefields and behind the lines. Official reports state that the Red Cross trained tens of thousands of nurses at that time, many of whom received war honors.

CONCEPT, STATUS, AND EDUCATION OF NURSES

From this outline it will be seen that nurses occupied a middle position on the medical ladder. Their preparation was considered a definite step toward qualification as physicians. Nurses, midwives, and *feldshers* were trained in middle medical technicums where technical subjects were supplemented by some general secondary education. The course was four years in length, the first two years in theory and the second two in about equal periods of theory and practice. Among the more academic courses were general science, history of communism, and Soviet economy. In 1933, in a total of 2000 hours of class work, only thirty were given to a course in nursing as such. All these curricula in the medical field were prepared by the Central Commissariat of Health in Moscow, as were the textbooks and journals and other literature translated into the various languages represented in the population of the Soviet Union. Students who went directly into medicine had to have ten years of schooling before being admitted to a four- or five-year medical course. After passing the state examination, students were·expected to work three years in their specialty wherever they were sent. On the lower level of the medical ladder were such groups as ward maids and orderlies, who had four years of general education and training of a more practical type.

In addition to the three vertical divisions there were three horizontal divisions of the medical industry, and all personnel including nurses were expected to have special preparation for *one* of the three. These were (1) child health and welfare, (2) general medical and prophylactic services, and (3) hygiene, which stressed community sanitation and epidemiology. Although all branches of medical work combined prevention and cure, the fighting of epidemics required trained mobile forces and special techniques. Precedence was given to such campaigns in the early days, and some striking results were reported in the control of typhus, malaria, bubonic plague, and other epidemic diseases. Although some parts of the country are still backward in medical facilities, rapid advances have been made in recent years. Most of the population now have access to free and relatively modern medical services, and reductions in sickness and death rates have been impressive. Physicians are in charge of most of the teaching and supervision of nurses, the result being that nurses are overloaded with medical functions and doctors with duties that in most western countries belong to nurse administrators and instructors.

Most western nurses who have visited Soviet Russia have been especially interested in the work for mothers and children which integrates legal, educational, and sociological and medical services. This division controls a vast network of day nurseries in factories, farms, and parks, as well as children's hospitals, clinics, and home visiting services. Nurses who serve here are part nurse and part teacher ("nurses with a pedagogical slant" as described to one visitor). The standards of service as well as the general attitude of these workers seem to be more like that found in western countries. In the medical division nurses work chiefly in hospitals and clinics, sometimes going out with physicians and surgeons for home visits. Though employed and paid by the state, they may take some outside private work in their off-time. The term "patronage nurse" is used for such workers.

Economic conditions correspond to those found in other industries. According to recent reports, nurses have a six-and-one-half-hour day in general hospitals and clinics, six hours in mental hospitals, a five-day week with pay about two thirds that of physicians, and two eight-day holidays each year. A large proportion are married and carry family responsibilities in addition to their regular work. Other so-called "voluntary" (but actually required) activities are noted later.

NURSES' ORGANIZATIONS

Before 1917 nurses, doctors, and other groups had their own independent unions or professional associations. After the communist regime was established, all workers in the same industry, whatever their rank or specialty, were required to join one large union. This is often called the vertical as opposed to the horizontal plan, in which each craft or profession is organized as a separate unit and all exist side by side. Doctors at first refused to join other medical and health personnel, but they were soon forced by economic pressure to comply. Since all members had equal status in the unions and the higher ranking members were outnumbered by the other groups, officers and influential delegates who represented the medical workers' union in discussing questions of national policy were often drawn from the base of the pyramid rather than from the apex. For example, it was not unusual to have a laundry worker or cook in the chair at a union meeting while the top surgeon and hospital superintendent sat in the rear.

Soviet unions differed in many other ways from the free unions of the western world. They were in no sense self-governing, since they were actually a part of the state machinery and subject to control by the higher authorities. Such unions were not allowed to bargain for better incomes or conditions or to strike. Their chief function was to stimulate production in their industry and to expose and correct conditions that tended to interfere with working efficiency and with the welfare and safety of the state. Their members, therefore, were encouraged to report all persons high or low who were guilty of graft, tardiness, slack or incompetent work, or deviations from communist principles. The unions employed many forms of discipline and indoctrination for such offenses, and in their comrade courts sometimes imposed heavy penalties for such crimes as accepting tips or fees from patients. They also developed a system of honors and special privileges for good workers. An ingenious scheme of publicity, such as the wall newspapers and bulletin boards seen in all industrial plants and many hospitals, featured both bad and good examples of conduct often with amusing illustrations and pungent comments.

Attendance at union meetings was compulsory, and much of what might be considered free time went into union projects which included recreational, political, and social activities of many kinds. All USSR citizens were supposed to do some voluntary "social work" to contribute to the general welfare. This might be helping to build the famous Moscow subway, aiding in the liquidation of illiteracy, or searching for spies and traitors. From these few examples it is evident that Russian nursing differs in many respects from western systems, which were based on Nightingale principles. Nevertheless, western nurses, such as Rebecca Timbres, a member of a Quaker group who served in Russia earlier, found many points of common interest.[2] The

²*We Did Not Ask Utopia.* See Bibliography, p. 362.

International Council of Nurses has made some efforts to bridge the gap, so far with little success. In the border countries to be considered next, all of which had some experience with modern western nursing before they were taken into the Soviet orbit, the differences tend to be less marked.

THREE BALTIC STATES

The peoples of the three Baltic Provinces, Estonia, Latvia and Lithuania, though conquered earlier by Russia and gaining their temporary independence only in 1918, were in general closer to their neighbors in Scandinavia and Germany than to the Russians. This could be seen in their nursing and hospital work which reflected the influence not only of the Roman Catholic and Lutheran sisterhoods but of the Teutonic Knights, many of whom had settled after the Crusades along the Baltic coast and the Gulf of Finland and had passed on their traditions to their descendents. When the Red Cross appeared in the 1860's it drew most of its volunteers from such families, and it was not surprising therefore that after World War I and the liberation of the Baltic Provinces this influence became dominant in nursing and hospital work.

LATVIA

Soon after 1918, when the new government of Latvia was formed, the Red Cross was made the official agency for all hospital nursing and welfare work and the premier's wife, Marta Celmin, a Red Cross nurse, was appointed director. She sought the advice and aid of the League of Red Cross Societies, which was then beginning its work and making a special effort to encourage the preparation of professionally qualified nurses. This led to the organization of a two-year Red Cross School in Riga (1921), which was intended as an example for others to follow. One of its able graduates, Justine Kushke, was sent to London as a student of the international course sponsored by the League of Red Cross Societies and returned to carry forward as far as was then possible the principles of modern nursing and public health work. She also helped to organize the Latvian Nurses Association. Since this was an integral part of the Red Cross structure and therefore not self-governing, it could not qualify for membership in the International Council of Nurses. It did, however, keep in touch with the ICN as well as with the League of Red Cross Societies and was developing along professional lines when in 1940 the short period of national independence came to an end and Latvia was incorporated into the Soviet Union.

LITHUANIA

In Lithuania the Red Cross had less of a monopoly in nursing, but the best-known school was developed at the Red Cross Hospital at Kaunas. The others were of the usual hospital type. The Lithuanian Nurses Association, organized in 1922, was making an effort to qualify for membership in the International Council of Nurses and had a representative in that body, but the task of bringing its schools and nurses up to an acceptable standard was difficult, especially since there was little support for such efforts in medical or other influential groups. As in Latvia, its people were scattered when the Baltic Provinces were absorbed by Soviet Russia.

ESTONIA

The people of Estonia were related to the Finns, and with the help and advice of these northern neighbors a small group of Estonian nurses had made a good fight for modern standards and for professional autonomy. The chief leader of the nurses was Anna Erma, a woman of strong character and good education who had been trained in Germany as a deaconess but had decided that a broader type of educational program was required to attract the better educated young women needed in modern nursing. After observing the nursing system of Finland, she sought the support of a number of influential professors in the medical school of the old Tartu University and with their help proceeded to build up an independent school whose students came from some of the leading families of the town. The university clinics supplied most of the clinical experience for the three-year course and the medical staff gave many of the lectures, but the teaching of nursing was carried on by nurses. Miss Erma also led in organizing a small group of nurses who stood for a self-governing profession, and this Association of Estonian Nurses joined the International Council of Nurses in 1933. Scholarships were raised to send some of their nurses abroad for postgraduate courses in Britain and America. Such preparation was chiefly in public health and school nursing, in which fields a good start had been made before 1940. When the USSR suddenly occupied Estonia and many prominent citizens were arrested, Miss Erma and some other leading nurses were warned and escaped to Scandinavia. Those who remained in the Baltic states shared the fate of their people, many of whom were deported and scattered throughout the USSR.

OTHER BORDER COUNTRIES

Farther south and reaching into the Balkan region were several other formerly independent nations which were drawn into the Soviet orbit after 1940. Many of their peoples were related to the Slavs, but they also had close ties with western Europe and had been influenced by western systems of medicine and nursing.

POLAND

Poland, a Roman Catholic country, had a good many nuns in hospitals and nursing work before World War I. Apart from the secular servant-nurses who did most of the hospital work, there were at that time numerous Red Cross volunteers. Among them were some exceptionally intelligent, patriotic young women who became interested in qualifying as professionals after observing the work of nurses who came from other countries to help their people. It was through a gift to the American Red Cross by an American nurse (Dorothea Hughes) that the first modern school of nursing was developed in Warsaw under an American nurse educator, Helen Bridge. This became the first State School of Nursing in Poland. It was organically and financially independent, leaving it free to secure whatever clinical and other opportunities its students needed in the hospital with which it was connected, but took no responsibility for nursing service in other hospital units. Within its own units, nursing service was covered by the school, with nurse instructors in charge. Modern health centers were also developed in Warsaw, and a good standard of public health nursing was established under the head of the city's health department, who was an enthusiastic supporter of these reforms. Such centers were also used by the school for the training of its nurses.

Substantially the same plan was adopted in the Jewish School of Nursing in Warsaw under another American nurse, Amelia Greenwald, the funds being provided chiefly by the American Joint Distribution Committee, a Jewish organization. These two schools directed by Zofia Szlinker and Sabina Schindler, respectively, were of a modern type and prepared a number of keen and capable nurses. Two Red Cross Schools which followed similar lines trained nuns as well as lay nurses. Graduates of all these schools worked together in building up modern nursing in Poland, in organizing the National Council of Polish Nurses, which became a member of the International Council of Nurses in 1925, and in securing nursing legislation for the whole country.

The indomitable spirit of the Polish nurses did not fail them when the country was occupied by Russia and Germany. Special attention has been given to rural areas, and, according to recent reports, there has been a great expansion of nursing schools and personnel in which leading Polish nurses have cooperated and have been allowed considerable initiative. There are now forty-eight basic schools and one post-graduate school. One of the former is a four year combined program of academic and nursing content. Short courses for practical nurses have also been organized by the Red Cross assisted with funds provided by the Ministry of Health, where a nurse, Jadwiga Izycka is now vice-director of middle medical personnel. Some nuns with nursing preparation were said to be continuing their work, though they were not allowed to wear religious garb or to belong to their motherhouses. The Polish Nurses Association reapplied for membership in the ICN in 1957 and was readmitted with an individual membership of 13,000 nurses at the 1961 Congress.

CZECHOSLOVAKIA

Czechoslovakia was formed after World War I by combining different fragments of several countries. Nursing was backward when President Masaryk took the helm in 1918, and his sister, Alice Masaryk, a Doctor of Philosophy, sought the advice of the American Red Cross about forming a new school to prepare *fuersorginnen* (part nurse, part social worker) on the German pattern. She was advised instead to develop a modern school for nurses, and at the request of President Masaryk an American nurse, Marion Parsons, and two assistants were sent over to start such a school. They remained until a Czech nurse, Miss Malcharova, finished her training in the Nightingale School in London and returned as director. Other promising Czech nurses were sent to Britain and America for advanced preparation. In the brief time they had before World War II they managed with help from their national Red Cross to lay a fairly good foundation in modern nursing service and education and to extend community nursing and health services. A nursing office was established in the Ministry of Health, with a Czech nurse in charge. They also formed the Nurses Association of Czechoslovakia, which joined the International Council of Nurses in 1933.

This work was disrupted by the war and contacts with the West were weakened by the growing orientation of the country toward Soviet Russia. Nurses, like other Czechoslovakian citizens, were divided in their sympathies. This was apparent when the ICN Congress met in 1947 in Atlantic City. The report of this group, which appears in the *National Reports* of that year, suggests a compromise that would allow the nurses association to retain its membership in the ICN and at the same time belong (as then required) to the Communist-controlled Central Union of Trade Unions. The revolution then imminent soon cut off all communication, and little is known of subsequent developments beyond the fact that nursing was reorganized to fit into the Soviet pattern of medical and health services then adopted. Recent visitors to Czechoslovakia report that many new hospitals have been built and that they have been integrated into the national health service, as have all other health agencies. Public health nursing is part of a service that includes many new health centers. Apparently, many nurses are employed in such activities, but little is known of their preparation, status, or duties.

HUNGARY

In Hungary modern nursing got its start after World War I as a direct outcome of the public health movement and was limited in general to this field. Dr. Bela Johan, a vigorous and able public health officer, helped to found the first modern nursing school in 1921 in close cooperation with the University of Debrecen. Another state school was located in Budapest under the State Institute of Hygiene. All nursing schools by law were directed by physicians, but well-qualified nurses held important positions in them and were influential in shaping their policies. They also helped to form the Hungarian Nurses Association, which joined the International Council of Nurses in 1933. This group was relatively small and had little influence on the hospital situation, in which untrained nuns, nurses, and attendants continued to operate much as in the older days. After the Communists took over in the late 1940's, the intelligentsia were displaced in most sections, many escaping to other countries. The Hungarian Nurses Association was dissolved, and apparently few members who originally represented the western concept of nursing have remained in the country.

Rumania

Rumania's story is similar in many ways. The first modern school (named Regina Marie after Queen Marie of Rumania, a granddaughter of Queen Victoria) was started in Bucharest after World War I under the Queen's sponsorship. It was later taken over by the Ministry of Public Health in order to prepare public health nurses. Dr. Eugenia Popa, a woman physician, was sent to the Yale School of Nursing (USA) to prepare as a public health nurse before being put in charge. Other schools in Cluj and Jassey were put under nurse directors who had had some preparation in London. Hospital nurses were trained in twelve state schools, which were on a lower level, and the two groups had little to do with each other. The Red Cross also represented a different group, mainly composed of intelligent and able women of the aristocracy, who, although they had received some training in hospital nursing, did not qualify as professional nurses. The Association of Trained Nurses, which became a member of the International Council of Nurses in 1937, tried to bring these nurses together and to create more uniform standards, but without much success. War conditions brought many dangers and hardships, and the separation from friends and supporters in other countries was keenly felt, but students and graduates of the three schools held together under their leaders, who kept their work going. After a brief period in 1947 when contacts with the West were reestablished at the ICN Congress, the doors again closed and here as in other border countries the Russian system seems to be dominant.

Bulgaria

In Bulgaria some attempts were made in 1900 by Russian Red Cross nurses to set up a one-year nursing program, but it was not until 1915 that a modern school was founded. At the request of Queen Eleanora, Helen Scott Hay and Rachel Torrance came from the United States to establish this American-type school in Sofia. Interrupted for some years by Balkan wars, the school was taken over in 1922 by the Bulgarian Red Cross, and Miss Torrance was called back to direct it. She and Hazel Goff, her successor, rebuilt the school and turned it over to two Bulgarian nurses, Nevena Sendova and Krustarka Pachedjieva, who had been sent to Teachers College in New York to prepare and who in succession directed the school's work. The graduates of this school led the modern nursing movement in Bulgaria and formed the Bulgarian Nurses Association (1924), which joined the International Council of Nurses the following year. As more schools began to develop, efforts were made to secure state laws governing nursing practice and education, but though the Sofia school was recognized by the Ministry of Education no nurse practice law was passed. Nurses came more and more under the direction of the State Department of Health, which favored the Soviet system. Since the war, when Bulgaria joined the Communist countries, direct contacts with the West have been cut off and little is known of later developments.

YUGOSLAVIA

The nursing history of Yugoslavia between 1918 and 1940 was much like that of the other Balkan countries, except Albania, where modern medical and health work did not secure much of a foothold. Under Dr. Stamper, an able state officer who is a well-known leader in public health work, and with the aid of the Rockefeller Foundation, two modern schools of nursing were started, one in Belgrade under Enid Newton, an English nurse, and the other in Zagreb under Dr. Marie Vietch. She, like Dr. Popa in Rumania, added a Yale nursing degree to her medical preparation and continued to focus her efforts on the promotion of nursing. The Zagreb school admitted nuns and secular nurses to its four-year course which included both hospital and public health nursing. A Yugoslavian Nurses Association was organized and affiliated with the International Council of Nurses in 1929 but dropped out after the Communist revolution, rejoining as the Federation of Nurses Associations of Yugoslavia at the Rome congress in 1957.

Little information was available about nursing in this country until 1956, when a Yugoslav nurse, Dina Urbançic, attended a World Health Organization conference in Geneva as a delegate from her country. Her report indicated that nursing patterns there had not diverged so much as those in other Communist countries, though the influence of the Soviet system was apparent. Middle medical programs of education were placed in secondary schools, but nurses were able to bring about some changes when they found that the fifteen year olds who entered the nursing courses were too immature to cope with the difficulties of nursing practice. Entrance requirements were raised to senior matriculation in some cases or programs were lengthened to include more general education before nursing subjects began. Three types of basic programs in nursing, which vary in academic standing, are found in Yugoslavia. A postgraduate course has been added to prepare nurse teachers and administrators as well as some clinical specialists.

With advances in hospital and public health work, the opportunities for nurses have widened. Many more nurses are needed to keep up with these demands, but standards have been well maintained on the whole. More time is being given to the mastery of the nursing art. Nurses taught this subject as well as the history and ethics of nursing, and when they discovered that doctors often failed to teach other subjects from the nurse's point of view they asked for more teaching by nurses. Since this called for special training, advanced courses were started for classroom teachers and ward nurses. Although nurse-directors of some schools have been replaced by doctors, the State Conference of Middle Medical Schools supported the nurses' plea for members of their own group in such positions. The big problem here as in most other countries has been the shortage of good nurses, and it was recognized that the prospects of building up a better qualified and more permanent nursing group of good morale would be improved where nursing could be clearly differentiated from medicine, with opportunities for advancement in its own field. Such reports as this are especially significant, since they show that when nurses of the East and the West have some opportunity to do their own thinking and planning they tend to reach much the same conclusions on at least some of the vital problems in this area.

It will be seen from this brief review of nursing in Soviet Russia and in several of the border countries that are operating more or less on the same lines that there are fairly marked differences between the systems and concepts of nursing of this group and of the others so far studied. These differences have their roots in precommunist patterns in eastern Euorpe and in the Communist system itself. Though much has been done to improve the health of the people in all these countries, it is difficult to identify nurses' special contributions or to know how much freedom they have to develop their own field of work. In Poland and Yugoslavia there seems to be a greater evidence of initiative and professional spirit among nurses and a desire to again unite with nurses of the world in studying their common problems and in improving their preparation and service as nurses. Evidence so far seems to indicate that nursing as such flourishes best when it is a para-medical profession, developing side by side with medicine with full cooperation and room for expansion and initiative.

SELECTED BIBLIOGRAPHY

Albin, Ellen. "Nursing in the U.S.S.R.," *Am. Jo. Nurs.*, August 1946, 525-528.

Anscombe, Ella. "A Brief Report of the Schools of Nursing in Bucharest, Roumania," *Int. Nurs. Bull.*, January 1942, 22.

Bridge, Helen L. "The Warsaw School of Nursing," *Int. Nurs. Bull.*, January 1924, 3-12.

[Bridges, Daisy C.]. "Poland, Report on a Visit by the Gen. Sec'y of the ICN," *Int. Nurs. Rev.*, October 1959, 25-31.

[————]. "Yugoslavia," *Int. Nurs. Rev.*, January 1959, 23-27.

Counts, George S. *The Challenge of Soviet Education.* New York: McGraw-Hill, 1957. Ch. 8.

Cramer, John Francis, and George Stephenson Brown. *Contemporary Education.* New York: Harcourt, Brace, 1956. Esp. pp. 401-405.

Holliday, Jane. "Glimpses of Nursing in Russia," *Nurs. Outlook*, September 1958, 496-497.

International Council of Nurses. *National Reports. 1933,* 11, 32, 37-38, 43-44, 46-48, 53-55, 61; *1947,* 58-61, 66-69.

Izycka, Jadwiga, "Nursing Education in Poland," *Nurs. Outlook,* June 1960, 304-307.

The Report of the United States Public Health Mission to the Union of Soviet Socialist Republics. Washington: Govt. Print. Off., 1959.

Sigerist, Henry E. *Socialized Medicine in the Soviet Union.* New York: Norton, 1957. Published in 1947 as *Medicine and Health in the Soviet Union.* New York: Citadel Press.

Szloch, Stephanie M. "Nursing in Poland—Before and During the War," *Am. Jo. Nurs.,* March 1947, 156-158.

Timbres, Rebecca (Janney) and Harry Timbres. *We Did Not Ask Utopia.* New York: Prentice-Hall, 1939.

Torrance, Rachel. "Nursing in Bulgaria," *Int. Nurs. Bull.,* January 1924, pp. 13-19.

Urbançic, Dina. "Nursing in Yugoslavia, 1956," *Am. Jo. Nurs.,* May 1956, 585-587.

CHAPTER 17

Asia

THE Asian peoples are justly proud of their ancient civilizations and of their early contributions to medical learning
which were outlined in Part I. Modern medicine, public health,
and nursing have come chiefly from contacts with the West
through colonial governments, missionary and humanitarian
agencies, and sometimes business and trading groups. Many
factors have tended to retard the progress of modern nursing in
this part of the world; for example, restrictions in women's
activities and education, poor economic conditions, and in
recent years sweeping political and social changes which have
often disrupted existing health services. Nevertheless, definite
progress has been made in a number of countries and a few have
made impressive records. Here three regions are considered: (1)
southwest Asia; (2) southeast Asia; and (3) northeast Asia.

SOUTHWEST ASIA

Most of the countries in southwest Asia (often called the
Near East, where three continents meet), can be considered an

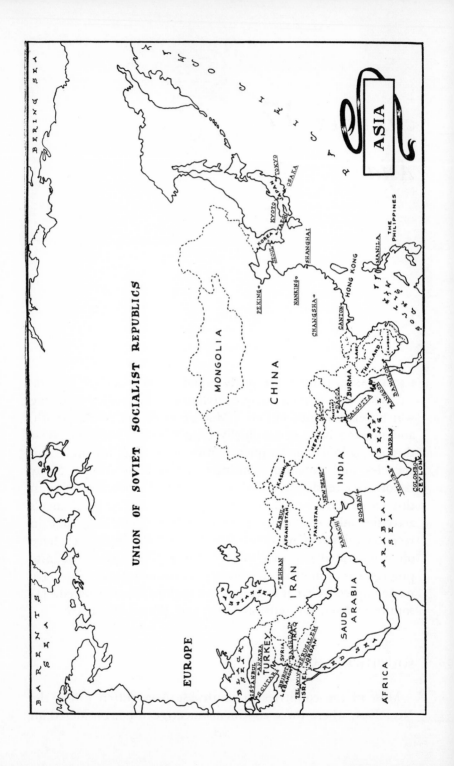

extension of the Moslem belt that stretches across North Africa from the Atlantic Ocean to Pakistan and India. Though their peoples belong to several different races and are politically divided, the great majority find a strong common bond in their Moslem faith, laws, and customs. This bond has been strengthened in recent years by a movement to revive the ancient culture and might of the Islamic peoples, to restore their national sovereignties, and to make them again a dominant power in this region. These ambitions and the influence in many cases of western education have led to fundamental changes in the old Kismet mentality that accepted disease and death as Allah's will and made little effort to relieve or prevent illness. The countries to be studied in this section of the chapter are Turkey, Syria, Lebanon, Israel, Jordan, Iraq, Saudi Arabia, Iran, Pakistan, Afghanistan, India, and Ceylon. Though Israel has been in recent times a Jewish state, it was for many years a part of this group of predominantly Moslem counrties.

TURKEY

Before World War I when the Old Ottoman Empire was defeated and broken up, very little had been done to modernize medicine and still less to develop nursing. A few western missions, chiefly from America, had included nurses and physicians, and German deaconesses had served in at least one Turkish hospital in Constantinople. In general, however, untrained men attendants were employed in such institutions. In 1923, when Kemal Ataturk and the young Turks created the Republic, they abolished polygamy, ordered women to unveil, and encouraged them to earn their own living as well as to vote and enter public life. Religious freedom was established and the power of the Moslem hierarchy was curbed. Girls of well-to-do families began to attend college and to enter some of the professions. A number studied medicine, but it took exceptional courage and pioneering spirit to go into nursing largely because of the stigma attached to manual work.

The first school of nursing to be established in Istanbul (1920) was in the small American Hospital later named for

Admiral Mark L. Bristol. Organized on American lines by Lyda Anderson, it attracted students of several nationalities, including a few Turkish girls. This school remained an American institution until a few years ago when it received recognition from the Turkish Government. The first Turkish school of nursing was opened by the Red Crescent in 1925 with the help of German and Austrian Red Cross nurses. Turkish physicians controlled both teaching and ward experience, which was available only in old type hospitals where conditions were far from modern. In 1936 Hazel Goff, an American nurse with wide European experience, reorganized the school, introduced a three-year course, and made some headway in modernizing the nursing service and the ward teaching; also in attracting some good candidates. She was followed by Turkish, Polish, and American nurse directors, the predominant influence being American. Finally, Asuman Türer, an attractive, well-prepared Turkish graduate of the school, was appointed (1948) after a period of study in the United States. With good support from influential Turkish groups, she was able to expand and strengthen the school's program and to build up its general reputation.

In 1927 Turkey had passed a law recognizing nursing as one of the professions and ten years later a government examination was required for admission to practice. A few state schools of nursing were also established on the apprenticeship basis in different parts of Turkey. These were open to boys and girls who had completed middle school (at about 15 or 16 years of age) and who were required to accept positions for at least six years after graduation wherever the State sent them. In 1959 only about 1000 nurses had completed such training, most of them men. After the World Health Organization established a regional office in Alexandria, Egypt and opened an advanced course for nurses in this area, the Ministry of Health sent a few Turkish nurses to prepare for more responsible positions. The numbers, however, were quite inadequate.

Meanwhile a Turkish Trained Nurses Association was organized in 1933 with Esma Deniz as president. A graduate of the Womans College in Istanbul and the School of Nursing in the American Hospital there, she had also taken advanced preparation in nursing at Teachers College, New York. Through the gift of a noble lady, the Association acquired an attractive headquarters. It soon began to publish its own journal and joined the International Council of Nurses in 1947 when its membership was about 100. In 1955 it invited the ICN to hold its interim meeting in Istanbul when there was a special celebration of Florence Nightingale's heroic work in nearby Scutari. This aroused much interest among members of the nurses' association and some public-spirited citizens of Istanbul. Shortly after a plan was made to build a Florence Nightingale Hospital and School of Nursing in that city. One of the leaders in this project was Mrs. Seden, a graduate of the American Woman's College and of the Henry Ford Hospital School in Detroit. With the aid of the Red Crescent and the International Cooperation Administration of the U.S.A. and also of Teachers College, Columbia University, a plan was developed for a faculty training project to prepare ten or more Turkish nurses who were to build up this school on a collegiate level with the general advice and cooperation of Dr. R. Louise McManus, then Director of Nursing Education at Teachers College. When the Florence Nightingale Foundation became financially unable to carry out its plans the Turkish Ministry of Health took over the project and this school was opened in the fall of 1961. In addition plans were made by the Ministry of Health to establish a School of Nursing and Health as an integral part of the University of Ankara. Some of the nurses who had been prepared in America were assigned to this University School which is also being developed with the cooperation of the same American advisors.

The main point to be stressed is that both schools will be breaking away from older patterns in nursing education and it is hoped will attract well qualified applicants who are expected to help provide needed leadership in nursing education and service in this country. Such evidences of professional spirit and initiative are especially notable considering the brief period since women's emancipation and the introduction of modern nursing in Turkey. The political instability of the country makes the task especially difficult.

SYRIA

Like most of its neighbors in Asia Minor this country was for centuries under the Turks and gained its freedom after World War I when Syria and Lebanon were united in 1920 under a French mandate. The French influence is still evident in nursing and hospital work in both countries. Roman Catholic and Protestant missionaries from France, Britain, Denmark, and the United States have small hospitals in Syria and have trained a number of native girls as nurses. Though the majority of the people are Moslem Arabs, Nestorian Christians have lived here since St. Ephrem's day (see pp. 47, 58), and it is from such families that most of the nurses are recruited. The National Hospital at Damascus has the only school officially recognized by the Syrian Government (1952). British nurses organized this school (1922), and recently a well-qualified Syrian nurse was put in charge.

Most of the nurses in this country work in hospitals and clinics, and very little public health work had been developed before the World Health Organization was formed in 1948. This body has done much in its direct contacts with governments to stimulate active public health programs and the recruitment and preparation of nurses and midwives for such service. It has also urged the appointment of a well-qualified nurse to the Ministry of Health to advise on nursing questions.

The course in public health nursing organized at Beirut, Lebanon (see p. 369) is open to Syrian nurses. This as well as the rural health demonstrations of the Near East Foundation and regional conferences of nurses did much to raise the standards of nursing service and education in Syria. In 1950 a national association of nurses was formed which was recognized as professional by the Syrian Government but did not qualify at that time for membership in the International Council of Nurses. It has an associate representative in that body, however, and is working toward full membership. The effects of the union of Syria and Egypt and Syria's subsequent secession from the United Arab Republic, make future nursing developments uncertain at the time of writing.

LEBANON

Here more than half the population is Christian, including Armenians and members of Syrian and Greek Orthodox
Churches. Though modern nursing was introduced nearly half
a century ago, its progress was hampered by political, racial, and
religious divisions within the nursing group and by the great
diversity of nursing standards and of basic concepts of nursing.
Of the four government-recognized schools of nursing, two were
French in language and pattern, one under French nuns and
the other under Red Cross nurses. There was also a Moslem
school for Arab-speaking trainees. The pioneer nursing school
of the Near East was established in 1905 in the American Hospital of Beirut and for years was led by Jane Van Zant. Later
it became a part of the American University of Beirut, with an
optional program leading to a degree. Though education among
Lebanese women was more advanced than in most countries of
this region, few in this group showed much interest in nursing.
However, students came to this educational center from many
lands, East and West, twenty-four countries being represented
among its alumnae. Few remained in Lebanon chiefly because
of the lack of openings for professional nurses. Contacts among
the four schools, their students and staffs, were few, and efforts
to find some basis of cooperation were not very successful,
often because of language and religious differences and the
lack of government interest in setting minimum standards of
nursing practice and education.

This was the situation in 1950 when the country became
fully autonomous and joined the United Nations and the World
Health Organization. On the advice of WHO experts, a public
health program was drawn up for the country and steps were
taken to prepare public health nurses and midwives to help
carry out plans for rural as well as city health centers. Public
health nurses from abroad were appointed temporarily to the
Ministry of Health to advise on and direct these activities the
first being an American, Mary Mills. A regional one-year training program was established at the American University of Bei-

rut in 1951, and by 1954 forty-eight nurses from eight different countries, including a number from Lebanon, had completed the course. An Arab nurse, Hilda Hakim, who was sent abroad for study, then replaced the American nurse (Margaret Willhoit) who had directed it up to that time. With the aid of the Near East Foundation and the U. S. Point IV Program, some rural health demonstrations were established. These helped to arouse interest and to create a demand for similar centers elsewhere. Plans were taking shape for nursing legislation and a nursing association for Lebanon was formed, which, like Syria's, had an associate representative in the International Council of Nurses. This is only one of many examples of the influence of international agencies in advising and helping not only to provide leadership but to defray initial expenses in such programs.

ISRAEL[1]

The old biblical land of Palestine, inhabited chiefly by Jewish and Moslem (Arab) peoples, was for centuries a part of the Turkish Empire. Before 1918 it was still in the dark ages as far as medical and health work was concerned. That year the first Zionist unit of twenty trained nurses entered Jerusalem with General Edmund Allenby and the British Army. Shortly after, Henrietta Szold, an ardent American Zionist and philanthropist, organized Hadassah (the American Women's Zionist Organization). The main purpose of this highly useful and influential group was to develop public health services and to train Palestinian nurses for both hospital and visiting nursing. Three nurses from the United States, the Misses Klombers, Kaplan, and Landsman, started the Hadassah school which was later named for Henrietta Szold. After 1936, Shulamith Cantor, an able Palestinian graduate of the Beirut Nursing School in Lebanon, was appointed director. With good support from Hadassah, standards were raised, and this school was able to keep pace with general developments in nursing education in the United States. It was made an integral part of the Hebrew University and

[1] This section applies also to Palestine up to 1948 when Israel became a separate nation.

Medical Center which were located on Mount Scopus some miles from Jerusalem. Later it had to move back to that city because of the Jordan-Israeli hostilities, which continued for years to make this fine building unsafe for use. It is now replaced by a new one in Jerusalem.

The British Government, which held trusteeship for Palestine from 1918 to 1948, had built hospitals largely for its own military and other personnel. The nursing was directed by British matrons and sisters who followed in general the system of their country. Jewish and Arab trainees, both men and women, were prepared for practical hospital service in these institutions. Palestine also had an important health agency, Kupat Holim, which grew out of the Workers' Sick Fund, a small health insurance project started in 1912. This fund, later taken over by the General Federation of Jewish Labor, supported many social and health services and had its own hospitals, clinics, and nursing schools which gradually spread over the country. In addition, a few Christian missionary groups of different sects and nationalities were located in Palestine, some of which operated hospitals and trained a few nurses.

Reorganization Under the Republic of Israel

In 1948, when the State of Israel came into existence, it proceeded to admit Jewish refugees in unlimited numbers from all quarters of the globe and soon faced a national emergency which in its complexity has rarely if ever been paralleled. Pouring into this small land from as many as thirty different countries were thousands of refugees of all ages and stages of civilization, many of them speaking strange languages, suffering from unfamiliar diseases, and knowing nothing about modern hygiene, sanitation, and medicine. The new State of Israel had already committed itself to a comprehensive socialized system of medical and health care for all its people. Its Ministry of Health immediately drafted all the health personnel available and proceeded to work out plans for doubling the number of nurses and auxiliary workers and utilizing as far as possible the newcomers who had previous preparation or the basic qualifications needed for such work. Mrs. Cantor was appointed head of the nursing department in the Ministry which was responsible for the recruitment and training of such workers, including all groups from nursing aides to nurse teachers, supervisors, and administrators. A large proportion of the new arrivals had to learn Hebrew, the official language of the country, as well as the technical content of their courses. At one time as many as ten different language groups were being taught in schools of nursing, some taking supplemental courses and others the complete nursing course.

By 1952 the three-year schools had increased to eleven, and six one-year assistant nurse programs were going on in addition to shorter programs for aides. The most serious shortages were in the higher posts, where complex adjustments had to be made almost on a day-to-day basis. The fact that the personnel represented almost every known system of medical and nursing care made human relationships as well as efficient service exceptionally difficult. It was obvious that some integration of these various systems would be necessary but this could not be attempted while the emergency was still acute.

Palestinian nurses were handicapped in dealing with this crisis chiefly because they had not yet organized themselves as a unified professional group. In the early days most of the nurses had joined the National Labor Federation, which was an integral part of the political and economic structure of the country and had responsibility for the health and welfare of workers through its insurance system and other economic plans. The federation had different sections for professional and practical nurses. Since the former group was not self-governing in the sense required for membership in the International Council of Nurses, it could not join that organization, but it had a national associate representative who reported regularly on nursing developments and attended meetings of the grand council. At the 1953 ICN congress this group qualified for full membership as the National Association of Nurses in Israel. The League of Nursing Education, another Israeli organization, was composed chiefly of nurse administrators and teachers, friends and supporters, lay and medical. Though useful and influential, the League could not speak for the entire group of trained nurses.

Since the regional office of the World Health Organization was set up for the East Mediterranean area, its nursing adviser has been available for advice and consultation and Israeli nurses have been well represented in regional workshops and conferences. With WHO assistance, a survey of nursing in Israel was made in 1951-1952 which focused mainly on nursing education both basic and postbasic. Special attention was given to the integration of public health and social content into the basic nursing curriculum. A longer study, in which nursing, medical, and other specialists participated, presented a comprehensive scheme for the reorganization and unification of nursing in Israel. This included plans for the aid of the Hebrew University in strengthening the basic and advanced programs of the Henrietta Szold School, also for the establishment of a school of nursing by the government.

Though the political and economic situation continues to be tense and difficult and relations between the new state and its near neighbors are still strained, many examples of racial, religious, and organizational cooperation are found. For example, the Hadassah school since leaving Mount Scopus has been hospitably housed in part of the Jerusalem Convent belonging to a French order of nuns. Visitors also speak of the fine spirit and good team work of Moslem, Christian, and Jewish students enrolled in the school. In spite of all the complications and hazards that this little country still faces, it continues to be a leading example of progressive policies and standards in nursing and health work in this part of the world. Recently the state schools have enrolled students from several African countries at the request of their governments.

JORDAN, IRAQ, AND SAUDI ARABIA

These three countries are predominantly Arab in race and Moslem in religion and have much the same historical and cultural background. For the most part nomadic, their people have few settled communities, and modern educational and medical facilities are still quite primitive, except in a few large centers. Conquered by the Turks and for many centuries a part of the Turkish Empire, these Arab lands were liberated in World War I and put under a British mandate by the League of Nations. As in Palestine, Britain built government hospitals where native attendants and nurses (chiefly men) were given practical training, and some beginnings were made in modern public health and educational programs. A few schools, hospitals, and clinics were developed also by foreign religious groups and in some cases by oil companies for their employees. In the last two decades more women nurses and midwives have been trained, but the supply is very small in comparison with the size of the area and the health needs of the people. The Arab part of Palestine now included in Jordan is relatively better supplied with hospitals and trained nurses, and the nurses there have had longer experience in both hospital and community nursing. Since 1948 about a million Arabs have been living in the refugee camps near the border and some of these people have been trained as nurses and midwives for such groups. A new school in Amman is now in charge of Adebih Mussalem, a Christian Arab.

In Baghdad, Iraq, the largest city in this area, once a great cultural center which supported medical schools and hospitals superior to any in Europe at the time, the chief school of nursing was opened in 1933. This school which offers a three-year program is connected with the Hospital of the Republic (formerly the Royal Hospital). Within the last few years it began to attract some Arab girls of good social position and education, and a few of its graduates have been sent abroad for advanced preparation. Another hospital and nursing school were organized recently at Jeddah in Saudi Arabia where a quarantine station has been established.

Here as elsewhere in the Near East the regional office of the World Health Organization and the United States Point IV program in this area have opened a new chapter in the field of health and welfare work. Governments were aided in carrying out surveys and demonstrations which have led to a great saving of life, especially among mothers and infants and sufferers from infectious diseases. Such campaigns, which dramatized the services of modern doctors, nurses and midwives, have increased the demand for such workers. Foreign nurses employed by international health agencies have done much to establish sound patterns of nursing education and service and to help indigenous nurses to organize themselves for mutual support and self government. A promising sign of progress is the admission of the Jordan Nurses Association as one of the new members of the International Council of Nurses at its 1961 Congress.

Other encouraging developments are the wider use of oil revenues for health and education and the rise of a new middle class which is demanding better conditions of living and a greater measure of self government. The isolation of these countries from other parts of the world has been greatly lessened in recent years, and better economic and educational conditions have contributed to a decline in the old fatalistic attitudes which so long obstructed progress in medical and health work. With the modern revival, however, political and nationalist tensions have increased, and the growing unrest in most of the Arab nations makes the future rather uncertain at the time of writing.

IRAN

Farther east is the old kingdom of Persia which has preserved its national independence and much of its ancient culture but has done very little to improve the health and welfare of its people. Though racially distinct from the Arabs, the majority of the Iranians are Moslems. Nearly a century ago western missionaries introduced modern medicine in a few spots but did not make much headway in promoting the training of doctors and nurses. Health conditions, especially in rural districts, are still quite primitive. In the 1930's a liberal government unveiled women, introduced compulsory education for girls and boys, and authorized the opening of four government schools of nursing under English and American nurses. These schools were barely started when because of World War II most of the foreign nurses were compelled to leave. In Teheran hospitals western-trained physicians and missionary nurses made some effort to train ward nurses and doctors' assistants, but facilities were lacking and the status of nurses was too low to attract suitable applicants.

Fortunately the ruling Shah, Mohammed Riza Pahlevi, and his twin sister, Ashraf, were deeply interested in health and welfare work and with other influential Iranians formed a voluntary association similar to the Red Cross which was called the Imperial Organization for Social Services of the Red Lion and Sun. In 1951 this society built a beautiful school of nursing with a nurses' home in Teheran and staffed it with a British matron and sisters. Though the entrance standard was equivalent to full secondary education, this school attracted more applicants than it could accept. It has had many ups and downs, however, caused chiefly by unstable political conditions which weakened the influence of the Shah and his family and led to the resignation of the British nurses who were replaced by others from Sweden. Other difficulties have arisen from the ill-defined role of nurses and the lack even of a suitable designation to indicate the range of their responsibilities and the dignity of their calling. The Ashraf nurses, however, have made a good name for themselves and have been the chief pioneers in both hospital and public health nursing.

Early in the 1950's the Ministry of Health, in cooperation with Point IV experts from the United States, began to develop a national rural health program in which mobile teams were employed. Nurses and midwives on these teams demonstrated methods of health teaching and helped to train health aides to work in the villages, particularly with mothers and children. An Iranian nurse, Fatemeh Salsali, has now been appointed in the Ministry of Health. Under the Iran Foundation a new school of nursing at the Nemasee Hospital in Shiraz is giving its students special experience and training in order to fit them to teach and supervise such auxiliary personnel and to carry on the nursing work in the health centers, which are part of the national health scheme.

The number of trained nurses and midwives is now said to be increasing in Iran (many of them trained in England). With the aid of World Health Organization regional advisers, their leaders have formed a national association, the Iranian Nurses Association, which has full membership in the International Council of Nurses.

PAKISTAN

Since most of Pakistan's nursing history is included in the story of India, this part will begin in 1947 when British rule ended and India was divided into two nations, the one predominantly Hindu and the other Moslem. Up to that time the Moslem families had followed most of their ancient customs, though a few of the younger women had emancipated themselves and were taking some share in community activities. Following partition, the tragic loss of life from bloody riots, and the lack of medical and sanitary facilities forced the government and community leaders to take immediate action. Few foreign nurses remained in either country, leaving about 750 trained nurses in Pakistan for a population of about seventy millions. Among them, only a handful had any administrative or teaching experience. There were 300 hospital schools of nursing in the entire area, most of which were disorganized. During this emergency valuable aid came from foreign missionary and other humanitarian groups, some of which stayed on to help reorganize hospitals and schools. The Pakistan Government also employed a number of British matrons and sisters who had been in similar positions in India and sent about thirty Pakistani nurses to Britain and Australia for special training.

Fortunately, it was not necessary to create much new administrative machinery, since registration laws governing the training and practice of nurses, midwives, and health visitors had been set up earlier in all parts of India with Provincial Nursing Councils to administer them. A new Central Council was appointed in Karachi, the capital, and plans were made to appoint a Pakistani nurse to the post of Nursing Superintendent in the Ministry of Health as soon as a suitable person could be found. Also previously organized were the provincial branches of the Trained Nurses' Association of India, which had nurse appointees on the Provincial Councils and some experience in dealing with such official bodies. In 1949 a Trained Nurses' Association of Pakistan was formed with a British nurse as president and with about 200 active members and 400 associate members, these chiefly among student nurses. This association took immediate steps to secure membership in the International Council of Nurses, of which it is now an active member, and to make its influence felt in plans for the new medical and health service. In making such plans the Pakistan Government had as a guide the results of the comprehensive national health survey of India made shortly before partition. This called for a large increase in all health personnel but especially in nurses, midwives, and health visitors. According to the estimates at that time, Pakistan would need 170,000 nurses for its population and did not have even one per cent of that number. It now has 2000 nurses.

Although the situation was extremely serious, the authorities had at least a skeleton health structure to build on and the shock of the national emergency had roused their people, particularly their women, to a new sense of their civic obligations. Many women who had emerged from purdah to share in the rescue work decided to discard the veil. A stimulating example was set by Begum Liaquat Ali Kahn, modern-minded wife of the first prime minister. As founder-president of the All Pakistan Woman's Association, she led many of her Moslem sisters into active participation in political and civic affairs and now rallied her followers in helping to staff schools, hospitals, and refugee enterprises with volunteers. Meanwhile, they secured recruits for training schools, where nurses, midwives, health visitors and social workers were prepared. This association also did much to secure a dignified status for such workers and to provide needed support for the schools.

The old prejudices against hand work did not disappear at once, and, as in India, the health visitor's role was often preferred to that of nurse or midwife. Some change in viewpoint was noted when a number of public health nurses and trained midwives from other countries began to arrive as members of health teams sent by the World Health Organization, the United Nations Children's Fund, and other international agencies to develop maternal and child-health centers in both urban and rural communities. Their example as well as the talks they gave in nursing schools and communities raised the prestige of their professions, and many girls were attracted also by the offer of fellowships for study abroad to qualify them for more advanced positions. Before long a postgraduate course was started in Karachi, and a College of Nursing was established in which a higher level basic program was given for girls with better education. These with junior and assistant nurses and two grades of midwives helped to meet the urgent need.

Though many problems remain here as in other countries of this group, a good beginning was made in breaking down centuries-old taboos and in laying the foundation for an effective nursing and health structure in this large and populous country.

AFGHANISTAN

Bordering Iran, Pakistan, Kashmir, Tibet and the USSR is this remote, almost inaccessible, and relatively undeveloped country of mixed races, most of them followers of Islam. Until 1950 there was little or no organized medical and public health work in the area. Then the government invited the World Health Organization to help survey its needs, to conduct anti-typhus and antimalaria campaigns, and, with the aid of the United Nations Children's Fund, to set up a pilot project in maternal and child health which was expanded in 1951. Plans were next made to start training schools in the capital, Kabul, for men and women nurses under the medical staff of Kabul University. Midwives were also prepared under the Ministry of Health. Since girls have only recently come out of purdah and general education is still at a rather early stage in this country, it is too soon to expect much initiative from this group. Under the leadership of regional staffs of WHO and allied groups and with the now promising improvements in general education, there are good hopes that health work, including nursing, will improve steadily. As to the system of nursing that will be adopted, much depends on whether the dominant influence in Afganistan will come from its powerful neighbor in the north, or from the western nations that have adopted the principles laid down by the founder of modern nursing.

INDIA

This large and important country, which up to 1947 included Pakistan, was for many years a part of the British Empire and was the first in Asia to benefit from the Nightingale reforms in nursing, hospital, and health work. As noted in Chapter 7, Miss Nightingale's discovery of the high mortality and morbidity rates of British soldiers in India led her to urge the establishment of a government commission to investigate health conditions in that country. She had a large share not only in writing the commission's report but in publicizing its findings and in helping to make its recommendations effective. Progress was slow, however, for many reasons, among them the limited funds available, the extremes of wealth and poverty in India, the wide variety of races, languages, religious beliefs, and castes, and the restrictions under which most Indian women lived. Although some of these conditions have improved in recent years, the problems facing health workers of all groups are still great and should be kept in mind in tracing the progress of modern nursing in India.

The first definite steps were taken in 1865, when in answer to a request from the Sanitary Commission for Bengal Miss Nightingale sent a detailed report entitled "Suggestions on a System of Nursing for Hospitals in India." [2] This contains a full outline of a scheme to train Indian women which followed the general plan of the then new Nightingale School in London. She even offered to help prepare nurses to start the new system, saying that though the supply was limited the school was "most anxious to send some seed." It was not until 1879, however, that the first contingent of British sisters arrived to staff the military hospitals in India. Shortly after, a plan for civilian hospitals and training schools was developed largely through Miss Nightingale's efforts to interest the governors of India in

[2] Reprinted in Lucy Ridgely Seymer, *Florence Nightingale, 1820-1910. Selected Writings* (New York: Macmillan, 1954), p. 228. See Bibliography, p. 121.

such work. Among these Lord Dufferin and his able wife were especially active and influential. With the aid of prominent Indians and British residents, a substantial fund was raised for the health of mothers and children and named for Lady Dufferin. Because men doctors are almost entirely excluded under the purdah system, this national association established cottage hospitals for women, in which women doctors and midwives as well as nurses were employed. The first of these hospitals (opened in 1886 at Cama, Bombay) was headed by Edith Atkinson, an English trained nurse, who organized a small school for the training of native nurses and midwives. Government and Lady Dufferin hospitals and training schools were followed by others established by Christian missionary groups of different denominations from Britain, America, and other countries.

Until the British left India, the majority of trained nurses came from these mission schools, which were directed in most cases by foreign superintendents and head nurses. It took some time to attract the better educated young women of the middle and upper classes into an occupation that most Indians considered menial and low caste. Among the first groups to overcome these obstacles were the descendents of Christian families around the Madras area whose ancestors were converted by apostles of the early Church many centuries ago. Parsee women around Bombay, whose ancestors came from Persia, were also freer from caste restrictions. A third group of Eurasians, who were of mixed western and eastern parentage, with no well-defined social status, were less restricted in their choice of occupations and when educated sometimes occupied important positions. An example is Edith Paull who became president of the Trained Nurses Association of India.

In more recent years Mahatma Ghandi's influence did much to weaken caste and class prejudices and to encourage men and women of all groups to share in nursing and other practical services which benefited themselves and others. According to his biographers, he was an excellent practical nurse and sanitarian, scrupulously careful in his diet and personal hygiene, and so strongly convinced of the need for cleanliness that he led his disciples in scavenging and cleaning up dirty, insanitary streets, public conveyances, and temples. Like St. Francis, he cared for lepers, nursed in plague hospitals, and even treated sick animals. He also stood for the emancipation of women. Rajkumari Amrit Kaur, a Princess who became the new India's first Minister of Health, was one of his disciples. It is significant too that the national fund in memory of his wife Kasturba is devoted to the training of village workers to lead in home health and better living.

Indian Health Services Since Independence

Ghandi's campaign led in 1949 to a more general movement to free India from colonial rule. This was successful, but it resulted also in the separation of India and Pakistan. For a time religious and communal conflicts brought serious loss of life in both countries. Four years earlier an important plan outlining a health program for India had been prepared by the Government Commission on Health Services and Development. This commission had as chairman Sir Joseph Bhore, a distinguished Indian judge, and the report whose first four volumes were published in 1945 is commonly called *The Bhore Report*. This was followed in 1951 by *The First Five-Year Plan*, which summarized the results of the program actually carried out and outlined the next steps to be taken. The commission, drawing on the experience of many countries, both East and West, and on all the health professions, presented an exceptionally objective, realistic picture of the whole situation, which is valuable as a guide to India's medical and health problems and to similar situations elsewhere.

The general scheme had much in common with those of other British Commonwealth countries which had nationalized their health services but was handicapped by India's seriously limited supply of trained nurses (the proportion of nurses to doctors was then six to ten). It was decided to proceed by stages, and though the long term goal was one nurse to 500 of the population the immediate goal was one to 40,000. The nurse supply was to be increased from 7000 to 80,000 in the next few years with the hope of reaching a million by 1970. Schools of nursing, which numbered 300 (most of them operated on the apprenticeship plan), were to be greatly expanded, their programs broadened and strengthened, and more emphasis given to disease prevention and public health nursing. The minimum standard of education (approximately that of school leaving at about fifteen years) was to remain, but better educated girls were to be recruited and prepared for teaching, supervision, and administrative posts in hospitals and community nursing services. Similar plans were made for training midwives and health visitors, and these programs and services were to be more closely coordinated with nursing in the future. Several kinds of auxiliary workers also were attached to the nursing services, and plans were made to give them more instruction in home nursing, hygiene, sanitation, and child care, also in teaching of these to the general public.

A total of four schools of nursing of a collegiate type provide basic and graduate nurse programs for applicants with better academic backgrounds and leadership potentialities, and it is hoped that similar schools will soon be developed in each of the Indian provinces. The school at Madras University is affiliated with the nearby Christian Medical College and Vellore Hospital. Its first educational director was Florence Taylor, a Canadian nurse who was followed by Annamma Matthews, a graduate of Vellore. The College of Nursing at New Delhi University was directed for several years by Marguerita Craig (an American). Her associate, Edith Buchanan (a Canadian), continues as educational director. Meanwhile Indian nurses who had gone abroad for postgraduate study were taking responsible positions in hospitals and schools of nursing throughout the country. They were appointed also to top posts under the national and provincial governments, the most responsible of which was chief nurse of the Central Nursing Council in the National Government filled by T. K. Adranvala, a well-qualified Parsee nurse, who had been the first Indian to be president of the Trained Nurses Association of India. Indian nurses also have important positions in the army, navy, and air services and in the provincial branches of the Trained Nurses Association of India, which are semiautonomous and function under their own paid officers. The Indian Nursing Council is responsible for recommending minimum nursing standards for the whole country and coordinating the work of the provincial councils which administer regisration laws and supervise schools in their areas.

Nurses' Organizations and Their Work

The Trained Nurses Association of India was first proposed in 1905 by a group of British matrons, chiefly those in government hospitals. A few years later it was expanded to include other trained nurses, the majority of whom were from English-speaking countries and were employed in mission hospitals. This group had formed a Nurses' Auxiliary of the Christian Medical Nursing Association which then affiliated with the TNAI. Nurses from Britain, Australasia and North America were fairly well represented in the new membership, and the policies and programs sponsored by the Nurses Association showed a mixture of such influences. One serious limitation in the early years was the relatively small number of Indian nurses and their inactive role. This was due in part to language differences, and to the limited general education and professional experience of most Indian nurses at that time. The TNAI launched *The Nursing Journal of India* in 1910 and joined the International Council of Nurses in 1912 as the first Asian member.

This world body soon became an active influence in stimulating national groups to look into the conditions and preparation of nurses and to work for a higher status for them. Studies were made by the TNAI that brought to light many bad conditions in both Indian and foreign-controlled hospitals and schools and these were reported to government officials with recommendations for improvement. A major activity was the campaign for legislative controls which led to nurse registration laws in all the provinces and to effective machinery for their administration. Qualified nurse-secretaries were appointed and nursing councils set up on which representatives of the nurses' association served. By affiliating the TNAI with the Women's Council of India, the understanding support of many well-educated, public-spirited, and influential lay women was secured. This did much to help change public opinion on the status and work of nurses. The Trained Nurses Association was also consulted and made many excellent suggestions when the new medical and health plans were being drawn up.

Although these recent requirements for expansion brought some decline in standards of service and education, one stabilizing factor was the relatively large number of hospitals and schools that remained under private (chiefly missionary) agencies. Though less independent than formerly, such groups have cooperated actively in the national plans and have often supplied needed leadership in introducing medical and nursing teaching on modern lines. Examples of medical centers under inter-denominational missionary auspices which have contributed substantially to the preparation of Indian doctors and nurses for their new responsibilities are Vellore in south India and Ludiana farther north. Miraj in west India is also cooperating with the government in preparing a similar center for Bombay state.

CEYLON

For more than a century a part of the British Indian Empire, this beautiful island became independent in 1948 and like India and Pakistan soon joined the British Commonwealth of Nations. Its people, who are predominantly Singhalese in race and Buddhist in religion, have had fewer caste divisions and are more homogeneous than those of India. Recently, however, the infiltration of workers from South India has resulted in communal clashes and some radical political movements have developed.

What has been said about the recent history of nursing in India applies in general to Ceylon. Its government has developed a new national health plan based on a study of the island's needs and resources. This plan includes an extension of preventive and curative services to meet the health needs of its nine million people and the preparation of much larger numbers of health personnel, including trained nurses. Of these there were only about 1000 when the plan was made, most of whom had rather limited general and professional education. In strengthening their system and preparing more and better nurses, the Ceylon Government has sought the advice and help of nursing and health specialists from the World Health Organization, the countries joining in the Colombo Plan, the Rockefeller Foundation, and the Point IV program of the United States. A new school of nursing of higher grade, connected with the University of Ceylon near Colombo, was organized by two American nurses, Dorothy Sutherland and Martha Crawford. It is attracting English-speaking students who qualify for university matriculation and are otherwise fitted to prepare for the higher positions in nursing. Three other schools whose programs are conducted in the vernacular are preparing nurses for staff positions in hospitals and community nursing services. Several Ceylonese nurses have been sent to Australia, New Zealand, and Great Britain for postgraduate work in tuberculosis and other specialties, and seminars and workshops have helped to upgrade and round out the preparation of local nurses. The nursing group has had help also in forming the Ceylon Nurses Association, which had about 250 members and was admitted to the International Council of Nurses in 1953. This association has carried out plans for state registration and other measures designed to raise nursing standards and to put this work on a professional basis. With good government support and fairly stable political and economic conditions, the outlook for modern nursing in Ceylon seems to be promising.

SOUTHEAST ASIA

Facing toward the Indian and Pacific Oceans are Burma, Malaya, Cambodia, Laos, Viet Nam, Thailand, Indonesia, and the Philippine Islands. Though they represent peoples of quite varied racial strains, religions, cultural traditions, and political affiliations, all except Thailand had been governed by western nations and had been directly influenced by their systems of education, medicine, and nursing. During the last few decades nationalist movements have led to the taking over of all of these countries by their own peoples and the setting up of independent governments. Although medical and health work has suffered a good deal, some of the foundations established by the western nations remained and the patterns of nursing reflected these influences. A few also show the influence of Communist Russia and China.

UNION OF BURMA

Earlier governed as a part of British India, this country was detached in 1937 and gained its independence in 1948. Its people, who are chiefly Malay and Mongoloid in origin and Buddhist in religion, have fewer class and caste divisions, are more homogeneous in language and customs than their neighbors to the west, and have much in common with the Chinese and Malay peoples in this region. As in other British colonies, modern nursing was introduced first in government and missionary hospitals and followed in modified form the system in the English-speaking countries. Though Burmese girls were in general freer to engage in such occupations, few of the better educated entered nursing in the earlier period. The situation changed, however, in the last two or three decades when Burma suffered invasions by the Japanese and Chinese armies and a serious civil war.

An American physician, Dr. Gordon S. Seagrave, head of a pioneer missionary hospital, in his book, *Burma Surgeon,* gives a vivid account of the work of these nurses during the war period and pays eloquent tribute to their courage, loyalty, and resourcefulness. Most of the hospitals and schools of nursing in Burma were seriously disorganized and their staffs were scattered. Help came, however, from many sources, including the World Health Organization and other agencies which brought doctors and nurses from various countries. Valuable advice was given on the reorganization of health work. A Ministry and Directorate of Health was set up, and plans for health and rehabilitation centers as well as for hospitals and the training of personnel were developed.

One of the most influential persons in mobilizing support and training workers in nursing and midwifery was Mrs. Aung Sang, widow of the first premier of Burma and herself a trained nurse. Well-prepared nurses from abroad made surveys and helped to organize health centers, particularly for mothers and children. Burmese nurses were sent to other countries for added preparation in the training and supervision of nurses and midwives. Especially helpful were the contacts established with the Philippine Islands, whose nurses were familiar with the problems of the area and had long experience in dealing with them.

During this period a national association of Burmese nurses and midwives was formed, and an associate representative was appointed to the International Council of Nurses to help it meet the requirements of active membership, which was attained as the Burma Nurses Association in 1961. A law recently passed controls the education and practice of nursing. Though still at an early stage in the organization of modern nursing in the country as a whole, the outlook for further development seems hopeful, provided peace is restored in that part of the world and economic, educational, and medical facilities are extended and improved. The health situation, however, has been serious. Life expectancy in 1958 was twenty-seven and seven-tenths years, the second lowest in the world. There is only one physician to every 10,000 of the twenty million population as compared with one to 7100 in India.

The Federation of Malaya and Adjacent Islands

Much the same story has been repeated in this long, narrow Malayan peninsula with the Island of Singapore at its tip and in other nearby regions such as Sarawak and North Borneo, the last three now forming a separate self-governing state. In all this region continued warfare and the influence of subversive groups have led to unstable conditions which have made it exceptionally difficult to maintain constructive health measures. Divisions due to the mixture of Malay, Chinese, Indians, and other races with their differing languages and cultures have also impeded cooperative action in health work as in other essential services.

Earlier, a number of modern government hospitals had been established by the British in the larger centers, and there were smaller missionary hospitals in different parts of the country under foreign-trained doctors and nurses. As elsewhere in this region, girls married early and had to be admitted, as a rule, at about fifteen years of age if they were to receive any training as nurses. In most cases their parents took them out of school when they found eligible husbands for them, and few completed their preparation. With such handicaps, it was difficult to build up a professional group capable of carrying on nursing services or filling responsible posts. For these and other reasons men nurses have had an important share in hospital work.

After World War II, during which most of the foreign nurses were evacuated, various relief and health organizations and the Colonial Office in Britain sent detachments of nurses to help in reconstruction. Courses were set up for assistant nurses, dressers, and *bedans* (midwives with elementary training who worked chiefly in rural districts). Some of the better prepared nurses and midwives from these eastern countries were sent to Britain or to Australia, New Zealand, or the Philippines for added training and experience to broaden their preparation and fit them for teaching and supervisory positions. The organization of the Regional Office of the World Health Organization in New Delhi provided a permanent nurse consultant in this general area who could advise and help these local leaders in their difficult task. A Malayan Trained Nurses Association was organized which brought nurses together for mutual help and the advancement of their work. This body under its president, Myra Wang, was recently admitted to full membership in the International Council of Nurses.

Singapore nurses are separately organized as the Singapore Trained Nurses Association, which became a member of the ICN at the 1961 Congress. One school of nursing, which provides full training, is recognized by the Singapore Nursing Board and the General Nursing Council for England and Wales.

Individual nurses who qualify may also secure reciprocity with the General Council for England and Wales. Such steps indicate that a beginning has been made toward a more permanent and stable status for nursing in this region.

THAILAND

This fabulous little kingdom (before 1948 known as Siam), has attracted much attention in the western world. It has also managed to retain its independence and to escape many of the wars and other troubles that have beset its neighbors. The Royal Family has taken an active interest in nursing and midwifery. In 1896 the Queen Mother established the first training school for midwives at the Siriraj Hospital, Bangkok. Other members of the Royal Family have become patrons of hospitals and schools of nursing and some have themselves taken training and assumed responsible positions in directing such work.

Before 1914 there were two schools of nursing, one under missionary auspices and the other at the Red Cross Hospital in Bangkok. Shortly after, a school of nursing and midwifery was opened in the Siriraj Hospital, with a well-known American nurse, Alice Fitzgerald, in charge. Several others were developed later, there being eight hospital schools and two which are affiliated with universities at the time of writing. Basic preparation takes two and one half to three years, and some schools offer an extra year for midwifery. This specialty, which in Thailand enjoys good standing, is often combined with nursing. Some Thai nurses have gone to the Philippines or elsewhere for more advanced training in these and other fields.

The Nurses Association of Thailand was organized in 1927 with the aid of western nurses, and a national associate representative from the group was appointed by that body to the ICN. This first step and other organizational developments led in 1961 to full membership in the International Council of Nurses. Consultants from the Regional Office of the World Health Organization have urged the government to appoint a nurse director and two assistants to the Ministry of Health to advise on nursing education and registration, to promote more advanced courses for nurses, and to provide modern textbooks and teaching aids. The association also helps to provide fellowships for study abroad to give promising Thai nurses an opportunity to broaden their outlook as well as to prepare them for more effective leadership at home. As a result some progress has been made in improving schools of nursing and in providing postbasic courses. Since the supply of nurses in this country as in many others is inadequate for the population of more than twenty million, further stimulus is needed to recruit candidates for nursing and to provide appropriate preparation for them.

LAOS, CAMBODIA, AND VIET NAM

The former associated states of Laos and Cambodia and Cochin-China, Tonkin, and Annam, now known as Viet Nam, were part of the French colonial empire. Their peoples are closely related by race, religion, and culture to nearby Thailand, and their governmental and other institutions, including those concerned with health and education, were patterned on those of France. Though there were some French nuns and lay nurses in the hospitals in the large cities such as Saigon and a few hospital schools which trained men and women nurses and midwives, the numbers and services of such workers were quite limited. These and other medical and health groups were seriously disorganized by the civil wars and the nationalist movements of recent years which resulted in the partition of Viet Nam and the exodus of many thousands from the Communist North to the South. A serious emergency developed which brought specialists from the World Health Organization and many other health and relief organizations to this overcrowded little country. After a brief survey of the health situation of South Viet Nam, a five-year plan was set up which focused on measures to control prevailing epidemic and endemic diseases and to improve the health and welfare of women and children. Professional nurses from several countries conducted demonstrations, developed health centers, and taught indigenous health workers of all grades. Some of the more promising of these were sent away for further preparation, and as elsewhere in this area an effort was made to bring nursing and midwifery into closer relationship both in service and training.

Similar programs have been started in Laos and Cambodia which were also greatly influenced by French systems of medicine and nursing. As to North Viet Nam, little is known, but it is assumed that Communist China has established its patterns of health work here as in other countries under its influence. Though efforts have been made to help the trained nurses in the other associated states to organize themselves and to get in touch with the International Council of Nurses, there is little evidence of progress at this time.

Before leaving the history of nursing in this part of the globe, a word should be said about a courageous French Army nurse, Généviève de Galard Terraube, who won the admiration of the world by refusing to leave her post during the siege of Dienbienphu in Viet Nam. This daughter of a long line of French aristocrats and soldiers exemplified not only the ancient knightly motto *noblesse oblige* but the best traditions of the modern nursing profession to which she belongs. An heroic figure of more recent years, and one closely associated with this part of eastern Asia, was the American doctor, Thomas A. Dooley. His example inspired many nurses as well as doctors to volunteer their services often in improvised jungle hospitals here and in at least eleven other countries. The work begun by Dr. Dooley is being carried on by MEDICO, a service of CARE, and the effort to boost health aid overseas is now receiving new and a greater emphasis through the consolidation of these two groups.

INDONESIA

Southeast of the Malay Peninsula and north of Australia lie the islands of Sumatra, Java, Bali, and many others formerly belonging to the Netherlands East Indies, which in 1950 became the Republic of Indonesia. Only a part of New Guinea remained under the Netherlands, the other half being assigned by the United Nations to Australia's trusteeship. The Indonesians are related to the Malay peoples scattered throughout this general area. Their earlier history, however, was closely linked with that of India and in recent times large numbers of Chinese, Indians, Eurasians, and other groups have been added to their total population of nearly one hundred million. The majority of Indonesians are Moslems, but many other religions are represented.

The Dutch Government and people did much to develop the economic resources of these islands and to build up the health, education, and well-being of their people. In addition to modern hospitals and health services under government control, there were some under missionary auspices (chiefly Lutheran). Many hospitals had schools of nursing which prepared young men and women for less responsible positions but rarely for administrative and teaching work, since registered nurses from the Netherlands usually filled these posts. Though national registration in Holland was open to Indonesian nurses, few were able to qualify because of language, educational, and other handicaps. There was a Java branch of the National Nurses Association of the Netherlands to which most of the registered nurses belonged and so were represented in the International Council of Nurses. Indigenous nurses were subject to special restrictions, especially as nationalist and communist movements became stronger.

When the Netherlands Government was finally forced to leave, the Indonesians who took over had little training in self-government or in positions of responsibility and serious confusion resulted in nursing, as in other fields of work. Intensive efforts were made to convince them of the superiority of the Soviet system of government and of medical and health work. After Indonesia joined the United Nations and the World Health Organization, advice was sought from these agencies and preliminary surveys were made which led to recommendations similar to those given in other countries of this general area. Reports indicate that some progress has been made in rebuilding nursing schools and services and in preparing leaders in nursing and midwifery. An Association of Indonesian Nurses has been organized and its president, Miss A. E. Kalangie, has been appointed a national associate representative affiliated with the International Council of Nurses. These steps would seem to indicate that some Indonesian nurses are anxious to join with other nurses of the world and to develop their work on a modern professional basis.

REPUBLIC OF THE PHILIPPINES

Also located in southeast Asia north of Indonesia are the Philippine Islands. In their racial origins and early traditions the people of these islands are closely related to those of Malaya, Indonesia, Thailand and other countries in this region. They were greatly influenced, however, by their Spanish conquerors, who remained more than four centuries, introduced their language and religion, intermarried with the Filipinos, and established many Spanish customs. Beginning with the Spanish-American War in 1898 when the United States took over this and some other parts of the Spanish Empire, the American influence has been strong, even though this country became an independent republic in 1946. One reason is that in these islands where there are nine different languages and ninety-five dialects, the introduction of English in the public schools gave the majority of people for the first time a common language (even though not the official one). This and the building of roads and the introduction of self-government are considered the great contributions of America. The form of government is also much like that of the United States. Most of the population is Roman Catholic, but there is freedom of religion, and substantial numbers of the people belong to Protestant, Moslem, and other faiths.

Until the end of Spanish rule, hospitals were administered chiefly by religious sisterhoods, with a low grade of servants doing the actual nursing and ward work. After 1900, trained nurses in the American Army of Occupation reorganized the nursing in several hospitals but did not attempt to train Filipino nurses until 1907. A year earlier a small nursing school had been opened in a Protestant mission hospital in Iloilo by Dr. Andrew Hall and his wife. Its influence was limited chiefly because of social and religious prejudices at that time and the immaturity and low educational standing of the girls who entered.

Much of the success of the first Manila school can be traced to the influence of a distinguished lady, Mrs. Jaime deVeyra, who was Mary Coleman, American dean of the Manila Normal School. She encouraged promising girls to apply by appealing to their patriotism and ambition for higher education. They were first given one year of preparation in the normal school and then sent into reorganized hospitals for two years of practical instruction and training. Since women nurses at the start were not allowed to care for men patients, a school of equal size for men was developed. These two schools were later combined and attached to the Philippine General Hospital, a new modern institution under the Bureau of Health. When women nurses began to care for both men and women, nursing became more of a woman's profession.

General Leonard Wood, who headed the government's medical and public health program, had much influence in gaining the support of the medical profession and the public for the new concept of nursing. Representatives of the Rockefeller Foundation also encouraged Filipino nurses to prepare themselves for positions of responsibility in various branches of nursing, and some of the more promising received scholarships for study in the United States. The group as a whole showed unusual self-reliance, initiative, and courage in opening up new schools and nursing services in different parts of the country. These qualities were traditional among Filipino women. When the United States announced its policy of turning over leading positions to Filipino nurses, most of the American nurses withdrew, but there were always a few in mission hospitals and in other positions, such as the Red Cross, who could give advice and help when asked.

They stood by, for example, in the early years of the Filipino Nurses Association (organized in 1923) when the young profession was taking its first steps in self-government and meeting a good deal of opposition. One critical issue was courageously faced when a student nurse who gave a fatal dose of medicine prescribed by a physician was threatened with a prison term. The nurses' association defended her in the courts and won after a stiff fight. It joined the International Council of Nurses in 1926 and launched its own magazine, *The Filipino Nurse* (now called *The Philippine Journal of Nursing*), in the same year. Many other successful achievements in nursing service, education, legislation, and other professional activities followed in the next few years when this new group was establishing itself, in most cases keeping close to the policies and programs of the sister profession in the United States. Qualified leaders, several with advanced preparation in American colleges and universities, continued to keep in close touch with nursing developments in the United States.

When World War II struck and this country was attacked and isolated, the Filipino nurses showed their courage, initiative, and stamina in many ways. Later, when peace came and the new republic became independent, the government and people were ready to back them in carrying through a number of important projects: the creation of a permanent nurse corps for the armed forces; the establishment in the new National Department of Health of a Division of Nursing Service headed by a nurse, Genera 'de Guzman; the realization of a long-cherished plan for a College of Nursing as a part of the University of the Philippines under Julita Sotejo (a lawyer as well as a nurse) who is Dean of this College; and the building in Manila of a fine new Nurses Club House and Professional Headquarters to replace the one destroyed in the war. They undertook many other tasks of reconstruction and faced many difficult problems, including a serious nurse shortage. As indicated earlier, they also gave substantial assistance to neighboring countries in southeast Asia, where nursing was in an earlier stage of development and pioneer nurses needed encouragment and friendship.

During recent years nursing progress has continued. For example, there are now ten or more colleges of nursing in the Philippines and many diploma programs requiring one to two years of college preparation for admission. Nursing continues to be one of the most popular vocations for women. One school alone reported recently a thousand applicants for a class of forty students. Several nursing texts have been written and though **a** shorter history of nursing in this country was published earlier, a group at one of the Colleges of Nursing is now at work on a longer history of nursing in the Philippines. These and many other evidences of the progressive spirit and practical achievements of the Filipino nurses will be found in *The Philippine Journal of Nursing* which continues to be a live professional organ.

NORTHEAST ASIA

The countries in this area include mainland China, Formosa, Korea and Japan, all related in race, religion, and culture but varying in national characteristics, language, politics, and other respects. Until about a century ago these ancient oriental nations were comparatively isolated from the western world and opened their doors very reluctantly to traders from Europe and America. Such groups were soon followed by Christian missionaries of various denominations, who established schools and hospitals as well as churches and introduced modern medicine and nursing. These new ideas had a powerful impact, especially the scientific, military, and technical knowledge of the West which led to the rapid modernization of all these nations and to many conflicts between East and West.

China

This immense country, which includes Inner Mongolia, Manchuria, and Tibet, covers a larger territory than Soviet Russia and exceeds it in population, estimated as over 700 million and multiplying rapidly. Until a few years ago, the social, ethical, and religious ideas and customs of the Chinese people were derived chiefly from the teachings of Confucius, but there were also followers of Buddhist and Taoist doctrines and, in recent years, a relatively small group of Christians. Traditionally, the family was the strongest social unit, but outside the home women's activities and influence were quite limited.

When the first trained nurse missionaries arrived in China in the late 1890's they found no organized system of nursing and not even a word for "nurse" in the Chinese language. Their efforts to train Chinese girls and some boys as nurses began shortly after 1900, when small schools were set up in mission hospitals in Foochow, Canton, Shanghai, and Peking. At first the probationers were drawn from the elementary schools, but when secondary schools were developed the standards of admission were raised and in general kept pace with those of the English-speaking countries from which most of the early nurse missionaries came. The first was Elizabeth McKechnie, a Canadian, who arrived in 1884 and started a small school of nursing. These schools varied widely in their training programs and methods, but as their directors began to meet in medical missionary conferences and to discuss such matters they saw the need for greater agreement. Soon they formed their own association, partly for mutual support but chiefly to develop a more uniform and effective system of nursing for China. In 1909 the Nurses Association of China began its work. Realizing the impossibility of securing registration laws at that time, this association became in effect the accrediting agency for such schools and not only conducted national examinations but gave its own certificate to the students who qualified. Other activities were the publication of the *Nursing Journal of China* as its official organ and the preparation of textbooks in the Chinese language.

Capitalizing on the traditional respect of the Chinese people for scholarship, this group embodied in the new word for "nurse" the symbol of the scholar. This did much to counteract the prejudice against nursing as a menial occupation and to justify the long period of training which in many cases was four years. This was no handicap in attracting and holding Chinese student nurses, since such a status was honorable and the ceremony of graduation with a certificate from the NAC was a very important event. The foreign nurses who at first comprised the NAC membership also began to bring in as members the better qualified Chinese nurses and to prepare them for their broader professional responsibilities.

In 1922, under its first president, Nina Gage, this association joined the International Council of Nurses, and in 1925 when the ICN was invited to hold its next meeting in China Miss

Gage was made president of the ICN.[3] Cora Simpson became the first paid secretary of the NAC. Her indefatigable efforts to extend its work, build up its branches, and develop its attractive headquarters in Nanking are described in her book *A Joy-ride through China.* Lillian Wu, American-trained director of the Red Cross Hospital School in Shanghai, was the first Chinese president of the NAC, and Mary Shih, who had taken a postgraduate course in New York, was the first Chinese secretary.

A new period opened in the 1920's when two collegiate schools of nursing were developed in China, the first under Nina Gage at Yali (Yale in China) College in Changsha and the second under Anna Wolf at the Peking Union Medical College and Hospital, which was largely financed by the Rockfeller Foundation. It was also affiliated with nearby Yenching College for Women and later with four others. All offered prenursing courses that admitted students to the PUMC school. Though this whole program was in English, postgraduate courses in Chinese were provided for nurses from other schools who needed to round out their backgrounds and to prepare for responsible positions in hospitals, nursing schools, and public health nursing services.

Considering the vast needs of China, the number of qualified nurses was very small, but the work was growing and many Chinese nurses gave excellent proof of their competence when they were suddenly forced to take over in the wars of the 1920's, at which time most foreign nurses were recalled. By 1930 the stronger national government then in control set up special Ministries and officials for such services as health and education. This led to the transfer of nursing schools from the general supervision of the Nurses Association of China to the National Department of Education, which evaluated them and administered the examinations and registration machinery. Since ninety per cent of the 300 schools of nursing in China at that time were under foreign auspices and about the same proportion of the 12,000 graduate nurses in China were prepared in these schools, such changes created some new problems for them

[3] Because of war conditions in China, the 1929 meeting was held in Canada.

and their graduates. The situation became more complicated when some of the leading Chinese physicians who had studied the Russian system began to plan for the rapid multiplication of nurses, midwives, and other "secondary medical personnel" who were to serve in the villages and rural districts under regional medical officers.

Before this plan could go into effect, the Japanese invaded China in 1937. For the next ten years health workers in occupied China were engaged chiefly in war work and in trying to solve the most urgent public health problems.

During the Japanese invasion, when most western nurses were called home, Chinese nurses administered nursing schools and hospital services and carried on the Nurses Association with great fidelity, courage, and resourcefulness. The secretary, Ravena Tien, literally held the fort at Nanking Headquarters, fighting almost singlehanded to keep the military from seizing the building and properties of the association. When the Ministry of Education could no longer do so, she and other nurses took over the hazardous task of conducting examinations and awarding certificates, going through the enemies' lines to reach those in the occupied territory. These and other stirring events are recorded in the *National Reports* of the International Council of Nurses Congress held in Atlantic City (1947), which was attended by several Chinese delegates. Shortly after they returned home the civil war began, and the Nationalist Government and army were forced to evacuate the mainland for Formosa, which they called Taiwan or Free China.

Reports from the Peoples Republic of China since 1948 have been fragmentary and often contradictory. Although several features of the Russian medical system have been adopted and some of the better qualified nurses have been pushed through a short medical training to meet the crying need for doctors, others seem to be still in charge of nursing schools and services. The traditional system of medicine (chiefly herb therapy and acupuncture) has been revived and is being incorporated with the modern system of medicine and nursing. Communist discipline, indoctrination, public self-criticism, and anti-western propaganda have had their effect on nurses who continued on the mainland. But from reports that have filtered through there are indications that some have not forgotten the Lady of the Lamp or their friends in other countries and are hoping some day to rejoin the International Council of Nurses.

TAIWAN

For centuries a part of the general domain of China, Taiwan (Formosa) was ceded to Japan in 1895 after the Sino-Japanese War and was returned to China in 1945 following the defeat of Japan. Shortly after (1947), it became the headquarters of the Nationalist Government in exile and was called Free China to distinguish it from the People's Republic. Medicine and nursing systems here had followed older Japanese patterns under which nurses were obedient handmaids to physicians instead of co-workers. Though a few Formosan girls had received western preparation at St. Luke's Hospital School in Tokyo, they had little opportunity at home to assume positions of responsibility in hospital or community health work or in schools of nursing. During the war period many hospitals were destroyed or badly damaged, and what there was of medical, nursing, and public health services was disorganized.

When the Nationalist Government officials and those of the National Defense Medical Center arrived in Taiwan they brought with them 200 well-trained Chinese nurses for the military hospitals and the staff and students of the associated School of Nursing formerly located in Shanghai. General Chow Mei-Yu, an exceptionally capable nurse leader and administrator, was in charge of both units. The first nurse in the world to receive the rank of General, her broad preparation in China and America fitted her well to carry the varied and heavy responsibilities that fell on her shoulders in both mainland China and Taiwan. In addition to her work in organizing and equipping military hospitals and reestablishing army nursing services, nursing school programs, residences for personnel, and the like, she and her associates concerned themselves with the health needs of the civilian population and the problems of nursing service and education in Taiwan.

The National Defense Medical Center (including the nursing school) was fortunate in having the interest and assistance of sympathetic friends such as those associated in the voluntary American Bureau for Medical Aid to China.[4] Started during the active war period, this organization continued to support many projects in Taiwan, and when the war emergency was over it took the initiative in working out a comprehensive health plan for that island. With aid from several of the United Nations' special agencies, the U. S. Point IV Program, and similar groups, a survey of the island led to an interrelated program covering nutrition, agriculture, and sanitation as well as medical, nursing, and midwifery projects. Included in this program were three modern schools of nursing, one of which provided training in midwifery and all stressed public health nursing. These schools had little difficulty in securing good students, but with a population of about eight million and an active body of around 600 nurses it was evident that it would take some time to meet the needs of the island.

In 1962 there were seven schools of nursing in Taiwan ranging from university to vocational status. The first collegiate school was started in 1947 under General Chow at the National Defense Medical Center in Taipei. In 1956 a four-year university school of nursing became a part of the Taiwan University College of Medicine in the same city. Its nurse director is Tao-Chen Yu and it had at the time of writing, 125 students.

Meanwhile, much was done to dignify the nurses' work and to improve their economic, ethical, social, and professional status. A Nurses Association of Taiwan was organized, its first president being Shuai Chu, who held an important position in the National Institute of Health. One serious difficulty is that the mainlanders and the islanders do not speak the same language, though they can read the same Chinese texts. There are other differences in background and viewpoint which will take time to overcome.

Among the projects that have been initiated by the Nurses Association of China assisted by some of their graduates living in the United States was the translation of recent nursing

[4] Headquarters in New York.

textbooks to supplement the very limited materials available for graduate and student nurses in Taiwan. Much has been done by the association to maintain the morale and solidarity of the nursing group, to develop refresher courses, and to keep up contacts with professional nurses in other countries. The yearly celebration of Florence Nightingale's birthday with tableaux and candle ceremonies and addresses by leading speakers helps to interpret the profession and its ideals to the public. Nurses of Taiwan have also shared in some important educational seminars that were attended by representatives of the profession from as many as twelve Pacific countries.

The newly organized nurses association, under the name of The Nurses' Association of the Republic of China, became a member of the International Council of Nurses at the 1961 Congress, with an individual membership of 1500 nurses.

JAPAN

The religion of Buddhism introduced into Japan many centuries ago stressed works of charity, including the care of the sick and wounded. This became a part of the national tradition, emperors and empresses often leading in such activities. During feudal times the role and status of women became more limited but the older traditions of service persisted. In 1853, when this country opened its doors to the outside world, a new era began and the process of modernization was seen not only in the armed forces but in medicine, sanitation, and to some extent in hospital work. In all these fields, including nursing, Japan tended to follow the German pattern. In public hospitals, for example, the medical head of each ward had full control over nurses and nursing.

In 1886 a Nightingale School was established in a small American mission hospital connected with Doshisha College in Kyoto. Linda Richards, the first American trained nurse, was sent by the American Board of Missions to organize this school. During her five-year stay she developed both hospital and district nursing and also trained head nurses. Though her American successor carried on the work for some years, financial and other difficulties led to the closing of the institution in 1906. A Japanese physician who had helped in this project continued the training of nurses and midwives (chiefly the latter) in his own private hospital, but apart from the uniform designed by Miss Richards few of the school's original features remained in later years. Another small school was started around the same time in Jakei (Charity) Hospital in Tokyo by Baron Takagi, a physician of fine character and high standing. In his studies abroad he had been greatly impressed by the English system of nursing and had secured the interest and patronage of the Empress in this undertaking. The school was organized by an American missionary nurse, Miss Lead, and a number of well-qualified Japanese girls of good social standing were admitted for training. From these a superintendent and head nurses were prepared to take over the work. A third school under an English nurse, Miss Welch, was organized about the same time at the Tokyo Imperial University Hospital.

In 1890 when the Japanese Government launched an ambitious military preparedness program, it followed the general plan of the German Red Cross in providing nurses for its military hospitals. A Red Cross hospital and training center were built in Tokyo, and the ladies of the Royal Family and Japanese nobility set an example for the nation by taking first aid courses, rolling bandages, and participating in other types of voluntary service. Younger members of respected middle-class families were urged to take the longer two-year course of training for Red Cross nurses and were then expected to pledge themselves to answer calls for military service in the ensuing twelve-year period. Head nurses were to have an extra year of training and to receive a higher rank. Though their status was much better than that of most nurses in civilian hospitals, Red Cross nurses, who were under strict military discipline, had little freedom or initiative.

During the wars with Russia and China, the Red Cross was greatly expanded and training centers were set up in the different provinces. Some units were sent to aid the Allies in World War I, and this experience together with the influence of the

League of Red Cross Societies led the organization to broaden the scope of its nursing program to include some forms of social service and community health work. An able Red Cross nurse, Matsuye Inowye, was sent to London in 1928 to attend the International Course in London, and on her return she became instructor in the Tokyo Red Cross Center, giving much of her time to the community health program. Efforts were made also to organize Japanese nurses in a self-governing association, but the Red Cross nurses were handicapped by their military regulations and such an organization did not materialize until later.

Though foreign missionary institutions were not generally encouraged at this time, an exception was made when in the 1920's the small St. Luke's Hospital in Tokyo built a large modern medical center under the inspiring leadership of Dr. Teussler, its medical superintendent, Alice St. John, director of the new school, and Ayo Araki, director of the Nursing Service. This became a joint effort of Japanese and American leaders in medicine and nursing. The new St. Luke's College of Nursing was recognized by the government as a special junior college and attracted a well-educated group of students from Japan and some adjacent countries. Its three-year program provided a broad and varied preparation designed for leaders in different branches of institutional and public health work. Demonstration and training centers were set up in city and country districts, where such students could get suitable experience in school health work and home visiting. These centers soon showed what could be done by well-prepared nurses to reduce sickness and death rates and to raise the whole level of maternal and child health. City and provincial public health authorities were just beginning to recognize the need for such workers when in the late 1930's the Japanese launched the disastrous military campaign in China which set back all progress for many years.

Before St. Luke's Hospital was taken over by the military and its nursing school was closed, efforts had been made to develop a national organization of Japanese nurses which could qualify for membership in the International Council of Nurses. St. Luke's and a few other schools had alumnae groups, and there were local organizations of nurses in such cities as Tokyo and Osaka. The Korean nurses had formed an active self-governing association before the annexation of that country to Japan in 1910, but it could not join the ICN because of Korea's loss of national status. Then, too, the dominant position of the Red Cross in the national nursing picture made it impossible to proceed without this group. After long and delicate negotiations, Miss Tagiwara, Chief Nurse of the Japanese Red Cross, was made president of her own group (replacing a military officer), and a federation was formed of this and other eligible organizations under the title, Nurses Association of the Japanese Empire. Miss Tagiwara was its first president, and on her death shortly after Miss Inowye took her place. At the ICN congress in Paris (1933) the new association was admitted, the Japanese and Korean representatives advancing hand in hand to the great delight of the audience. It had just begun to knit its widely different units together when the war started in 1937, and activities were discontinued until after the defeat of Japan in 1945 when Korea regained its status as a nation.

During the war nurses and nursing standards in Japan were seriously disorganized and general conditions were chaotic. Many hospitals and schools were destroyed, legal regulations were ignored, and morale was low. Economic conditions were such that all kinds of nurses, trained and untrained, were employed in menial services, if at all, and much of the ground gained in preceding years seemed to have been lost.

Postwar Developments

A new era began, however, with the American occupation when nurse officers were attached to the General Headquarters' Staff and were given exceptionally good support in helping the Japanese reestablish their nursing and health structure on a sound and permanent basis. Captain Grace Alt, who headed the nursing staff during most of this time, was well prepared by her previous experience in a mission hospital in Korea and by her wide knowledge of recent developments in nursing service and education.

In the reconstruction of the Japanese Government's Division of Welfare Ministry, Mrs. Grace Seki Hora was appointed chief nurse, the first woman to hold this official position in Japan. This nurse had built up a successful visiting nurse service in Osaka, like the Henry Street Nursing Service in New York, where she had received part of her training (the rest at Teachers College). For this and her work as the first nurse in government service she has received high honors from the Japanese Government and other organizations. She gives full recognition to the General Headquarters Staff and especially to Captain Alt for their help and support without which the rapid and extensive improvements in the status and preparation of Japanese nurses and midwives would have been impossible. Among these were (1) full high school education for students in schools of nursing in place of elementary education or two years of high school, (2) three years of training in schools designated by the Minister of Education or by the Welfare Minister, in place of two years in schools designated by prefectural governments, (3) six months' additional training for public health nurses and midwives after registration or licensure, instead of two years' training in all.

In these reforms good support was given by graduates of the St. Luke's and Red Cross Schools, who were better prepared for positions of leadership. By combining Red Cross and St. Luke's facilities, a demonstration school was started which received official recognition as a college of nursing. Later the trend toward connections between nursing schools and higher educational institutions became more marked, several becoming parts of schools of medicine and one of a division of home economics. All are recognized by the Ministry of Education. Japan had, in 1961, 110 schools of nursing under the new regulations and this number is increasing. Refresher courses for all grades of nursing personnel and midwives have been organized and students are sent from all parts of Japan for supplementary training, several going abroad on Fulbright scholarships. An important part of this educational program is the publication of textbooks, pamphlets, films, and other appropriate visual aids, many of which are translations and adaptations of existing American materials. Nurses and midwives are taught how to use these aids and how to carry on health teaching in the hundreds of health centers that are set up throughout the country.

The fact that Japanese women are now admitted to full citizenship and are encouraged to take an active part in civic and national affairs has helped greatly in these reforms. It took some time, however, to arouse the interest of nurses and midwives in creating their own organizations. During the war these groups had been controlled by medical men who gave the members little or no voice in their management. Miss Inowye, who was elected to sit in the House of Peers, helped to bring about this amalgamation and for a time was president of what was called the Japanese Midwives, Clinical Nurses and Public Health Nurses Association (later changed to Japanese Nursing Association). Though small at the start, it reached in five years a membership of more than 80,000 and carried on an active campaign for legislation (passed in 1947) providing for the inspection of nursing schools and the licensing of those who passed the national examination. It should be noted also that the Japanese Nursing Association became an active member of the International Council of Nurses in 1925. It now has a fulltime executive secretary and office staff and publishes a monthly journal, *Kango*.

Western nurses who have worked closely with Japanese nurses and midwives are full of praise for the way in which they have handled their difficult postwar problems. They have shown not only good judgment, determination, and fortitude but a fine spirit of cooperation and a capacity for hard work which promises well for the future of nursing in this country. It would be a mistake to assume, however, that their problems are all solved. Many physicians still prefer semitrained nurses who have had two years of training and are paid less, and here as elsewhere the increasing demand for nursing service exceeds the supply of better prepared nurses. It should be noted also that physicians still hold the directorships of most Japanese schools of nursing. These are only a few of the difficulties that Japanese nurses have to meet in their efforts to become a self governing profession.

KOREA

Though Korea's vulnerable location has exposed it to many invasions by powerful neighbors, its people have maintained their own national character, language, and culture and have fought valiantly for their political independence. The old system of medicine was similar to that in China and Japan. It was not until 1884 that Dr. Horace Allen, an American physician to the foreign legations, was requested by the Royal Family to open the first modern hospital for Koreans in Seoul. Under the leadership of Dr. O. R. Avison who came to Korea in 1893 to direct the Royal Korea Hospital, this institution was enlarged and later became known as the Severance Hospital. Its nursing service was organized by Anna Jacobson, a Norwegian nurse trained in the United States, who arrived in 1895. Three years earlier two British nurses, the Misses Heathcote and Webster, had come to work with the Anglican Mission in two small hospitals, one for women and children and one for men. In 1905 the first Korean school for nurses was opened by Dr. Mary Cutler and Margaret Edmunds (a Canadian nurse) at the Methodist Woman's Hospital. This was soon followed by a school at the Severance Hospital under Esther Shields, an American nurse who had come to Korea in 1897. Before long they were joined by Australian nurses and by some of other nationalities.

Many difficulties had to be overcome before these schools could attract suitable applicants and develop anything like common standards of training. Among the handicaps were the bad reputation and low status of such service in Korea, the very elementary education of girls, and the different systems of nursing represented by the foreign nurses themselves. At first only girls of Christian families were admitted, and because of inadequate basic education the early courses which combined general and nursing education were often six years in length. This time was reduced to three years when general educational standards improved.

As in China and India, the foreign nurses organized (1908) a group of their own, which was at first called the Nurses Association of Korea. Its main purpose was to confer on their common problems and to develop greater uniformity and effectiveness in their schools and nursing services. In 1910 when the Japanese annexed Korea the name was changed to the Association of Occidental Nurses of Korea, and in 1923 it was again named the Nurses Association of Korea, at which time Korean trained nurses joined the group. Had Korea not lost its national status, this organization would have been eligible for active membership in the International Council of Nurses. However, under the leadership of Elizabeth Shepping, it was represented at the Montreal meeting of the ICN in 1929 and was given associate status. The two Korean nurses who attended were cordially welcomed, and before long they and others of their group were holding responsible positions in the Nurses Association of Korea. This organization has since acquired full membership in the ICN.

After annexation, the Japanese Government began to take control of Korea's internal affairs. Although it allowed the foreign-directed hospitals and schools to continue their work, it also built a number of public hospitals where Korean nurses were trained according to the Japanese system of that period. In addition, the Japanese Red Cross founded hospitals and schools of nursing similar to those in Japan. In 1930 there were seventeen nursing schools of these types and eight under mission boards. The differences in entrance requirements, ethical standards, economic conditions, nursing service, and training were marked and the two groups found little in common. Serious difficulties arose when laws were passed requiring Korean as well as Japanese schools to give courses in Shinto Ethics, participate in national religious ceremonies, and follow the government syllabus for nurse training. Nurses who wanted to practice were required also to register with the police department after passing a very elementary examination. Though the mission schools conformed, they also maintained their own higher standards, which then were much like those in English-speaking countries. This was a very difficult period for Korean nurses and also for the friends who stood back of them. It helped however, to build up the unity and stamina needed for the years ahead.

World War II and Postwar Period

It was here in northeast Asia that war broke out in 1937 and during the period from 1941 to 1945 foreign residents in Korea were forced to return home. When the government took over their hospitals and schools, standards slumped badly, and well-prepared Korean nurses and doctors were unable to do much under war conditions to remedy the situation. Missionary physicians and nurses who returned after peace was declared found that the achievements of half a century had been nearly wiped out, but they soon began to rebuild. In these efforts toward reconstruction they had the aid of the United States Government, then occupying Japan, and of many other friendly countries and organizations. Their troubles were not over, however, because Communist forces were soon mobilizing in the North, and in 1950 a civil war broke out which developed into an international East-West conflict resulting in the almost complete destruction of the country, tragic suffering, and great loss of life. In 1954 an armistice was signed, but Korea was divided and almost bankrupt. Most of its public institutions and homes were shattered or disorganized and its population of about eight million had little or no regular medical and nursing care. Help was given by such organizations as the United Nations Korean Reconstruction Agency, and the American Korean Foundation, and a good beginning was made in attacking the most serious epidemic diseases and in rehabilitating the large numbers of crippled war victims and orphaned children. After the fighting stopped medical and nursing personnel from the allied military services located in Korea gave much of their time to civilian reconstruction. But the need for health personnel of all kinds remained acute and funds were required to reopen and equip medical and nursing schools and to get hospitals back into working order.

Among the nurses of other countries who took a lead in mobilizing available resources and personnel for nursing and health services and helping to plan countrywide programs, Captain Grace Alt and her colleagues from the Headquarters of

the American Army in Tokyo should be given special mention; also Susan Haines of Tasmania, Australia, who had wide
experience in the United Nations Relief and Rehabilitation
Administration as well as in the World Health Organization
and served as Chief of Nursing Affairs of the United Nation's
Korean Reconstruction Agency. Recovery in nursing, as in other
health services, has been slow, but the achievements of South
Koreans who have worked under great hardship and personal
sacrifice compare favorably with those of other countries who
have gone through similar experiences.

Among the Korean leaders were Ok Soon Hong, Chief of
Nursing Affairs in the Ministry of Health, who did much to
reorganize nursing services during the postwar period. Another
was Frances Lee Whang, President of the Korean Nurses
Association at that time. Recent reports indicate that good
progress has been made in the later period under the leadership
of Korean Nurses. At the present there are twenty-one three
year diploma schools of nursing and five connected with colleges or universities. One of the outstanding leaders in education is Shin Young Hong, now Chairman of the Department
of Nursing at Yonsei University, who has held other important
positions in Severance Hospital, Ewa Woman's University and
the Government Bureau of Nursing and has studied abroad in
Australia and the United States.

A recent report by Mildred Adams of Indiana University who
served as advisor to Korea under the ICA (International Cooperation Administration) in 1959, gives a promising picture of
progress; as does also the report of a nursing team from Minnesota University, sent to Seoul in 1957. Student nurses now have
their own association and are showing keen interest in the progress of nursing in their country.

Considering all the differences between the Orient and the
Occident in religious beliefs, social traditions, and inherited
systems of medical and health work, the modern nursing move-

ment, though very uneven, has shown many bright spots. Though much can be said against the colonial system and the war evil, they, as well as world trade and travel, Christian missions, the Red Cross, the woman's movement, national and international agencies, and civilization in general have contributed to the introduction of modern nursing in this vast area as in other parts of the world. Even catastrophes which have disrupted nations have sometimes brought reforms in nursing and an aroused interest on the part of the public and of governments leading to a much better appreciation of this type of national and international service.

SELECTED BIBLIOGRAPHY

Anderson, Lyda W. "Some Points on the American School for Nurses, Constantinople," *Int. Nurs. Bull.*, January 1924, 20-21.

Cantor, Shulamith L. "Nursing in Israel," *Am. Jo. Nurs.*, March 1951, 162-163.

Clarke, Avis. "Goodwill Mission to China," *Nurs. Times*, March 16, 1956, 215-218.

Craig, Margaretta. "The College of Nursing in New Delhi," *Am. Jo. Nurs.*, April 1951, 238-239.

Devi, Lakshmi. "Twelve Years of Nursing in India (1943-1955)," *Int. Nurs. Rev.*, October 1955, 49-52.

Fine, Jacob, "The Development of Medicine," *Atlantic Monthly*, November 1961, 137-139.

Fineman, Irving. *Woman of Valor: The Story of Henrietta Szold, 1860-1945.* New York: Simon and Schuster, 1961.

Fujikara, Yuka Yasui. "Public Health Nursing in Japan," *Am. Jo. Nurs.*, November 1956, 1416-1419.

Galt, Edith J. "Korea's Midwives," *Am. Jo. Nurs.*, June 1957, 755-757.

Gould, Etta M. "A Pilot Study in Modern Israel," *Can. Nurse*, March 1957, 214-217.

Hill, Elizabeth. "Nursing Education Seminar in Formosa," *Am. Jo. Nurs.*, October 1953, 1188-1191.

Hodgman, Gertrude E. "Nursing in Formosa," *Am. Jo. Nurs.*, July 1953, 838-840.

International Council of Nurses. *National Reports. 1933,* 22, 26-27, 51, 52, 63-64, 67-68; *1947,* 28-29, 36-39, 70-73, 74; *1949,* 33-37, 68-72, 98-100, 101-104, 108-110, 114-116; *1957,* 20-22, 48-50, 61-63, 64-66, 81-82, 83-84, 98-100; *1961,* 12-13, 36-37, 38-39, 42-43, 49-50, 51-53, 56-58, 70-72, 83-85, 86-87, 90-91.

Japan. Ministry of Health and Welfare. *Report on Nursing and Midwifery in Japan.* Tokyo: Ministry of Health and Welfare, Nursing Sect., 1953.

Lin, Evelyn. "Nursing in China," *Am. Jo. Nurs.*, January 1938, 1-8.

Lucka, Mildred Vivienne. "Korea: A Challenge to Western Nursing," *Am. Jo. Nurs.*, Oct. 1946, 668-670.

M. Claire, Sister and Sister M. Laetitia. "Nursing in India and Pakistan," *Am. Jo. Nurs.*, June 1949, 359-361.

Moore, W. Robert. "Thailand Bolsters Its Freedom," *Nat. Geog. Mag.*, June 1961, 811-849.

Nutting, M. Adelaide, and Lavinia L. Dock. *A History of Nursing*. New York: Putnam's, 1907-1912. 4 vols. Vol. IV, Ch. VI, pp. 307-322.

Salsali, Pari Fatema. "Iran's Nurses," *Am. Jo. Nurs.*, May 1961, 99-101.

Seagrave, Gordon S. *Burma Surgeon*. New York: Norton, 1943.

Shanks, Mary D., and Faith A. Selden. "Nursing Schools in Japan," *Am. Jo. Nurs.*, June 1952, 698-700.

Simpson, Cora E. "Examinations for Nurses in China," *Int. Nurs. Rev.*, May 1950, 236-242.

———. *A Joy Ride Through China for the N. A. C.* Shanghai: Kwang Hsueh Pub. House, n. d.

Smith, Emily Myrtle. *Taiwan Nursing Report*. Washington: Dept. of Health, Education and Welfare, Public Health Service, 1954.

Sotejo, Julita V. "New Trends in Curricula for Schools of Nursing," *Can. Nurse*, December 1953, 929-932.

———. "The Nursing Profession in the Philippines," *Int. Nurs. Bull.*, Winter 1948, 6-7.

Spencer, Barbara. *Desert Hospital in China*. New York: Roy, n. d.

Stephenson, Temima. "Nursing in Burma," *Int. Nurs. Rev.*, May 1930, 296-299.

A Survey of Nursing and Nursing Education in Mission Hospitals and Schools of Nursing in India—1946. Mysore: Wesley Press & Pub. House, 1947.

Trained Nurses Association of India. *Handbook of the Trained Nurses Association of India*. Delhi: TNAI, 1951.

Türer, Asuman. "The Red Crescent School in Istanbul," *Am. Jo. Nurs.*, May 1938, 298-299.

Turnbull, L. "Nursing in the Western Pacific Region of the World Health Organization," *Int. Nurs. Rev.* April 1958, 13-16.

Whang, Frances Lee. "The Advance of Nursing in Korea," *Am. Jo. Nurs.*, July 1954, 818-819.

WHO Regional Office for South East Asia. *Report on Seminar on Categories and Functions of Nursing Personnel*. Delhi: Patialsi House, 1957.

Widmer, Caroline Ladd. "Nursing in Syria," *Int. Nurs. Rev.*, February 1956, 12-27.

Wilkinson, A. *A Brief History of Nursing in India and Pakistan*. Madras: Diocesan Press, 1958.

Zeitlin, Rose. *Henrietta Szold: Record of a Life*. New York: Dial Press, 1952.

CHAPTER **18**

Central and South America and the Caribbean Islands

CONSIDERING first the conditions in this region that have tended to advance or retard the modern nursing movement or to modify it in various ways, one notes such geographic and physical features as the location of many of the countries in or near the equatorial region, the relative sparsity of inhabitants in much of the interior because of unsuitable climate or tropical diseases, and the concentration of most of the population in coastal cities or within one or two hundred miles of the coast. Though air travel and modern sanitation have opened up more of the interior of South America, living conditions there are still difficult if not impossible for all but primitive peoples.

As to the origins of those that make up the population of this vast region, it is difficult now to distinguish one from another because of the great mixture of races, including the descendants of the early Aztecs and Indians, Spanish and Portuguese conquerors, imported African negroes, and in later years, Asian and European settlers from many countries. South Americans, in general, are remarkably free from race prejudice and readily assimilate such diverse elements. Other important influences that came from southwest Europe were the two-class system,

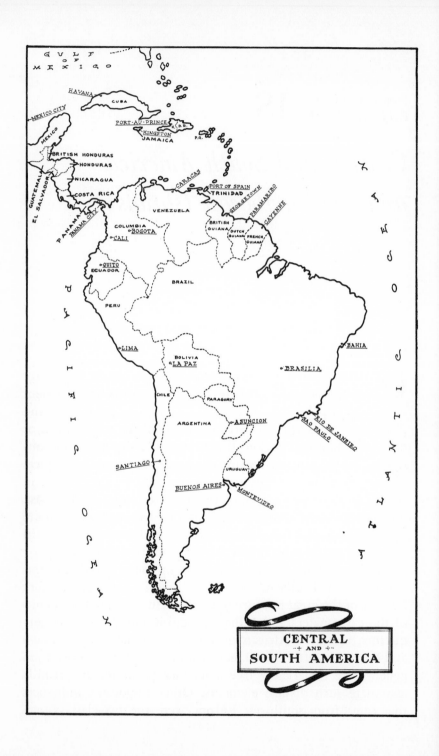

CENTRAL
+ AND +
SOUTH AMERICA

which divided people into high and low, rich and poor, leisured and working classes, the prejudice against menial work, the dominant position of men in the family and outside, early marriages and the close chaperonage of girls (of the upper classes). These were also predominantly Roman Catholic countries in which the clergy and religious orders had much power. Then, too, many physicians had received their training in French and German public hospitals and tended to favor the nursing systems in those institutions. Obviously, all of these were important factors in the efforts to establish modern nursing in this hemisphere.

Politically, Latin America is composed of twenty separate continental, isthmian, and insular republics, colonies and dependencies, stretching from the United States-Mexican border in the north to the Drake Strait in the south. There is a long tradition of revolutionary activity in many of these countries which has come down to modern times. Despite the rich natural resources and the great wealth of a very small minority, malnutrition and disease are widespread and death rates are high. The prevalent diseases include tuberculosis, hookworm, yaws, and others common in tropical and subtropical countries.

Reforms in hospital, public health, and nursing work have been retarded in this region not only by the lack of well-qualified leaders but by the persistence of many social customs, traditions, and attitudes which tend to restrict women in their choice of a career such as nursing. At present, the most critical shortage of health personnel is that of well-prepared nurses and nursing *auxiliares*. As in Europe, dedicated religious sisters and amateur nurses who served in the Red Cross and similar organizations often had a much better social standing than those who were paid for such service. Until quite recent times, poorly paid servant-nurses did most of the housework and nursing in hospitals, the general administration of both being as a rule under the religious sisterhoods. Neither group had any real preparation for nursing. Only charity cases were sent to hospitals, for most families cared for their own sick at home; in the wealthier families by servants and among the poor by women members of the family as a rule.

BEGINNINGS OF NURSING REFORM

The first known attempt to introduce the Nightingale system into Latin America came at the beginning of the twentieth century when, in response to a request to the Founder, a party of British sisters arrived in Buenos Aires, Argentina, to start a school. According to her biographer,[1] this plan did not materialize, and when word came that the nurses had decided to marry and remain there Miss Nightingale washed her hands of the whole scheme.

In 1908 a small school was started in Panama City in the Santo Tomás Hospital, then under the administration of the Sisters of St. Vincent de Paul. The first nurse-director was Miss Brake-meier, a well-educated German school teacher who had been trained as a nurse in the United States and remained in the Panama school for ten years trying to attract and prepare suitable Panamanian girls as nurses, but without much success. In recent years this school has been revived and reorganized and has done much to introduce modern nursing in the Isthmus.

In 1912 another group of English nurses was sent to Monte-video, Uruguay, at the request of Dr. Carlos Nery, Director of the City Department of Charities, who had visited Britain and planned to introduce the Nightingale system into the public hospitals. He started a school in his own small private hospital and continued it under graduates of the first class, he himself serving as director. Though some of these nurses did good work, his plan to extend the system into the public hospitals did not succeed at that time, and his own school declined after his death. At the time of writing, however, it is one of the recognized schools in this country.

Other beginnings in modern nurse training were made by mission hospitals, most of which were sponsored and supported by North American Protestant groups and directed by qualified nurses. There were also some independent private hospitals established by British and American residents holding diplo-matic or business positions in Latin America. These were chiefly

[1] Sir Edward Cook, *Life of Florence Nightingale*, Vol. II, p. 412.

for the use of their own families and employees. Though such hospitals prepared a few local nurses and gave an example of higher standards of nursing, they did little to weaken the prevailing servant-nurse system in the large public hospitals.

The earliest example of reorganization in such institutions in this area came as a result of the Spanish-American War (1898-1899). When the United States Government took over the public hospitals of Cuba for its troops, several were reorganized by American nurses. Before Americans left Cuba, a few schools had been started, some textbooks translated into Spanish, a registration law passed, and a nurses' association organized. After Cuba became independent, however, there was little public support for such reforms, and the small group of trained nurses in the Cuban Nurses Association was unable to make much headway against the strong political, medical, and labor groups that opposed the new concept of nursing. These factors as well as the general instability of the government help to account for the slow progress of modern nursing in Cuba.

In spite of similar conditions in Puerto Rico, which remained under the U. S. Government, good progress was made. The developments there are described in the chapter on the United States (see pp. 233-234).

BRAZIL

Brazil, the largest country on the continent, has a population of approximately seventy million. Its health and medical problems are related to the topography; most of its people live on the broad plateau in rural areas, in tropical forests, and in coastal cities. On the plateau the chief health problem is malnutrition; in the forests the primary diseases are those of the tropics: dysenteries, intestinal parasites, trachoma, leprosy, and malaria. In the urban areas rapid strides are being made to meet health problems of various kinds. The medical and health services are comparable to those of similar cities in the United States and other countries and include rehabilitation of the physically handicapped, who are numerous in this whole area.

This country, whose official language is Portuguese, was the first in Latin America to give modern nursing a secure position in its system of public health and education. The entering wedge came in World War I, when young physicians interested in public health began to go north to the United States for study. Here they were impressed by the emphasis on health teaching in tuberculosis and similar cases. One of them, Dr. Carlos Chagas, National Director of Public Health in Rio de Janiero, then approached the International Health Board of the Rockefeller Foundation with a request for aid in preparing health visitors to teach in the homes of tuberculosis and other patients. Ethel Parsons, a well-qualified public health nurse who was sent to study the situation, agreed to stay and help with the plan for brief training of health visitors on condition that a permanent school of nursing be established to prepare fully qualified nurses. She was later made Chief of the Nursing Service in the National Health Department, said to be the first position of its kind on record.

With the help of the Rockefeller Foundation and the support of influential physicians and lay citizens, the Ana Neri School [2] was organized in 1923 in Rio de Janiero by a group of North American nurses. They were soon joined by Brazilian nurses, some of whom had received their entire nursing preparation in North America and others who had been sent there for post-graduate study. This school, although remaining independent of hospital control, provided clinical nursing experience in both hospitals and public health agencies. It had its own school and residence and was affiliated with a government hospital. Special attention was given to the character and social development of its students as well as to the three-year program of nursing theory and practice. Full secondary education was required for admission and students were carefully selected. The first three directors from the United States (Clara Kieninger, Lorraine Denhardt, and Bertha Pullen) laid the foundations on a sound basis. The school then came under the direction of an able Brazilian nurse, Rachel Haddock Lobo, who in her own experience had gone through all the stages of nursing develop-

[2] Named for a famous war nurse of Brazil.

ment, starting as an amateur in her home community, assisting religious sisters in hospital work, volunteering as a Red Cross nurse for war service, then receiving two years' training in the school of the *Assistance Publique* in Paris and later supplementary and advanced preparation in Philadelphia and New York. The early death of Mrs. Lobo was a heavy loss to the school and to nursing in Brazil.

By a decree in 1943 this school's control was transferred from the National Department of Health to the University of Brazil, and in 1942 it became an integral part of that university, remaining under nurse administration and leadership and having its own faculty and budget. This was something quite new in Latin America, though some medical faculties had previously formed classes for so-called nurses (*infermiera*). These were primarily doctors' assistants who did very little real nursing or teaching.

In 1939 Brazil passed a federal law making the Ana Neri standard a requirement for all registered nurses. This was modified later to allow two levels of preparation, one for registered nurses (a 36-month course) and the other for *auxiliares* (18 months). The Nursing Education Act was passed in 1949, and in 1955 a new law provided for three levels of nursing education including these two, the second for high school graduates, leading to a diploma, also a four-year program requiring seven years of secondary education for entrance and leading to a degree. *Auxiliares* may qualify for registration by supplementing their general education and nursing program. Between 1945 and 1956 the number of schools on the higher level increased markedly, and at present there are many such schools, a number being connected with universities. Outstanding among the university schools is a large one at São Paulo connected with a 2000-bed teaching hospital and the medical school of the university. This school, whose first director was Edith Fraenkel, has recently been under the leadership of Maria Rosa Sousa Pinheiro who has added courses for qualified graduate nurses.

The Red Cross also began to support schools for professional nurses after 1940 when the League of Red Cross Societies held its congress in Latin America. Though six-month Red Cross courses are still given to *visitadores* who help in some community projects, these workers are no longer in competition with trained registered nurses. The Sisters of Charity were also beginning to prepare nuns with full nursing qualifications. Through the influence of the Institute of Inter-American Affairs, Sister M. Olivia Gowan, dean of the School of Nursing of the Catholic University of America in Washington, D. C., had visited Brazil in the '40's and had conferred with influential Roman Catholic leaders on nursing questions. Arrangements were made for some of the better educated sisters to attend the Catholic University and to observe nursing in the United States, thus opening up channels for further exchanges in the future. Although the older hospital orders did not share actively in this program (they were gradually retiring from the public hospitals), some other sisters' groups with long nursing experience and better preparation established their own hospitals and schools and contributed to the general advance of nursing in Brazil.

Meantime, the Ana Neri graduates had formed an alumnae association (1926) which soon evolved into the Brazilian Nurses Association and was opened to all qualified registered nurses without respect to nationality or creed. In 1929 it became a member of the International Council of Nurses. Its magazine is called the *Revista Brasiliera de Enfermagen*. The meeting of the ICN in Brazil in 1953 did much to arouse popular interest in professional nursing and to bring together the professional nurses of South America.

In 1959 the School of Public Health of the University of São Paulo, Brazil, started a postgraduate course for public health nurses. Other progressive steps included the establishment of a postbasic course in obstetrical nursing, as well as one for instructors in schools of nursing. Among the agencies that have helped with this and other nursing projects in South America are the W. K. Kellogg and Rockefeller Foundations, the Institute of Inter-American Affairs, and the Pan American Sanitary Bureau (recently renamed the Pan American Health Organization, which is the regional office for the Americas of the World Health Organization—PAHO/WHO), and the League of Red

Cross Societies. A recent activity has been the international workshop for the study of nursing needs and resources held at the School of Nursing of the University of Bahia under the direction of Maria P. Tito de Moraes, a well prepared Portuguese nurse and WHO consultant. A nurse in the Ministry of Health helps to interpret nursing to the government. Such activities carried on by leading nurses of the country indicate that modern nursing is now well established and has a promising future.

In reporting the progress of nursing in Brazil special recognition should be given to the exceptional influence and activities of Agnes W. Chagas, now nursing consultant on the staff of the Pan American Health Organization which covers a wide area. Born in Bahia, Brazil, of North American parents, she later married the son of Dr. Carlos Chagas whose sponsorship of modern nursing in Rio de Janiero was referred to earlier. After graduating from Russell Sage College, U.S.A. she entered the Ana Neri School of Nursing in Brazil and later took advanced courses in Toronto and New York. She was thus exceptionally well qualified not only in nursing but in the languages and cultures of her adopted country and of its neighbors. She also is familiar with the resources and conditions of the hemisphere as a whole. Her reports are therefore of special interest in connection with the summaries here given of nursing in this region.

CHILE

This country on the western coast, with its geographic contrasts, its mixed population (many of north European origin), its relatively large middle class, and its stable democratic government, like its neighbors is growing rapidly, chiefly because of the declining death rate. Laws have been passed providing for women's suffrage, compulsory education, a modern system of health insurance and social security covering more than half the population. Reasonably good conditions for health workers are found in spite of recent economic setbacks which affect schools and health agencies. Though many hospitals and health services have not been fully modernized, they have been greatly improved in recent years largely as a result of advances made in nursing education and in various fields of service. Rehabilitation of the crippled has been added to the care of the sick and injured, the prevention of disease and the teaching of health. There is also an increasing awareness of the urgent need to prepare more public health nurses and auxiliary nursing personnel if public health programs are to be expanded and improved.

One of the oldest and best-known schools of nursing here is connected with the National University of Chile in Santiago (one of two university schools in that city) and is administered by its Faculty of Medicine. Under Dr. Gonzalez, a woman physician, who directed it for several years, it gradually evolved from a largely theoretical and didactic type of submedical program to one that is well balanced in the theory and practice of nursing and in its emphasis on both prevention and cure. Nursing students are fully matriculated and meet the same educational standards as those required for admission to the medical school. Like other schools in the country, it now has a four-year program and nurse teachers and supervisors have a much larger share in instruction. The director is now a nurse who has the chief responsibility for the school's administration.

This university school, in cooperation with the Chilean Association of University Nurses, is authorized by the government to register nurses and to approve the schools whose students are eligible for registration. The requirements have been substantially raised chiefly by the efforts of its graduates. For example, a clear distinction has been drawn between those who have completed a period of residence with a full program of theory and practice and those who, under the older extern system of the Red Cross, claimed much the same status as fully trained nurses. There are other schools, all of which are recognized by the National University of Chile, having the same entrance requirements and curricula, their final examinations being given by the university. These schools are said to compare favorably with similar schools in other countries. A number of Chilean nurses have been sent abroad for postgraduate study and are now holding positions as directors and instructors in such schools and in public health nursing programs.

Chile has recently developed postgraduate courses which are attracting nurses from other Spanish-speaking countries. The opportunity is welcomed by many nurses who do not speak English and who find that they are more at home in a Latin American country. Through the cooperation of the Institute of Inter-American Affairs and the local group in Santiago, the Quinta Normal Health Center, serving a population of approximately 118,000, has been established. Students from some of the schools of nursing acquire field experience here and participate in clinic activities and home visiting.

The graduates of the recognized or approved schools have formed a national organization, the Chilean Association of University Nurses, which became a member of the International Council of Nurses in 1953. In addition to its support of accreditation of schools, it has done much to improve the nursing care of the public and the living and working conditions of its members. These and other activities indicate a determined effort by Chilean nurses to raise the standards of service and education in their country.

PROMISING BEGINNINGS ELSEWHERE IN SOUTH AMERICA

Though the following countries are at an earlier stage of nursing development, recent studies indicate that social and health leaders are aware of the need to improve such services and have begun to develop a few modern schools of nursing. Most of these have been established with the aid of foundations and other international agencies interested in medical and health work.

The findings of a recent survey of schools of nursing in Latin America, made in 1959 by the Pan American Health Organization, under the direction of Agnes W. Chagas, provided a basis for defining what a school of nursing is and minimum standards for such schools. These are: (1) recognition of the school by the government of the country in which it is located; (2) six years of general education as a prerequisite for admission; (3) a nursing course of at least three years' duration; (4) supervised clinical experience; and (5) three or more fulltime nurse instructors on the faculty. The report published in 1960 showed that 110 Latin American schools of nursing met these standards. Other criteria generally considered are the passage of suitable laws governing the qualifications and practice of nurses, also the creation of national nurses organizations and the eligibility of these for membership in the International Council of Nurses.

COLOMBIA, PERU, ARGENTINA, VENEZUELA, AND URUGUAY

Judging by these standards Colombia, Peru, and Venezuela in the north and west and Argentina and Uruguay in the south and east have made a good beginning in developing nursing along modern lines. All of them have laws controlling nursing education and practice. Nurses are organized and with the exception of Peru and Argentina, all are members of the ICN. These two have associate representation and hope soon to be full members.

Colombia has several schools that meet the stated requirements. Three of these are university schools, two in Bogotá and one in Cali. The latter has had good support from the Rockefeller Foundation, while the other two are connected with the National and Catholic Universities in Bogotá.

Peru is another country that has made definite progress in recent years. All but two of its schools are in Lima, the capital. Though it has no university schools, the National School of Nursing in Lima offers courses for graduate nurses and another school which has had good support from the Rockefeller Foundation is preparing qualified graduate nurses as teachers. The quality of applicants to all such schools is steadily improving as is the status of nursing in the country and the qualifications of nurses. Health centers are being extended throughout

Peru bringing their services to more and more people and providing field training for public health nurses.

Another activity of the nurses association was the sponsorship, with the assistance of the Peruvian Government and the Pan American Health Organization, of a workshop (1952) in which nurses from ten Latin American countries participated. As in other Latin American countries, the nurses of Peru have engaged in a comprehensive study of needs and resources in the field of nursing. This activity was assisted by various national and international agencies.

Venezuela has a number of schools meeting the specified standards, two of which are in the capital city of Caracas. One, the National Nursing School, is described as self-governing and as supported by the Ministry of Health and Social Assistance. There is an increasing tendency in these schools, as in others in this southern continent, to appoint nurse directors. The nurses of Venezuela have been trying for some time to establish modern nursing on a firm basis and to this end have sent many graduate nurses to North America to prepare for positions of leadership.

In Argentina, where nurses are now beginning to give more emphasis to education and community service, nine years' preliminary education are required for entrance to the schools. The students at the University of Buenos Aires have a good educational background, and all schools there are said to be well supplied with desirable applicants. Many steps are being taken to raise the level of education in all parts of the country, one being the recent establishment of a Center of Nursing Education in Buenos Aires, which serves the nurses of the entire country. New legislation is now being studied by the Nurses' Association.

Uruguay, though slow in developing, is now reported to be making good progress. A new school established at the National University in the capital city of Montevideo has provided a modern program for nurses and the necessary facilities for it, including a library directed by a trained librarian. This school is about to establish courses for the preparation of graduate nurses as teachers and administrators. The school founded by Dr. Carlos Nery in Montevideo, mentioned earlier (p. 418), is meeting the required standards. Modern nursing in this small country gives promise of developing satisfactorily in the near future.

ECUADOR, BOLIVIA, PARAGUAY, AND THE GUIANAS

In other countries of South America, Ecuador, to the north and west, and Bolivia and Paraguay, in the central part of the continent, modern nursing is still at a rather early stage of development. With the assistance of national and international health bodies, however, they are moving forward.

In Ecuador, which has been strongly influenced by North America since the 1940's, the School of Nursing at the National University in Quito, the capital city (one of four meeting the standards), has been completely reorganized to provide preparation for professional nurses in general practice, public health nursing, and auxiliary work. Educational programs have united nursing by nongovernmental and governmental groups, utilized the resources of both, and broadened public support of the concept of nursing as a profession.

Bolivia maintains a small number of schools with acceptable standards at La Paz, the capital. Here, also, a children's hospital, recently built and equipped, functions as a training center for pediatricians, pediatric nurses, and social workers. The declared objective of the Nurses' Association, as in other countries, is the improvement of nursing service and education.

Paraguay reports that the statutes controlling the preparation of nurses and their practice are now undergoing a thorough revision. A few of its schools meet acceptable standards.

In the Guianas (British, Netherlands [Surinam], and French) the pattern of nursing in general resembles that of the mother country. British Guiana, which recently became an independent nation within the British Commonwealth, has three schools of nursing with basic programs of three years, which are financed wholly or in part by the government. The British Guiana Nurses Association, organized thirty years ago, attained full membership in 1961 in the International Council of Nurses.

Netherlands Guiana and French Guiana each benefits from assistance by the home government, in nursing as in other health activities.

MODERN NURSING IN CENTRAL AMERICA

As was stated earlier in this chapter, the first steps taken to establish modern nursing in Central America came in the isthmian state of Panama at the beginning of this century. Another country in this immediate area, in which nursing began early, was Mexico, the home of the first hospital established in the Western Hemisphere, the Hospital of the Immaculate Conception (Hospital of Jesus of Nazareth), founded in Mexico City in 1524 by Hernando Cortes.

The history of the modern nursing movement in Mexico, like that of other countries in this part of the world, records the cooperation of nurses, the government and various agencies, national and international, such as the League of Red Cross Societies, the Institute of Inter-American Affairs, and the Rockefeller Foundation. Basic nursing was given assistance by the League of Red Cross Societies at the time of World War II. Among the large number of schools, perhaps the best known are the University of Mexico School and the Red Cross School, both in Mexico City. There are several other well-established schools that offer programs for basic students, a number of them associated with universities. Graduate nursing education started after World War I when public health nursing education was initiated. The first course was offered in 1935 by the University of Mexico School of Nursing with the help of the Rockefeller Foundation, which granted scholarships to Mexican nurses for study in the United States. Since that time the numbers of public health nurses have increased considerably. Through the cooperation of the Institute of Inter-American Affairs and the United States Government, a few graduate nurses were sent to the United States in the 1940's and 1950's for one-year courses in administration, supervision, and teaching in hospitals and schools of nursing.

Conferences of nurses of the Western Hemisphere, such as the Congress of Nurses in Mexico City in 1956, planned by the Pan American Sanitary Bureau (now PAHO), and the United States-Mexican Border Public Health Association conference in Lower California in the same year, have been held at various intervals under the sponsorship of national and international agencies. At these conferences nurses have had an opportunity to discuss their common problems and to reach some agreements as to plans for their solution. The Mexican Nurses Association, with its 800 members, became fully affiliated with the International Council of Nurses at the 1961 Congress.

EL SALVADOR, GUATEMALA, HONDURAS, NICARAGUA, AND COSTA RICA

In other parts of Central America substantial cooperation of various agencies has helped to promote modern nursing. All these countries now have nurses' associations devoted to the improvement of conditions in the field of nursing and of the nurses' preparation. El Salvador has been able to improve its schools and extend its services, particularly those of public health nurses, many of whom work in the health centers. At the Najapa Clinic, for example, doctors, nurses, and auxiliary workers are being trained in fairly large numbers for service in this little country. New legislation for the control of nursing education and practice was reported to be under consideration at the time of writing, here as well as in Guatemala and Paraguay. El Salvador's nurses organization now has an associate representative in the International Council of Nurses. A new school in Costa Rica has been developed with the assistance of WHO and it is hoped that this will have university status. Some nurses have been given scholarships for study abroad, to prepare them for teaching and supervision. Though this school is still young, it seems to be developing well. Progress in public health services is seen at health centers such as the one at Xochimilco, where clinics are conducted and where public health nurses have an opportunity to teach.

In these Central American countries such beginnings are

definitely encouraging. The future depends on many factors, the will of the nurses themselves to improve the situation and the help and understanding of governments, health agencies, citizens and neighbors who are in a position to help.

THE CARIBBEAN ISLANDS

Leaving continental Central and South America, we now come to the islands of the Caribbean, where the chief influences, as on the continent, have been those of Britain, France, Spain, Portugal, and the United States. In general, the pattern of nursing care in the islands follows fairly closely that of the colonizing country, as does also the stage of nursing development.

The earliest non-Latin group was the result of colonization by Great Britain. The population of the British West Indies includes peoples of many races, the majority of whom are of African descent, though there are also substantial numbers of East Indians and some Chinese. The white minority, at first, held most of the positions of responsibility in these islands. But as in British Africa and Asia definite efforts are now being made to train indigenous peoples for leadership not only in government but in medical, nursing, educational, and other fields of service. In 1958 ten island territories in this region under British Sovereignty (including Jamaica, Trinidad, Tobago and Barbados) decided to unite in a self governing group called the Federation of the West Indies. Since that date Jamaica has decided to withdraw from the federation and is now an independent unit.

JAMAICA

In this island, which has the largest population of the British West Indies, the story of modern nursing and hospital development is much the same as in other British colonial territories. Various agencies, governmental and private, some of which were missionary groups, built hospitals, large and small, before 1900, and started the training of native helpers. Schools of nursing were the next step, those in rural communities being quite small, as a rule, and limited in their clinical and other educational facilities. Matrons and staff nurses were drawn from among British nurses or from those of well-to-do Jamaican families who had gone abroad to study nursing in Great Britain or the United States. When public health services were organized, a demand came for more broadly educated nurses to organize and carry on this work. The public health program was an outcome of a study of endemic diseases, such as hookworm, yaws, malaria, and tuberculosis, made in the 1930's under the auspices of the Rockefeller Foundation. A public health nursing service was established in the Department of Health, and a training school to prepare sanitary inspectors and public health nurses was set up in 1943. Some Rockefeller fellowships were given to prepare nurses for leadership in this field. The department now has a large staff and carries on an active and effective program throughout the island.

Further steps were taken in the 1940's and 1950's as a result of the report of the Anglo-American Commission which studied various aspects of health and welfare in the West Indies and made some important recommendations. One was for the establishment of a regional university and medical center in Kingston to serve the British West Indies and to prepare doctors, nurses, and other health personnel for service in this general area. This center has done much to modernize medical and health work generally. The school of nursing, though belonging to the University College Hospital, is not of university status, but it is recognized as a good modern hospital school.

Meanwhile, a Jamaica General Trained Nurses Association was organized in 1946. Its first president, Nita Barrow, later became matron of the University College Hospital and now holds an important position in the government. The primary purpose of the Association is to raise the status of nurses in Jamaica. Largely as a result of its efforts, a registration act for general trained nurses was passed in 1951, its standards being such that Jamaica registrants could have reciprocal registration in Britain. The accrediting body, another group, is the General Nursing Council for Jamaica. The Association, which has about

600 members, was accepted for full membership in the International Council of Nurses in 1953. It now has several branches and is engaged in various activities for the improvement of nursing service and education and the status of nurses. It has sponsored short courses for nurses at University College of the West Indies, and in 1958 promoted the establishment of a district nursing service known as the Hyacinth Lightbourne Nursing Service. Its most recent project is the publication in June 1961 of its official journal, *The Jamaican Nurse*, edited by Gertrude Swaby. Attractive in appearance and substantial in content, it is further evidence of the initiative and unity of Jamaican nurses. Other activities of the Association are the building of a headquarters opened in 1960 and named Mary Seacole House after the Florence Nightingale of Jamaica whose story is told in the December 1961 issue of *The Jamaican Nurse*. This reports also the thirteenth annual summer school for graduate nurses.

Much credit should be given the Jamaican government for its policy with respect to the advancement of its people. It allows no restrictions based on race, sex or religion and encourages all of its citizens to develop whatever abilities they may have for leadership. This is seen in nursing where two outstanding West Indian nurses after additional preparation in England, Canada and the United States have been appointed to responsible government positions, Nita Barrow as Principal Nursing Officer in the Ministry of Health and Eva Lowe as Assistant Officer in that division. With increasing educational opportunities many local student nurses are now able to enter schools with full secondary education and often have had additional study on a collegiate level before or after this period. These and other developments indicate that nursing is moving definitely toward professional status in Jamaica.

TRINIDAD AND TOBAGO

Some of the other islands in this area have much the same history as that of Jamaica, but on a smaller scale. In British Trinidad and Tobago, for example, definite progress has been made within the last few years. There are two basic hospital

schools with almost 400 students enrolled, approved by the
Nursing Council of Trinidad and Tobago, and a post-basic
course of one year for health visitors, sponsored by the Health
Department and approved by the Ministry of Health. Nursing
education and practice are regulated by the Nurses' Registration Ordinance of 1950 and subsequent legislation. The name of
the Trained Nurses' and Midwives' Association, changed now to
indicate its strictly nurse membership, is the Trinidad and
Tobago Registered Nurses Association. With E. Hargreaves as
president and Mrs. V. Awon-Khan as secretary, it conducts its
business from the office of the Nursing Council in Port-of-Spain.
Through the effective cooperation of its officers and members,
it became a member of the International Council of Nurses in
1957. The islands now have over 1000 professional nurses.

HAITI

The Republic of Haiti, an independent country of French
and African traditions, has shown progress in the establishment
of modern nursing in some of its aspects. One example is the
school of nursing connected with the General Hospital at Port-
au-Prince, where nursing standards are said to be upgrading,
and which meets the specified standards. This has been made
possible through the assistance of the Office of Inter-American
Affairs in program planning and new and remodeled buildings.
Recent notice has been drawn to this republic by the work of
Dr. William Larimer Mellon, Jr., and his wife Gwen. A hospital
inspired by the work of Dr. Albert Schweitzer and built in 1954
by Dr. Mellon, with the assistance of the Haitian Government,
lies hidden in a jungle valley. A community project, it differs
from Dr. Schweitzer's in some of its features. It has a staff of
highly trained professional personnel, who receive salaries in
keeping with their preparation and service and who have excellent living and working conditions. The group includes both
American and native nurses, as well as *auxiliares,* or nursing
aides, and dentists. Though isolated, this hospital is proving to
be an asset in setting good standards in health work in this area.
The practice of nursing in Haiti is under the Minister of Educa-

tion and the University of Haiti. At the time of writing there were approximately ninety registered professional nurses in the country. The National Association of Licenciate Nurses of Haiti is a member of the International Council of Nurses.

ORGANIZATION OF CARIBBEAN NURSES

Instead of trying to summarize a few facts about other islands in this region a brief account will be given of this interesting and important development. In 1957 a Nurses' Conference, organized by the Certified Nurses and Midwives Association of Antigua, an island of the Leeward group under the jurisdiction of Great Britain, was called to discuss problems of concern to the nurses of the Caribbean Islands. Delegates attended from British Honduras, Grenada, Martinique, Puerto Rico, the American Virgin Islands, St. Kitts, and St. Vincent. This led to the organization of a regional group called the Caribbean Nurses Organization which is to meet biannually. The second meeting was held in St. Kitts in August 1961 and was attended by 49 delegates, coming from 17 areas of the Caribbean, some as far distant from one another as 1000 miles. Nevertheless they were united in their aims and efforts, all anxious to discuss their mutual problems and to share their experiences and aspirations. Their theme "Planning for the Future" brought out a wide variety of topics. One stimulating paper on nursing research led to the appointment of a committee on the subject. This and other topics indicate that nurses in this area are keeping abreast of their neighbors on the mainland of North America as well as of Great Britain. It may be noted that lay members took an active part in many of the discussions at this meeting.

This brief survey of nursing in Central and South America and the Caribbean Islands has noted the part played by various individuals, beginning with Florence Nightingale, and by agencies, missions, foundations, and national and international organizations. It has also illustrated the concern of nurses themselves for the quality of nursing service and education and the welfare of those giving the service. Studies and conferences from time to time have revealed the strength and weakness of nursing in this area and have led to suggestions for improvement.

The studies and observations of Agnes W. Chagas, and others familiar with the situation in this part of the hemisphere, indicate that although the modern nursing movement has been relatively slow in developing in most Latin American countries a good beginning has been made in many countries while some have made substantial progress. Among the problems that seem most critical at the present time is the difficulty of securing well-qualified applicants for the schools of nursing and better prepared faculties. As in many countries, some schools and hospitals still do not measure up to acceptable standards; a large majority of hospitals lack trained personnel, and some lack suitable physical and clinical facilities. In spite of this, however, the chief leaders in this area agree on what constitutes good nursing education and service, and some headway has been made in securing government support for needed improvements. Considering the problems they have had to face and the lack of resources of all kinds, the fact that most of these countries have one or more modern schools of nursing which meet acceptable standards and are making definite progress toward the extension of modern nursing services to larger proportions of the population is encouraging.

SELECTED BIBLIOGRAPHY

Americas. Vol. I, No. 1, March 1949-   Successor to the *Bulletin of the Pan American Union.*

Chagas, Agnes W. "Modern Nursing in Latin America," *Am. Jo. Nurs.,* January 1953, 34-36.

———. "Notes on Nursing Legislation in Latin America," *Int. Nurs. Rev.,* February 1960, 32-35.

———. "Trends in Nursing in the Region of the Americas," *Int. Nurs. Rev.,* April 1958, 21-23.

Colby-Monteith, Mary. "Nursing in Mexico," *Am. Jo. Nurs.,* July 1940, 746-754.

[Dourado, Haydie Guanses, and Maria de Lourdes Verderese.] "Nursing Education in Brazil," *Int. Nurs. Rev.*, July 1958, 32.

England. Colonial Office. Committee on the Training of Nurses for the Colonies . . . Report . . . Presented by the Secretary of State for the Colonies to Parliament by Command of His Majesty August 1945. London: HMSO, 1945.

Facts on Health Problems. Health in Relation to Social Improvement and Economic Development in the Americas. Washington: PAHO/WHO, 1961.

Fisher, Anna M. "Nursing in El Salvador," *Am. Jo. Nurs.*, June 1955, 682-684.

Gibson, Eunice. "The Barbados Nurses Association," *Am. Jo. Nurs.*, January 1945, 16-17.

International Council of Nurses. *National Reports. 1933,* 3-5, 33; *1947,* 48-49; *1949,* 62-67, 95-97, 105-107, 111-113; *1957,* 13-15, 23-25, 58-60, 96-97; *1961,* 10-11, 33-34, 46-48, 68-69, 88-89.

Linke, Lilo. "Ecuador's National School of Nursing," *Am. Jo. Nurs.*, August 1955, 968-970.

Nutting, M. Adelaide, and Lavinia L. Dock. *A History of Nursing.* New York: Putnam's, 1907-1912. 4 vols. Vol. IV, pp. 288-307.

O'Hara, Hazel. "Public Health Nursing in Latin America," *Pub. Health Nurse,* February 1950, 73-78.

Olds, James M. "Country Doctor—Jungle Style," *Today's Health,* July 1958, 28-33, 43-46.

Pinheiro, Maria Rosa Sousa. "Nursing Problems in Brazil," *Int. Nurs. Bull.*, Summer 1953, 2-8.

Scofield, John. "Haiti—West Africa in the West Indies," *Nat. Geog. Mag.*, February 1961, 227-259, 240-243.

Seel, Sir George. *Development and Welfare in the West Indies.* London: HMSO, 1952.

Stoegerer, Beatrice J. "A Good Neighbor Fellowship Program," *Am. Jo. Nurs.*, July 1948, 440-443.

10 Years of Cooperative Health Programs in Latin America: An Evaluation. Conducted by the Pub. Health Service Dept. of Health, Education, and Welfare for the Institute of Inter-American Affairs, 1952. Ch. 8.

"Thiry Years of Nursing in Haiti," *Am. Jo. Nurs.*, October 1949, 643-644.

CHAPTER 19

Africa

Second only to Asia in size, this continent covers more than a fifth of the earth's surface and has a population of more than 225 million. Except for the area north of the Sahara Desert and along the coast or in the southern temperate zone, this vast continent was largely unexplored and inaccessible until quite recent times. It is now opening up rapidly and attracting much more attention from all quarters of the globe. Geographically, Africa is a land of contrasts, of beautiful mountains, vast deserts, hot, moist jungles, and fertile plains. Much of the interior is uninhabitable except by natives of the country, and health hazards are formidable, especially in the equatorial region. The two main groups of native Africans are the Negroes who live chiefly between the equator and the Sahara and the Bantus who in comparatively recent times have spread southward as far as the Cape of Good Hope. Two fairly large groups of Asian origin are the Arabs (located chiefly in northern and northeastern Africa) and the natives of India who have settled more in the south and southeast. In addition, there are many white settlers, generally classified as Europeans, and other groups of mixed heredity who are called Coloreds.

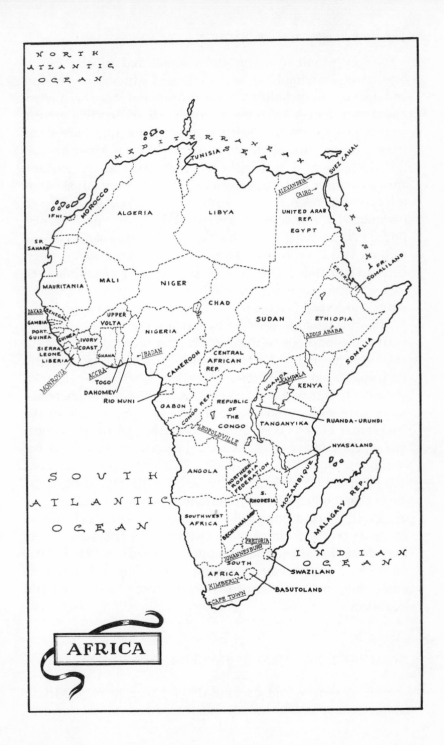

AFRICA

Though primitive beliefs and customs and tribal forms of organization are found in large sections of Africa, modern ideas and institutions including schools and hospitals have been introduced by colonial governments, industrial and trading groups, and in many cases by Christian missionaries who have come from different parts of the world. In recent years Africa has also felt the impact of such political movements as nationalism, anticolonialism, and communism, all leading to organized efforts toward independence. Many former colonies have now achieved nationhood and a large measure of self-government. The new slogan "Africa for the Africans," is speeding up changes on the map of Africa and is having a powerful influence on the international situation. Among the nineteen new members admitted to the United Nations in 1960-1961 were eighteen African states, and several that are now colonies, protectorates, or United Nations trusteeships expect to have that status soon.

Health conditions in this vast area are much the same as in other continents that lie for the most part in the tropical and subtropical zones. The most prevalent diseases are leprosy, malaria, dysentery, yaws, bilharzia, tuberculosis, and trachoma. Some countries are now reporting encouraging results in the eradication of several of these diseases. Malnutrition is widespread, chiefly because of the lack of protein in the diet. Other conditions such as poverty, poor housing, insanitary practices, and inherited taboos and customs stand in the way of efforts by medical and other workers to introduce preventive and curative measures. Witch doctors still have much influence, and even in the more civilized communities charms and fetishes are widely used. Instead of attempting to suppress the native medicine man, some efforts are now being made to secure his cooperation in establishing more modern methods of disease prevention and treatment.

DOMINANT INFLUENCES IN AFRICAN NURSING

Nursing systems and stages of development in these African countries vary widely and are influenced here as elsewhere by prevailing cultures and systems of government, the position of women, the traditional roles of the two sexes, and the opportunities for general and vocational education as well as for the employment of nurses. Even in countries that are now self-governing, the influence of former colonial governments such as Britain, France, Belgium, Spain, and Portugal tends to persist in medical and nursing patterns and systems of education and in the languages used in schools and hospitals. In many parts of Africa missionaries have been the first to set up hospitals and clinics and to train African midwives and nurses. Since these mission groups have come from different quarters of the globe, they also represent the systems and stages of educational and health work of their own countries. In recent years, however, largely through the influence of the World Health Organization and various foundations interested in international health, a good beginning has been made toward the exchange of ideas and methods among workers of different nationalities and countries.

An outstanding example is the first regional conference on African nursing held in Kampala, Uganda, in 1953.[1] This was attended by forty participants representing eighteen governments south and east of the Sahara, medical missions in this area and the professions of medicine and nursing. Preceding the conference, a survey of nursing in fifteen countries in this region was made by Jane McLarty, nurse consultant for WHO in that area, who had had wide experience as a matron in South Africa as well as good basic preparation in Britain. The survey focused on the health needs of the African peoples and the preparation of nurses of all races to meet such needs. Though differing widely in their languages and cultures and in their concepts of nursing and its relation to medicine, those who participated in the discussions made many helpful suggestions on the selection and preparation of nurses for service in Africa, the essential functions of nurses, and the importance of good basic as well as vocational education to fit them for the various types of work they were expected to do. Three African nurses who were pres-

[1] *African Conference on the Development of Nursing Education in Countries South of the Sahara.* Sponsored by the World Health Organization, Kampala, Uganda. 1954. Mimeographed.

ent made a valuable contribution by telling of their own experience in trying to bridge the gap between their homes and villages and the hospital world with its strange and to them often fearsome ways. The account of this conference in the *Chronicle of the World Health Organization*[2] presents a good introduction to this survey of nursing in Africa, which starts in the far south and moves northward along the east and west coasts and through central Africa across the Sahara to the Mediterranean. In this brief survey attention is given chiefly to the countries in which modern nursing has been introduced and has made a good start.

SOUTHERN AND EASTERN AFRICA

THE REPUBLIC OF SOUTH AFRICA

The Union of South Africa became self-governing in 1910, eight years after the Anglo-Boer War in which Britain defeated the Transvaal and the Orange Free State. It remained a member of the British Commonwealth until 1961, when it chose to withdraw from that affiliation. Thirty years before the union in the British Colony of Good Hope the first Nightingale schools for nurses in Africa were established by two members of Anglican nursing orders. The first was Sister Henrietta Stockdale who started a school in the early 1880's at Carnarvon Hospital in Kimberley. Shortly after (1886) Sister Mary Agatha of the Sisterhood of All Saints began to train nurses in the Somerset Hospital, Cape Town. These two sisters were also the moving spirit in getting the first registration clause included in a Medical and Pharmacy Act in 1891. Accompanied by sixty-five of her fellow nurses, Sister Henrietta appeared at the Cape Parliament to present this request and quickly won the support of both legislators and physicians. Though this was the first legal control of nursing in the world, it was many years before nurses were given representation on the Medical Council, which administered the act, and still longer before they secured their own act.

[2] *Chronicle of the World Health Organization*, January and September 1954.

After the Union of South Africa was formed, the four provinces administered their own hospitals and schools of nursing. English was the language used in such schools, but before long others were established for those speaking Afrikaans.[3] Many schools are bilingual, and separate schools which train non-Europeans are as a rule mainly English-speaking. At first the matrons and sisters in charge were European (chiefly British), but they were gradually replaced (except in the largest institutions) by non-Europeans. Some small mission hospitals are affiliated with large hospitals in order that students may qualify for the requirements of the South African Nursing Council.

All of the main fields of nursing have developed here. Midwifery has been closely related to nursing from the first, and many nurses qualify in both fields. Tuberculosis, which has been the most common of the fatal diseases among non-Europeans, has responded to better housing and working conditions. Smallpox and malaria have been similarly checked. District nursing, which developed under the King Edward VII Order of Nurses, now because of lack of funds functions only in a few outlying districts, mainly in the Cape Province. Some of the larger cities have district or visiting nurses attached to hospital staffs who make home visits and give nursing care when necessary. Plans for the near future include district nursing services in all provinces, their staffs to include both European and non-European men and women graduate nurses.

In the Cape, as in New Zealand, registration preceded professional organization. The South African Nursing Association was formed in 1914 with the help of physicians, one of whom, Dr. Tremble, continued for years to advise the nurses and to edit their journal. In 1922 the Association became an active member of the International Council of Nurses. Among its nurse leaders, Bella G. Alexander, Scottish-trained matron of the Johannesburg General Hospital, was especially well known, having held many important positions in national and international nursing organizations. Nurses worked for many years to get representation on the Medical Council which administered

[3] Afrikaners or white natives of South Africa who were of Dutch or Huguenot ancestry.

the registration act. They finally succeeded (1928) in securing two places in a total of twenty-seven. Their efforts to raise minimum requirements for schools were not successful, partly because of medical conservatism and also because of the wide variation in hospital and educational facilities of city and rural communities. In 1936 registered nursing schools were graded, the better ones (Class I) offering a three-year course and those with more limited clinical and other facilities (Class II), four years. A period of supervised practice following registration was required for both.

Though the highly controversial issues of apartheid are not discussed here, they should be kept in mind in considering the problems met by nurses in South Africa. This applies also to the rather arbitrary laws and policies concerned with labor which have had a direct influence on nursing. For example, in 1942 a crisis was precipitated by an aggressive trade union which threatened to absorb nurses and midwives and to compel them to adopt the standard union type of closed-shop organization. Securing legal advice and with the active support of a woman member of Parliament, the Nursing Association applied for and received a government charter which gave it the right to represent its members for purpose of collective bargaining and other vital interests. They also prepared a new nursing bill which became law in 1944.

This act, known as the South African Nursing Act, created two statutory bodies: the South African Nursing Council, concerned with the training, examination, and registration of nurses, and the South African Nursing Association, whose responsibility it was to raise the status of the nursing profession. The nurses of South Africa functioned under this act until 1951, when in carrying out the official policy of apartheid it was proposed by the Minister of Health that the membership be limited to nurses who were South African citizens and Europeans. The association, with the approval of representative non-Europeans, then proposed that there should be an advisory board of the latter group. The new act, passed in 1957, created two groups which functioned separately, one for Europeans and one for Bantus and Negroes. Although membership in the association is still multiracial, the act in practice is disadvantageous to non-European nurses in various ways. Miss M. G. Borcherds, who has been President of the South African Nursing Association during this trying period, has shown much courage in standing up for the principles of the International Council of Nurses which opposes the segregation of nurses on racial or religious grounds.

Until 1929 there was no lack of applicants for the schools of nursing in South Africa (approximately 100), and no plans were made to train assistant nurses. At that time a reorganization of schools was undertaken to lift nursing out of the apprenticeship stage into the professional category by improved standards, such as the establishment of nursing colleges in each province and by centralized teaching. Students were rotated according to a "block" system, not being attached to one hospital, but going from one hospital to another according to their need for clinical experience. Midwives' training was also strengthened. The majority of basic nursing schools are now associated with a nursing college, which functions as an educational center or teaching department, providing theoretical instruction for students and maintaining close collaboration with the clinical practice. Another forward step was the improvement of facilities for the preparation of nurse leaders and specialists. University education helped in this respect, as, for example, at the University of Witwatersrand in Johannesburg and the University of Pretoria, where facilities were offered for certain nursing specialties, including teaching and administration. From these and other developments it would appear that organized nurses here have been active and influential and have managed to make progress in spite of the many controversial issues in which this group has been involved.

RHODESIA AND NYASALAND

This federation is now virtually a self-governing part of the British Empire. A vote in 1961 provided a new charter which will give more direct African representation in the Legislative Assembly. General conditions are much the same as in the Republic of South Africa, though here medicine and nursing are at an earlier stage of development and political issues apparently are less acute. Various types of personnel are trained for medical, midwifery, and nursing work, and facilities for nurse preparation are expanding, especially in mission hospitals. Because of the inadequate preliminary education of girls, many men are admitted to these schools. Aside from the question of suitable applicants, the most serious problem is the shortage of qualified instructors.

Associations of fully trained nurses have been developed in both Northern and Southern Rhodesia and have been admitted to membership in the International Council of Nurses, Northern Rhodesia in 1953 and Southern Rhodesia in 1949. Laws governing the practice of nursing have been passed in Southern Rhodesia, and registered nurses, if they qualify otherwise, are eligible for practice or admission to more advanced courses in Britain. *The Northern Rhodesia Nurses Association Journal* was established in 1957. Legislation for Northern Rhodesia and Nyasaland has been under consideration. Though many of the positions of leadership are held by Europeans (mostly British), the minimum standards are the same for all. The World Health Organization is working with the nursing groups to help improve nursing standards and conditions in this part of Africa.

KENYA

Farther north, in Kenya, the proportion of European residents decreases, and the preparation of indigenous personnel for health services, chiefly among their own people, presents somewhat different problems. In this connection a study made a few years ago by Dr. Janet (Welch) Mackie, an English physician and public health specialist, is of interest. The study, which included Kenya, resulted from extensive social and anthropological observations of native cultures of a large area of Africa. The practical and farseeing suggestions made, although not fully adopted, have had a definite influence on the policies of Kenya and of some other countries in which matriarchal forms of organization exist. Here the older women especially did much to further the plan for nurse and midwife training once they saw its advantages. Institutions under both missionary and governmental auspices were also influenced by this study. Ten years later, in 1951, the education of nurses in Kenya was placed on much the same basis as the education of teachers. By this time secondary education for girls was more readily available, and the advantage of a longer period of schooling was recognized by many of the native inhabitants themselves. The value of nurse training was also seen as a means of raising the general standard of living and even of providing suitable wives for public officials!

The legal control of nursing in Kenya rested with the Kenya Registered Nurses and Midwives Council, which used the British syllabus and training scheme, thus making reciprocity with that country possible. Midwives and student nurses were associate members of the council. At the time of writing, two schools of nursing, administered and financed by the Kenya Government General Hospital and European Hospital Association, were giving full general nursing education. Europeans were admitted to these schools.

Believing that the International Council of Nurses would afford valuable assistance in solving the various problems in this rapidly developing country, with its increasing number of registered nurses from three different racial groups (European, African, and Asian), the Trained Nurses Association of Kenya applied for and secured membership in that organization in 1961.

With the assistance of the World Health Organization, a number of health centers have been established to provide service to an increasing number of people in the area and an additional field for practice for graduate nurses, especially those in public health. But though offering good facilities, they suffer from staff shortages. Here, as in other countries that have been administered by Britain, the nursing service of the Colonial Office in London has been helpful in giving advice and in supplying needed personnel. Nairobi, the capital city has some excellent hospitals and training schools for nurses and other health workers of different races. The Mau Mau troubles have tended to disrupt such activities in recent years and to create greater racial tensions.

UGANDA

Directly west of Kenya, this British Protectorate has many points of interest, including Lake Victoria Nyanza, the second largest fresh water lake in the world, explored by Henry M. Stanley in 1875. This country, whose population is chiefly Bantu, has a longer history of training women nurses and midwives than many other African territories. A recent educational department report shows that higher education for girls is developing, and it is hoped that a fair proportion of the better educated may be attracted into nursing and midwifery. Such changes are slow, however, because of the social prejudice against this work and the early marriage age of most girls. The mission schools seem to have an advantage with reference to recruitment because education, although subsidized by the government, is largely in their hands. Courses for nurses and other health personnel are given in both mission and government hospitals, and at the present time it is necessary also to provide instruction in English in some of these schools. A beginning in university education for nurses has been made at the Mackerere Medical School located in Kampala. Mengo Mission Hospital, one of the pioneer mission hospitals, has had courses for midwives and nurses for many years, and clinics have opened up a field of practice for public health nurses. Since 1950 the World Health Organization has sent students here from other African countries, such as Ethiopia, which have had a shorter experience in developing their health services and in training health workers.

ETHIOPIA

A neighboring country that seems to be making definite progress in establishing modern nursing is the Kingdom of Ethiopia, (formerly Abyssinia). The emperor, Haile Selassie I, is the 225th Solomonic ruler, claiming descent from Solomon's son and the Queen of Sheba. Although some of the inhabitants are Moslems, the majority are Christians belonging to the Coptic branch of the Eastern Church. The emperor and empress have been especially interested in nursing and hospital work, possibly because during their exile in London in World War II their daughter Princess Tsahai trained as a children's nurse. Her death occurred shortly after their return to their homeland, and one of the newer hospitals was built in her memory.

Though the morbidity rate is still high in rural Ethiopia and health services are weak outside the capital, Addis Ababa is well supplied with hospitals. In 1952, with the aid of western missionary groups, the Red Cross, the World Health Organization, and others, four nursing schools were organized. English, American, and Swedish nurse directors and staffs have pioneered in the organization of these schools, and despite differences in background they have apparently succeeded in avoiding serious disagreement on standards and programs that would hinder the development of a national pattern. Some of the more promising nurses who have been trained there have been sent to New Zealand, Canada, and other countries for more specialized preparation.

The Ethiopian Nurses Association became a member of the International Council of Nurses in 1957. These are all promising indications that modern nursing has made a good start in Ethiopia and that the evolving system there will combine the good features of several existing national plans and will also be adapted to the conditions and needs of the country.

ANGOLA AND MOZAMBIQUE

In this southern portion of the continent of Africa are two countries, Angola (Portuguese West Africa), and Mozambique (Portuguese East Africa), one a large area in the west on the Atlantic coast and the other in the east on the Indian Ocean. A new law, now in the process of preparation, is designed to grant constitutional equality to all races and colors, and to give more self-determination to all Portuguese territories. These reforms are being introduced in the midst of rebellion in some parts of these colonies. Health services are somewhat elementary here, compared with those in neighboring states. "Bush" hospitals, both Roman Catholic and Protestant, and clinics have been established. Plans include the building of hospitals and the training of nurses and other health workers. Provisions for health are said to be a little more advanced in Mozambique than in Angola, clinics and hospitals having been provided in greater numbers. In Luanda, capital of Angola, the hospital dates back to 1888. It provides care for all races and maintains a school of nursing at which various classes of workers are trained. The nursing program is available to both European and non-European students and is similar to that in Portugal. In spite of these indications of interest, it cannot be said that the modern nursing movement has made appreciable headway in these countries.

There are other protectorates, territories, and islands under various political administrations in and around east-central Africa, among which might be mentioned Tanganyika, where training centers for nurses and other health personnel are making progress, Somalia, whose people are chiefly Moslem and where such training of health workers is just beginning, and Ruanda-Urundi, where some activity in the field of nursing preparation has been noted. In the countries in this area nursing development is still at an early stage.

CENTRAL AND WEST AFRICA

REPUBLIC OF THE CONGO (LEOPOLDVILLE)

The former Belgian Congo (capital, Leopoldville), which became independent in 1960, was brought to the attention of the outside world in the middle of the nineteenth century by the explorations of Henry M. Stanley and Dr. David Livingstone. In 1908 it became a Belgian colony. Its several provinces produce large amounts of mineral ores and are covered extensively by tropical forests. Since independence, it has been torn by widespread violence and pillage. There have been serious food shortages, and its people, chiefly Bantu-Negro, have suffered from malnutrition and disease. In addition to those who practice the native religions, there are many Christians, predominantly Roman Catholic. Most of the schools are mission-operated.

Considerable expansion of hospitals and in the training of various grades of indigenous workers for the care of the sick (chiefly medical assistants, men nurses, and health inspectors) has taken place in recent times. The Belgian system has been followed as a rule, though some mission hospitals have been established by missionaries from other countries. Special efforts are being made to train women nurses and midwives by the use of several philanthropic funds for this purpose. The need for better applicants among African girls and for nurse teachers to assist in this training is now beginning to be recognized. A school of nursing has been established with the help of the Rockefeller Foundation at the newly organized University of Louvanium in Leopoldville, an institution identified in the minds of the people as distinctly Congolese in character. The Rector, who recognizes the urgent need to educate Africans, both men and women, for positions of leadership, has encouraged suitable nurses to secure such preparation. This university has remained open during all the uprisings, and it is hoped that it will play an important part in the development of leaders for the new republic including those in the field of nursing.

WEST AFRICA

Former French West Africa comprises a union of seven constituent territories, all of which have voted for independence within the French Community except French Guinea. The health of this vast area has benefited in the past from several programs. In Dakar, once its capital, an ever broadening program in serum and vaccine production is maintained by a branch of the Pasteur Institute. There are many hospitals, medical centers, dispensaries, health units, and maternity centers staffed by French-trained physicians (of high caliber in most cases), nurses, and midwives. Beyond the city of Dakar, the country is largely rural. Health centers and leper colonies are staffed as a rule by men nurses who have been trained for this work, and a few dispensaries and maternity centers are run by African doctors, midwives, and men and women nurses. A public health program which envisions hospitals and health centers for the entire area is being planned. Until fairly recently nurses were trained by the government for work in both urban and rural areas. The facilities in Dakar include a midwifery school and a nursing school, the latter opened in 1951. Teaching is done by physicians, religious sisters, and lay teachers (*monitrices*). The students are African men and women and European women, including religious sisters. The course of training follows the state training courses for nurses in France, and those who qualify are equal in professional status to their colleagues in that country.

EQUATORIAL AFRICA

Extending farther into the interior is former French Equatorial Africa, now four independent republics within the French Community, where the desire for learning is causing a reorganization of the federal and territorial system of education. Though the number of girl students is still relatively small, it has shown a marked increase in recent years. The Institute of Central African Studies exerts a powerful influence in teacher training. As in West Africa, a Pasteur Institute and a number of medical and maternity centers and leper hospitals are in operation. Public health measures have been introduced, and the public health battle is gradually being won by doctors, nurses, and midwives. Mobile units which visit the outlying areas also play an important role. The inhabitants of these countries are beginning to show appreciation of modern methods of caring for the sick and of educating personnel (nurses, hygienists, and laboratory technicians), as exemplified by the newer hospitals and health centers.

This part of Africa is perhaps best known to the world through the work of Dr. Albert Schweitzer, medical missionary, philosopher, writer, and musician. His rural hospital at Lamberéné has become famous, chiefly through the writings of those who have visited and observed it. Though often criticized because of its lack of modern technical and scientific medical and nursing care, it has served those who utilize its facilities in other ways, and the founder has impressed everyone with his zeal in putting into practice in everyday living his humanitarian and ethical principles.

NIGERIA

In this part of western Africa are Nigeria and Ghana, two countries whose health systems have been influenced by Great Britain. The Federation of Nigeria, the larger of the two, became an independent nation within the Commonwealth in 1960. It has had the assistance of Great Britain in preparing its people for self-government and in building up its educational, health and other services and is regarded by many as a leader among the new African nations. Modern nursing began here about 1900 under British nurses, and until World War II training was provided in government hospitals on an apprenticeship basis. Preliminary schools were later introduced in each of the regions where sister tutors gave systematic instruction to students of nursing and midwifery. These trainees were then transferred to regional hospitals, where they were taught by ward sisters and medical officers. Nigeria now has approximately forty schools of nursing in which students are prepared not only for general nursing but also for public health and psychiatric nursing and midwifery. In Ibadan, in the Western Region, the University College Hospital trains nurses to meet the requirements of the General Nursing Council for England and Wales. Miss L. M. Bell, the first director, a nurse in the Nightingale tradition, recruited the first class, which was required to pass the School Certificate Examination and other exacting requirements before entrance. They came from all regions, tribes, and family backgrounds, but all met the discriminating standards. It is planned that this school will help to provide well-trained Nigerian teachers of nursing for this area. Also, a post-basic course for nurse teachers is being planned. The northern part of Nigeria, in which a large proportion of the population is Moslem, has been slower to develop modern nursing chiefly because of the traditional position of its women and other influences that have tended to retard the education and professional preparation of nurses.

The Professional Association of Trained Nurses of Nigeria is relatively small because of the difficulties of communication and of making personal contacts where travel is exceptionally slow. It became a member of the International Council of Nurses at the 1961 Congress. In this vast tropical country, which is changing rapidly, rural health groups are dealing rather successfully with some health problems, but they have a long way to go in covering the total health needs. A good beginning has been made, and help is forthcoming here as elsewhere from the World Health Organization and other international agencies.

GHANA

This country (formerly the Gold Coast), with the encouragement of the British Government, delayed independence until trained leaders and administrators were ready to replace those from Britain. After becoming a republic in 1960, it remained within the Commonwealth. It had joined the United Nations in 1957.

Modern nursing was introduced here at the turn of the century by British matrons and sisters. Partly because of the tropical climate, the need not only for African nurses but for African leaders of nursing was soon recognized. Until quite recently African nurses, men and women, were trained by the apprenticeship method for regular hospital service. When the number of British matrons and sisters became limited in World War II, the government decided to experiment with a nurse training college, admitting only the better educated girls and starting them at once in a broad-gauge program that prepared them as nurses, administrators, and teachers in schools, hospitals, and public health services. This plan proved so satisfactory that an attractive, well-equipped building was erected near the Gold Coast Hospital at Accra. The college was independent in administration and clearly differentiated from the hospital. Its program attracted a superior type of applicant, and a second college of the same kind was planned. Here, as in some other parts of British Africa, in which programs for nurse leaders exist, a close connection is arranged with teacher training colleges and universities, the education of nurses being rated comparable with teacher education.

The fields of practice showing the greatest recent development have been psychiatric nursing, public health nursing, and midwifery. Preparation is provided for two types of nurses: State Registered Nurses and Qualified Registered Nurses. The graduates of the program for Qualified Registered Nurses, trained in less advanced schools, are expected to meet the nursing needs of the country as a whole, and their course is simpler in character than that for State Registered Nurses. Both groups of nurses are eligible for preparation as midwives and health visitors. State Registered Nurses are able to meet the requirements of the General Nursing Council for England and Wales, the majority being in this class. The Nurses' Board of Ghana was established by the Nurses' Ordinance of 1946 in which both categories of nurses are recognized. The Association of State Registered Nurses of Ghana was admitted to membership in the International Council of Nurses in 1961. The government has recently asked the World Health Organization for an experienced nursing administrator to act in an advisory capacity on nursing matters. Developments in Ghana are being noted with interest by many who believe that African nurses, given the opportunity, can assume leadership in their own field and measure up to their professional responsibilities.

LIBERIA

This republic on Africa's west coast came into existence in 1822 when the American Colonization Society began sending freed American slaves to Africa's "Grain Coast." Its government is patterned after that of the United States, and Monrovia, its capital, is named for President Monroe. The prevailing diseases are those of a tropical country. A public health program and a new school of nursing are being assisted by the World Health Organization, with additional help by the Point IV, U.S. government Foreign Aid Program. Negro nurses had an important share in establishing modern nursing practices in Liberia; the first trained nurse was Mrs. Jackson, a Jamaican graduate of the Lincoln School of Nursing in New York, sent in 1902 by the Baptist Church to assist in the improvement of nursing standards in this country. In 1903 a training school for nurses was started at Phoebe Hospital, now located at Zorzor. Several similar schools were developed later under missionary nurses, both white and colored.

A governmental program, which gave full recognition to nursing, was the result of a public health mission under Doctor John G. West of the United States Public Health Service, who was sent to Liberia during World War I primarily to improve health conditions in the Liberian militia and among employees of the rubber plantations then supplying war needs. With this mission went several well qualified Negro nurses, headed by Mary L. Mills, the first of her race to hold such a post in United States Government service. In addition to the establishment of health centers (some far up in jungle country), the mission was concerned with preparing permanent public health personnel. Out of this came the founding of the Central School of Nursing as a part of the Tubman Institute of Medical Arts, a government institution situated in the capital. First under Mary Mills and later under her assistant Clara Beverley, this school developed a health-centered educational program and proceeded to recruit and prepare Liberian high school graduates for the more responsible positions in the national nursing service.

The Liberian National Nurses Association was organized with the assistance of these nurses and later became a member of the International Council of Nurses (1957). Steps were taken in 1934 to revise the Medical Act, which had given full responsibility to a medical board for licensing nurses to set standards and hold examinations. Instead, the Liberian Nurses' Examining Board was established in 1950. The fact that women were voting citizens and that nurses had been given excellent status in government service helped to strengthen the position of nurses in Liberia. Nevertheless, much of the country is still in a primitive stage of development and has a long way to go before modern health services and trained nurses can be provided for the population as a whole.

NORTHERN AFRICA

Most of the countries that lie between the Mediterranean Sea and the Sahara Desert and extend from the Atlantic Ocean to the Red Sea are linked ethnically, politically, and culturally with the rest of the Moslem world, and their indigenous peoples hold much the same viewpoints on religious, social, and political questions. There are differences, however, in governmental policies and programs concerned with health and other matters. Morocco and Tunisia, which had been under French administration but are now self-governing, and Libya, formerly Italian, have health systems similar to those of their former colonial governments. Algeria, at the time of writing, a part of the political entity of France, also follows the French system. Recent unrest and open warfare in many of these sections have tended to upset health work. Then, too, because of the prevailing lack of education for girls and the prejudice against nursing or any similar occupation for women, men with full preparation as nurses are in the majority. This is in marked contrast to the situation existing in the countries in which British influence has been strong. Midwifery enjoys a higher status than nursing among women who are willing to undergo two or three years' training. In these countries doctors assume chief responsibility for most of the teaching, though they are sometimes assisted by religious sisters or secular nurses. Although many hospitals still train auxiliary personnel in the old way, the trend is toward better organized schools connected with hospitals or situated in some of the larger centers. In these institutions several different classes of health workers are prepared, some of them for the mobile units that have played a vital role in campaigns against epidemic and endemic diseases.

THE UNITED ARAB REPUBLIC (EGYPT)

This republic (Egypt) is perhaps the oldest and one of the best known lands of the African continent. Its archaeological records date back to at least 4000 B.C., and a high civilization of rulers and priests dominated the country in its early history. In 1914 Egypt became a British protectorate and in 1933, a republic. Women voted for the first time in Egypt in 1957. An extensive public health and sanitary program in the modern sense does not exist in this country. Efforts are being made, however, to extend clinic and hospital facilities to all areas. Training for health personnel is deficient, partly because of the weaknesses in educational programs. In this area the United States Operations Mission is assisting in the establishment not only of primary and secondary education but also of vocational training. Of special note is the work of the United States Naval Medical Research Unit in Cairo, which is carrying on basic research in the prevention of disease.

Probably the best known nursing school in northern Africa is attached to the large Kasr-el-Ainy Hospital in Cairo, which has attracted and trained a rather cosmopolitan group of applicants. Administered for many years by a British matron and sisters, it was later put in charge of an Egyptian matron and staff and has succeeded in enrolling a number of well-educated Egyptian girls. This effort has the support of leaders in the Egyptian women's movement, which has been quite active.

A new modern school of nursing, the Higher Institute of Nursing, was established in Alexandria in 1955 with the assistance of the World Health Organization. It is the result of long-term planning by the Egyptian Ministry of Health, the medical faculty of the University of Alexandria, and the World Health Organization, its object being to raise health standards. The program leads to a baccalaureate degree and includes instruction in public health as well as in other aspects of nursing. In the beginning nurse educators provided by WHO composed the teaching staff. Fellowships have been supplied for trained women from Egypt to go abroad to qualify for teaching positions when the present staff is withdrawn. In 1958 enrollment included students from Egypt, Iraq, Syria, the Sudan, and Jordan. These students have good academic backgrounds, and it is hoped that they will assume leadership in their own countries after the completion of the course.

Fifteen other schools, of which four are entitled university schools and eleven private and mission schools, follow a standard curriculum under the Ministry of Health. The Egyptian Nurses Association, with its 400 individual members, was admitted to the International Council of Nurses in 1961.

The foregoing brief picture of nursing in some African countries illustrates the point that, aside from education, health is Africa's greatest problem. The two are closely allied and both present almost insuperable difficulties. In most countries there is a system of hospitals and dispensaries for the treatment of the most prevalent diseases. Many recently built hospitals compare favorably with good hospitals everywhere but their effectiveness is too often lessened by the lack of properly trained physicians, dentists, and nurses. Contributing factors are the political upheavals in many of these lands and the fact that in some countries the education of girls and the preparation of women for such vocations and professions is not favored. The complexity of the problem was well demonstrated at the African Conference on Nursing Education referred to earlier. Here, as in Asia, we find many transplanted European and North American nursing systems which are often in conflict with one another and are not easily adjusted to the situations in underdeveloped countries. In recent years much more attention has been given to the development of nursing programs and services to meet the needs of the individual countries following certain general principles recommended by such international bodies as the World Health Organization and the International Council of Nurses. In spite of these variations, it is encouraging to note the amazing developments taking place in some areas. Those who work with African girls report that they adapt themselves well to nursing, and in many instances when given opportunity and encouragement have shown that they are capable of leadership as well as skilled service in this and allied fields.

SELECTED BIBLIOGRAPHY

Advisory Committee on Education in the Colonies. *Memorandum on the Education of African Communities.* London: HMSO, 1935.

African Affairs. Journal of the Royal African Society, 18 Northumberland Ave., London, W. C. 2, England.

African Conference on the Development of Nursing Education in Countries South of the Sahara. Sponsored by the World Health Organization. Kampala, Uganda. Geneva: WHO, 1954. Mimeographed.

"Africa New Star in History," *Sat. Rev.* July 19, 1958, 8-21.

"Africa South of the Sahara," *Atlantic Monthly,* April 1959, 4, 6, 8, 29-94.

Beverley, Clara J. "Nursing Schools in Liberia," *Am. Jo. Nurs.,* August 1947, 530-531.

Borcherds, M. G. "The South African Nursing Act, *Int. Nurs. Rev.,* July 1958, 33-43.

Chronicle of the World Health Organization, January and September 1954.

Collis, Robert. *African Encounter: A Doctor in Nigeria.* New York: Scribner's, 1960. Pp. 90-100.

Colmers, Elizabeth. "Nursing Education in Some South African Territories," *Nurs. Outlook,* August 1953, 466-467.

Cousins, Norman. *Dr. Schweitzer of Lambaréné.* New York: Harpers, 1960.

Creelman, Lyle. "Nursing in the African Region," *Int. Nurs. Rev.,* April 1958, 19-20.

————. "Nursing in the World," *Can. Nurse,* September 1958, 814-819.

Horley, George. *Native African Medicine.* Cambridge: Harvard University Press, 1941.

Houghton, Marjorie. "Nigeria's First Teaching Hospital," *Nurs. Times,* January 3, 1958, 13-16.

International Council of Nurses. *National Reports, 1933,* 30-31, 59-60; *1947,* 42-43; *1949,* 51-55, 75-77, 117-120; *1957,* 85-87, 88-89; *1961,* 21-23, 54-55, 64-65, 73-74, 75-76, 92-93.

Jenkinson, Vivian M. "The Nursing Colleges of South Africa," *Nurs. Times,* Vol. LI, No. 7, 1955, 175-176.

A Journey to Africa. Report of the Exec. Sec'y of Int. Council of Nurses, 1954, 7-13. World Health Organization in Kampala, 1954, 13-15.

Mackie, Janet W., and Olive Baggallay. "Nursing Education in Africa," *Am. Jo. Nurs.,* August 1954, 984-985.

Magnussen, Eli. "Nursing in Ethiopia," *Am. Jo. Nurs.,* March 1953, 296-297.

Mills, Mary. "Nurse Training in the Gold Coast," *Nurs. World,* January 1952, 14, 49.

"Nursing Education in Egypt," *Int. Nurs. Rev.,* May 1930, 291-293.

"On WHO's Tenth Anniversary," *Am. Jo. Nurs.*, May 1958, 706.

Report of the Special Study Mission to Africa, South and East of the Sahara. Washington: Govt. Print. Off., 1957. House Report No. 307, 85th Congress, 1st Session.

Scanlon, David G. "African Education From Bush School to University," *Sat. Rev.*, August 19, 1961, 34-35, 50-52.

Searle, Charlotte. "Nursing Education in South Africa," *Int. Nurs. Rev.*, May 1957, 49-62.

———. "A Review of Nursing Education in South Africa," *Int. Nurs. Bull.*, Winter 1953, 5-10.

Swindall, Hermione S., and Marguerite L. Burt, "A Beginning in Ethiopia," *Am. Jo. Nurs.*, May 1961, 82-84.

"University College Hospital School of Nursing, Ibadan, Nigeria," *Nurs. Times*, February 10, 1956, 139-147.

Welch, Janet (Mackie). *Nursing Education Related to the Cultural Background in East and Southeast African Colonies.* New York: Kings Crown Press, 1941. Mimeographed.

[World Health Organization]. *Public Health Work in Africa Ten Years of Progress.* Brazzaville: French Equatorial Africa, n. d.

CHAPTER **20**

Major International Agencies and Trends

PRECEDING chapters in Part II have followed the modern nursing movement into many parts of the world and have noted various kinds of agencies that have helped or hindered its advance in the geographic sense and in that of its strength, effectiveness and influence. Some of these agencies or instrumentalities for action were local or national in scope; others took in a much wider area. Some were individuals who provided leadership and guidance on a wide scale, others were international organizations, institutions, parallel movements, or similar agencies. It would be a mistake to assume that all were united in their aims, programs, and activities. Many conflicts have been noted, sometimes between rival individuals and groups, and often between differing national concepts and systems of nursing. Wise and competent leadership was a primary need in getting the movement started, but financial and moral support was essential in establishing schools and services, maintaining sound standards, protecting learners and workers from exploitation, and promoting the continued growth and progress of modern nursing. This chapter rounds out and relates some of the agencies mentioned in earlier chapters which had on the whole a constructive and potent influence on the world movement. Beginning with individual leaders few movements have been as fortunate as this one in its founder who for many years was also its chief leader. Florence Nightingale was not only a world-famous and popular heroine but a dedicated genius and born reformer whose vision took in the globe. She was no amateur in nursing, having served an extended and varied apprenticeship and given years of study to the subject. In spite of poor health, she was able to continue into her 70's her varied roles as organizer, master builder, publicity and public relations expert, secretary-general, and presiding officer of the international headquarters of the modern nursing movement which for many years was located in her sickroom. From here poured forth a steady stream of letters, memos, articles, pamphlets, and other writings packed with advice and specific directions to her nurse missioners at home and abroad, to governors of various countries, health officers, and other influential persons. The amazing thing about this fabulous invalid is that her fame has continued to grow since her death in 1910, and biographies are constantly appearing which reveal new aspects of her complex personality and her wide influence. The latest publication which nurses of the world have helped to promote is *A Bio-Bibliography of Florence Nightingale,*[1] prepared by a well-known librarian, the late William J. Bishop. This book contains abstracts of about 15,000 letters and memos as well as of many printed books and pamphlets. Together they are said to exceed in number and variety any known collection left by a famous person.

Why this remarkable leader failed to create a permanent foundation to carry on her work has puzzled many. According to her official biographer, Sir Edward Cook, she feared that such an organization would stereotype and standardize the movement and so impede its progress. This was her chief objection to the International Council of Nurses, launched at first to promote the movement for state registration of nurses. Too remote from the situation at that time to realize the dangers of the horde of unregulated pseudo-schools which had been allowed to mul-

---

[1] First volume published by Dawson's of Pall Mall for the International Council of Nurses, 1962.

tiply and rather critical of some of the new nurse leaders and their methods, she lent her support to their opponents. In spite of this, she retained her strong hold on the young profession she had done so much to create, and with her little lamp became the symbol of modern nursing throughout the world.

Although many individuals too numerous to mention here continued to play an important part in nursing leadership, organized groups became the means through which most of their efforts were channeled. The first were centered around the early schools and were composed of their own officers and graduates. Then came local, state, national, and international groups, which varied in their functions and characteristics. Here chief attention is given to international agencies that have had a marked influence on nursing in many parts of the world.

THE INTERNATIONAL COUNCIL OF NURSES

This Council could not have appeared when it did if nurses of several countries had not previously organized national groups and developed a number of outstanding leaders who had experience in such matters. It was decided that membership would be corporate rather than individual and at first (until 1904) on a provisional basis. However, the representatives meeting in July 1900 approved the constitution and by-laws and elected the first officers who were Mrs. Bedford Fenwick (Britain), president, Lavinia L. Dock (U.S.A.), secretary, and Mary A. Snively (Canada), treasurer. This was the first international professional organization on record, though there had been conferences and committees of such groups before.

The preamble to the constitution (quoted on p. 170) indicates the liberal spirit of its founders. The decision was made to bring together in international union fully trained nurses who in their own homelands had developed or were endeavoring to develop professional self-government and to admit to membership only national associations founded on that declared basis. In each country the Council sought the group allied to it in action and spirit, not caring how weak or small this might be, provided it stood for a free professional status for nurses and its voting members were qualified trained nurses. Only one such association from each country was to be admitted, so it became necessary for existing national groups to consolidate or federate if they wished to belong to the ICN. As noted in earlier chapters, associations that had started with mixed membership, which included physicians, laymen, and sometimes royal or wealthy patrons, had to reorganize, some giving their non-nurse members honorary titles but no vote. Those which had included midwives who were not also trained nurses gave them associate membership as a rule. Individual nurse members of non-qualified associations could attend meetings as visitors or fraternal delegates. No doubt Mrs. Fenwick's earlier experiences with mixed groups influenced these decisions and accentuated the determination of these professional women to manage their own affairs and to set their own standards.

Though the ICN insisted on the principle of self-government by duly qualified trained nurses, it did not impose any uniform pattern of organization on national associations. Its policy was to foster individuality and to encourage the application of broad principles in the manner best suited to the conditions and needs of the country and its stage of nursing development. Thus its national members represent many different patterns of organization, some being federations of a large number of smaller groups, such as alumnae, and others being much more homogeneous and better integrated.

The Council from its inception associated itself closely with the women's movement, stressed the duties of nurses as citizens, and passed resolutions supporting the enfranchisement of women. It took a firm stand on religious and racial discrimination and welcomed qualified nurses of all creeds and colors. Such social questions as the tabooed subject of venereal disease were openly discussed in its meetings, and its members did not hesitate to speak out on other controversial issues. For example, it opposed totalitarian tendencies—political, economic, and religious—which in certain countries made it almost impossible for nurses' organizations to maintain their own identity and independence. After its experiences with Nazi, Fascist, and Communist forces in World War II, the ICN decided (1947) that membership should be open only to self-governing associations that were nonpolitical and nonsectarian in character. These are only a few examples of the strong convictions and courageous spirit of those who built up this organization and established its traditions.

Before 1923 there was no paid secretary or official headquarters for the International Council of Nurses.[2] Christianne Reimann of Denmark was the first fulltime executive secretary and the first ICN office was set up in Geneva. During the following years it was moved to London, then (for the war period) to New Haven and New York, and then back to London. Here the executive secretary and her staff of fulltime assistants carry on a wide variety of activities which include the operations of an information bureau and a clearing house of professional information. They answer innumerable inquiries coming from active members, and associate representatives working toward full membership and from student groups. Inquiries come also from governments and diplomatic departments and from a long list of international organizations with which the ICN is affiliated. Among these are the World Health Organization of the United Nations, the League of Red Cross Societies, and other international associations representing medical, hospital, and similar groups. Since 1950 the ICN has taken over from the International Refugee Organization for Displaced Persons, its responsibility for keeping a register of its nurses, and the placement of these nurses. Further, it prepares and issues a wide variety of publications, including the *International Nursing Review*, the proceedings and reports of ICN congresses, and special studies by its committees and staff.

The planning of the ICN congresses in cooperation with the hostess countries is an important activity of the headquarters staff. These congresses have been held as a rule at four-year intervals (except during the two World Wars). The admission of new members is always a dramatic and stirring occasion, often

---

[2] Lavinia L. Dock's exceptional contribution as the first secretary has been noted on pp. 171-172.

attended by royalty, foreign ambassadors, and other distinguished guests. National flags, costumes, and music add color and interest to the proceedings. The regular sessions, though less colorful, give an impressive evidence of the unity and common problems of nurses the world over. The chart (pp. 468-469) summarizes some important facts about these ICN congresses, including the names of ICN presidents and executive secretaries who have given much of their lives to this work. The wide influence and prestige of this organization is due in large measure to these officers. Those who have shared in the work of its committees can testify to the interest and value of such an experience. Though the staff now carries on a large share of the ICN's work, voluntary assistants are still needed and contribute much to the Council's total program.

Since 1957 the International Student Nurses Unit has provided for membership of national student groups from countries having membership in the ICN. This makes it possible for students to attend meetings of the ICN and to share in many of its privileges. Those who may be traveling in Britain are also welcome visitors at the London headquarters, where they get an impressive picture of the wide range of activities carried on there by the international staff. In addition to written advice and help to national organizations wishing to qualify for memberships, the ICN has done much to help such groups by inviting their officers to ICN meetings where they come into direct touch with experienced leaders and are encouraged to take the first steps toward membership.

In her brief address at the Fiftieth Anniversary meeting in Stockholm, in 1949, the ICN secretary, Daisy Bridges, summarized the outstanding events in its history, winding up with an answer to her own question, "What then is outstanding in all this record?"

> Surely that our Council was founded in a century when professional work for women and organization for such work was all but unknown; that it has earned and retained the support and loyalty of nurses the world over; that it has survived two World Wars and built up bonds of friendship and fellowship which neither wars nor the repercussions of wars can sever;

SUMMARY OF MEETINGS OF THE
Prepared by

CON-GRESSES	DATE	PLACE	COUNTRIES REPRESENTED	MEMBERS PRESENT	WATCH-WORD	PRESIDENT
I	1901	Buffalo, U.S.A.		2000	*Work*	Mrs. Bedford Fenwick, England
II	1904	Berlin, Germany	9	95	*Courage*	Mrs. Bedford Fenwick, England
Interim	1907	Paris, France	15	3–400		Miss S. B. Gahey, Australasia
III	1909	London, England		5–600	*Life*	Mrs. Bedford Fenwick, England
IV	1912	Cologne, Germany	23		*Aspiration*	Sr. Agnes Karll, Germany
	1915	San Francisco, U.S.A.		Bd. of Directors		Annie Goodrich, U.S.A.
Interim	1922	Copenhagen, Denmark	10			Mrs. Henny Tscherning, Denmark
V	1925	Helsinki, Finland	33	1049	*Peace*	Baroness Sophie Mannerheim, Finland
Interim	1927	Geneva, Switzerland	34	700		Nina Gage, China
VI	1929	Montreal, Canada	36	6213	*Service*	Nina Gage, China
VII	1933	Paris, France Brussels, Belgium	42	2284	*Concordia*	**Mlle Leonie Chaptal, France**
VIII	1937	London, England	43	3362	*Loyalty*	Dame Alicia Lloyd-Still, England
IX	1947	Atlantic City, U.S.A.	40	6700	*Faith*	Effie J. Taylor, U.S.A.
Interim	1949	Stockholm, Sweden	41	4000		Gerda Hojer, Sweden
X	1953	Petropolis, Brazil	25	1300	*Responsibility*	Gerda Hojer, Sweden
XI	1957	Rome, Italy	57	3140	*Wisdom*	Mlle Marie Bihet, Belgium
XII	1961	Melbourne, Australia	31	1300	*Inquiry*	Agnes Ohlson, U.S.A. Mlle Alice Clamageran, France (Pres. Elect)

INTERNATIONAL COUNCIL OF NURSES
Hazel A. Goff

SECRETARY	TREASURER	HEADQUARTERS	OFFICIAL ORGANS AND EDITORS
Lavinia Dock, U.S.A.	Mary A. Snively, Canada	London, England	*British Journal of Nursing* and *The American Journal of Nursing* served as the official organs.
	Margaret Breay, England		
Christiane Reimann, Denmark			*1923—ICN Newsletter*
1925: First paid secretary Christiane Reimann	Dame Ellen Musson, England	Geneva, Switzerland	*1926—ICN Bulletin* Christiane Reimann (Ed.) (Published in English, French and German)
			1930—ICN Bulletin became *International Nursing Review* Christiane Reimann (Ed.)
1934: Anna Schwartzenberg, Austria		London, England	*1934—*Anna Schwartzenberg (Ed.)
1939: Calista Banworth, U.S.A. 1943: Anna Schwartzenberg, Austria		1939: New Haven, U.S.A. 1944: New York, U.S.A.	*1939—*Publication Suspended *1944—*Publication Resumed
1948: Daisy C. Bridges, England	G. E. Davies, England	1947: London, England	*1948—*Daisy C. Bridges, (Ed.)
			Susan King Hall (Ed.)
	Marjorie Marriott, England		Marjorie L. Wenger (Ed.)
Helen Nussbaum, Switzerland			

and in so doing has become an instrument in the cause of peace and good will; that it has allied itself with great and beneficent self-governing and highly organized professional groups in world deliberations.

THE INTERNATIONAL RED CROSS AND
THE LEAGUE OF RED CROSS SOCIETIES

Before summarizing the history of the Florence Nightingale International Foundation, which is now an integral part of the International Council of Nurses, a brief account should be given of the relations of organized nurses with the Red Cross, which was a partner in this tribute to the founder of modern nursing.

Though Henri Dunant, the Swiss founder of the International Red Cross, got his inspiration from Florence Nightingale's work in the Crimea, he apparently did not know much about her ideas on nursing. In any case, in presenting his plan for the care of the sick and wounded in time of war and disaster, he did not mention women nurses, trained or untrained. Men stretcher bearers and dressers were to serve, and though called volunteers they were in Switzerland recruited from hospitals and paid for their services. However, in most countries that signed the Geneva Convention (after 1864) "voluntary" meant unpaid and as a rule amateur nurses. This led to some confusion and conflict between the two parallel movements. Except in Britain and its dominions, where trained nurses were part of the army and navy services, most national branches of the Red Cross were at first expected to provide voluntary workers.

For fifty years there was no organization in which such policies could be discussed, the only central agency being a self-appointed committee of twenty-five Swiss citizens with headquarters in Geneva. This group acted as guardian of the Geneva Treaties and carried out their specific provisions. During World War I, when civilian populations as well as wounded and imprisoned soldiers became a major problem and when the relationships of trained professional nurses and untrained volunteers were often strained, the need for clarification of these issues was recognized by leaders in all the groups concerned. This led in 1919 to an important meeting in Cannes, France, of delegates from national Red Cross Societies, out of which came the decision to form the League of Red Cross Societies as a voluntary federation of national associations. The member groups had two main purposes—to improve their own services by interchange of information and to provide a channel for mutual help in time of war and disaster. They also decided that much more attention should be paid to continuous community services of various kinds. This was a broader interpretation of the original purposes of the Red Cross, which were the mitigation of suffering, the prevention of disease, and the maintenance of health, such services being as a rule on an emergency basis.

With the organization of the LORCS and the setting up of its large headquarters, first in Paris and later in Geneva, the work of Red Cross Societies, both national and international, was expanded and much was done to strengthen the preparation of nursing personnel—professional and nonprofessional. Member countries include Moslems, who use the term Red Crescent, and one (Iran) whose society is called the Red Lion and Sun. Many of these societies have been inspired and helped to develop their nursing work on a modern basis. In some of the member countries (such as France, Germany, Greece, Norway, Italy, Switzerland, Turkey, and Japan) the Red Cross conducts and supports regular schools for professional nurses, and in several parts of the world it has pioneered in public health nursing by establishing the first demonstration of such training and service. The LORCS also clarified the distinction between trained professional nurses, Red Cross aides, and other auxiliary workers and in general endorsed the standards of basic professional preparation recommended by the International Council of Nurses, distributing through its national societies publications of the ICN dealing with such standards.

The nursing bureau of the League of Red Cross Societies at its headquarters was put under a fully qualified professional nurse, the first appointee being Alice Fitzgerald (U.S.A.). She had much to do with the development of what was called "The

International Course" in London, to which many nurses were sent to round out their preparation for positions under Red Cross Societies of different countries. Since 1940 the Director of the Nursing Bureau has been Yvonne Hentsch, a Swiss professional nurse whose many qualifications include a wide knowledge of languages, national cultures, and nursing systems. Reference has been made in preceding chapters to the influence of this bureau, which keeps in touch with nursing activities and personnel in many countries and does much to interpret to lay workers the newer developments and viewpoints in professional nursing and to maintain contact with such groups through *The Information Bulletin for Red Cross Nurses.* The increasingly cordial relationships between professional nurses and Red Cross volunteers are due in large measure to such influences and to the joint tribute to Florence Nightingale undertaken by the ICN and the LORCS.

THE FLORENCE NIGHTINGALE INTERNATIONAL FOUNDATION

The first suggestion of an international memorial to Florence Nightingale was made shortly after her death in an article in *The Johns Hopkins Nurses Alumnae Journal* (December 1910), written by Adelaide Nutting, then Professor of Nursing Education at Teachers College, New York. In 1912 at the Congress of the International Council of Nurses in Cologne, Germany, Mrs. Fenwick moved and Miss Nutting seconded a motion that a fund be raised for this purpose, and the two were appointed on a committee to study and present such a plan. Among the many suggestions made for the memorial, the one most favored was the endowment of a Chair in Nursing Education in the University of London. It was soon found that the University charter presented legal obstacles, and the matter was dropped until after World War I when ICN activities were almost entirely suspended for nearly ten years.

Meanwhile, quite unrelated to these proposals, the League of

Red Cross Societies started in 1920 the International Public Health Nursing Course in London, referred to in the last section. From King's College the course was transferred to Bedford College for Women (another part of London University), where it became a special unit, distinct from the regular college program. As stated in Chapter 10, the College of Nursing cooperated in providing much of the teaching and field work directly concerned with nursing. Later the program was enlarged to include courses in nursing administration and nursing education, and the work was strengthened by the appointment of a fulltime nurse director, Olive Baggallay. The British Red Cross provided an attractive residence where all students were required to live. Though this was one of the most valued of their educational experiences it limited the number of students to twenty-three yearly. The fixed national quotas and the wide diversity of students' basic preparation also presented difficulties in promoting the scheme.

In the early 1930's when the LORCS found that it could no longer carry on this project, the joint boards decided to sponsor an endowed trust called the Florence Nightingale International Foundation, such trust funds to be used for post-basic education in nursing. National committees composed of representatives of the Red Cross and nurses' organizations proceeded to meet their quotas towards the £200,000 endowment fund and to raise money for national Florence Nightingale scholarships to enable nurses from their countries to participate in the international course. After a careful study, it was decided that the Foundation should become associated with the ICN, with its own director and with a special council to plan its activities. The Council existed from 1949 to 1957. It made and published studies of post-basic and basic programs in nursing. In a second reorganization the Council was replaced by the ICN Education Committee and the income from the trust now goes to support special projects.

Such a living memorial seems especially appropriate for the Founder of modern nursing, who was herself an internationalist far in advance of her time in statistical and other studies and also an educator both of nurses and the public. *A Bio-Bibliography of Florence Nightingale,* referred to earlier, is one of the major studies carried on under the fund and several others on nursing education have been issued.[3]

OFFICIAL INTERNATIONAL HEALTH AGENCIES

Since 1920, when the League of Nations was established, nurses have been associated with various health projects, but the nursing profession was not officially represented until the World Health Organization of the United Nations began its work in 1948. Largely because of the influence of Dr. Thomas Parran, American chairman of the committee that planned WHO, nursing was recognized from the start as an integral part of the new structure. Olive Baggallay, a British nurse and former director of the Florence Nightingale International Foundation, became first chief of the nursing section and Mary Lambie of New Zealand was the first chairman of an Expert Committee on Nursing, a series of which has been organized on special subjects. Nurse specialists who were invited to serve (without pay) also met from time to time to advise on special problems. The International Council of Nurses was one of the first voluntary organizations to be recognized and given consultative status. When six regional offices of WHO were set up in Europe, Africa, East Mediterranean, Southeast Asia, the West Pacific, and the Americas, respectively, each of these had a chief nurse in charge of its nursing section and many other nurses were employed for field projects and other special assignments.

Fortunately for nursing, several officers of WHO, in addition to the first Director General, Dr. Brock Chisholm, came from countries where nurses held responsible positions in government health services and where nursing was recognized as one of the allied health professions. As nurses began to function in committees, conferences, and field services, the attitudes of most

---

[3] Others are: *Post-Basic Nursing Education,* by Yvonne Schroeder and others; *An International List of Advanced Programs in Nursing Education 1951-1952; How to Survey a School of Nursing,* etc. See Bibliography for details.

former opponents changed and nurses themselves had to revise some of their ideas and methods as a result of the new experiences and professional problems. These included not only strange diseases, varying cultural patterns, and diverse governmental policies, but new concepts of health work as defined in the World Health Organization charter.

Even in the few years it has been in existence WHO has had a powerful influence on nursing. It has dramatized the nurse's role as a professional teammate of medicine and public health and has succeeded in persuading many governments to establish divisions of nursing in their health departments. When fully qualified indigenous nurses are not available to put in charge of such divisions, authorities are advised as a rule to employ suitably prepared nurses from other countries on a temporary basis and to delegate to them chief responsibility for the promotion of recruitment and educational programs and for advice and assistance on other matters concerned with nursing. Often regional nurses are selected and sent abroad for further study in order to qualify.

For World Health Day, April 4, 1954, the theme selected was "The Nurse—Pioneer of Health." There were many tributes to world nurses and to the founder of modern nursing whose work in the Crimea a hundred years earlier had started the movement. At that date 140 nurses of twenty-two different nationalities were working on WHO projects in thirty-one countries of the world. But this did not fully represent the contribution that was being made by WHO to world nursing. The World Health Assembly, which is the executive and policy-making body of WHO, seeks the advice of the nurse secretariat and of Expert Committees on Nursing on many important matters having to do with that field of service. These committees make formal recommendations and refer them back to the assembly which may or may not endorse them but does consider them and often takes action supporting the recommendations. The publication of the Expert Committees' reports also brings to the attention of health officers and others who influence nursing policies in different countries the recommendations made and the evidence to support them. Similar publicity is given to regional conferences and seminars on nursing, such as those discussed in preceding chapters dealing with Asia, Africa, and Latin America.[4]

Among other publications of WHO which have had an important influence on the development of world nursing should be mentioned the guide for nursing surveys by member governments, prepared by Margaret Arnstein, Chief of the U. S. Public Health Service Division of Nursing.[5] This has been used also by regional nurse consultants in studying the nursing resources and needs of the member countries in various parts of the world.

Such illustrations, as well as those included in the last few chapters, give a general idea of the way in which WHO functions and the influence it is having on world nursing and world health as well as the reciprocal effect of nurses on WHO. It should be noted that this organization not only initiates and carries out projects but is a directing and coordinating agency in the field of world health and thus greatly extends its scope. The following tribute by Dr. Hyde, Chief of the U. S. Public Health Service's Division of International Health, is quoted from the *WHO Chronicle,* which is published monthly and contains much valuable material on the activities of this organization and of the various agencies that are cooperating with it:

> The job of the World Health Organization is not . . . to stand alone and do the whole job of international health. Rather its job is to mobilize the great forces that are available; to give the lead to us all.
>
> It is doing this. It is increasingly setting the sights for all agencies, pointing up opportunities for social and economic advancement through health improvement. It has brought about jointness of operation in place of what could have been duplication and waste.
>
> In health, it is fair to say that under the leadership of the World Health Organization the various national and international programs have become, in a very real sense, a single,

---

[4] See *Technical Report Series* reports in Bibliography.
[5] Margaret G. Arnstein, *Guide for National Studies in Nursing* (Geneva: WHO, 1953), *WHO Bull.,* Suppl. #7.

unified movement with a common goal and common methods of attaining that goal.[6]

Within the United Nations are several other agencies whose work is closely related to that of the World Health Organization. Chief among them are UNICEF (United Nations International Children's Emergency Fund), which concentrates on the welfare of children and expectant mothers; UNESCO (United Nations Educational, Scientific and Cultural Organization), which is especially active in educational and cultural programs, including campaigns to overcome illiteracy and establish sound systems of education; FAO (Food and Agricultural Organization), which is primarily concerned with questions of food and nutrition and the improvement of agricultural methods; and TAB (Technical Assistance Bureau), a part of the Economic and Social Council which provides technical assistance for some health programs as well as for industrial, agricultural, and other projects.

Another unit of the United Nations Economic and Social Council (ECOSOC) is the Commission on the Status of Women which has done much to secure a better status for women workers in general and has put special emphasis on the rights of women as citizens. The fact that since 1945, sixty-five countries have taken action granting or extending full or limited political rights to women is believed to be largely the result of the active campaign carried on by this commission. The International Council of Nurses secured a place on the Consultative Register of the Economic and Social Council which entitles it on the invitation of the Secretary General to submit resolutions. The first such occasion occurred when attention of the member states was drawn to the importance of ensuring (*a*) wider recognition for the professional status of nursing and (*b*) legal protection for this status, with suggestions that nongovernmental associations cooperate with governments and professional nurses' associations for these purposes. Effie J. Taylor, a former president of the ICN, was the official observer for the Council at that time and was present with other nurses representing WHO and LORCS. Commission members paid tribute to nurses

[6] *Chronicle of the World Health Organization,* June 1954, p. 214.

and stated that to recognize the dignity of this profession meant
a step forward for all women.

INTERNATIONAL HEALTH AGENCIES
OF NATIONAL GOVERNMENTS

Most of the nations represented in the United Nations are
associated in the World Health Organization and contribute
directly to its funds, its pool of medical, sanitary, and nursing
information, and its other professional and technical resources,
including trained personnel. But some national governments
also conduct their own international programs or unite with
other countries in carrying on cooperative programs. Two examples are given here, one being the United States, which has a
variety of such agencies, the oldest being the Pan American
Sanitary Bureau (now called the Pan American Health Organization), an outgrowth of a conference of public health officers
of the Americas that began in 1881. In 1902 this organization
was set up in Washington as a permanent international bureau
with a steadily enlarging program which includes nursing
activities.[7] Around 1950 this became also the regional office of
the World Health Organization for the Western Hemisphere,
and its nursing director, Agnes W. Chagas, then became head of
the expanding nursing division whose work in Latin America
was discussed in Chapter 18.

Great Britain has a longer record of constructive health work
in other countries, its nursing reforms beginning with Florence
Nightingale's efforts to educate colonial officials in nursing,
sanitation and other health matters ("Governess of the Governors of India" was the title given her by her friend Benjamin
Jowett). This led to many health projects for the people of the
British colonies as well as for the military and other personnel
who served in those far countries. In 1940 a separate Colonial
Nursing Service (named later for Queen Elizabeth) was set up
under the able direction of Florence L. Udell. The reports of
this service and of the Medical Department of the Colonial

[7] See *Health Abroad* and other publications listed in Bibliography for details.

Office, of which it is a part, give many impressive examples of the pioneering work of its nurses in many different countries.[8]

In 1945 an important publication was issued (*Report of the Committee for the Training of Nurses for the Colonies*), which reflects the changing policies of the British Government with respect to colonial health services in general as well as those especially concerned with nursing. The emphasis throughout is on the health needs of the populations of these countries and the responsibility of nurses of the Colonial Nursing Service and other agencies, such as missionary societies for the preparation of indigenous nurses for the less responsible posts in their own countries and also for positions of leadership. Equal status with nurses of the mother country is given to those who hold such positions and have similar preparation either in Britain or in their own country. Included also are many points about how to adapt teaching methods and programs to the cultural backgrounds of the people and to conditions that affect nursing service and education.

This report led to plans for additional preparation of nurses of Queen Elizabeth's Colonial Nursing Service, and of others expecting to serve overseas, also to provisions for reciprocal registration and certificate courses for qualified nurses coming from colonial territories. Preceding chapters dealing with Asian, African, and Caribbean countries note the influence of these new policies on the development of nursing, especially in the British territories, and other international health agencies in the World Health Organization and other health projects.

PRIVATE FOUNDATIONS ACTIVE IN WORLD NURSING

This is another group of agencies that has given invaluable support to modern nursing in many parts of the world. The pioneer in this field is the Rockefeller Foundation, chartered in

[8] See B. A. Bennett, *A Guide to Professional Nursing: Nursing, Midwifery, and the Allied Professions* (London: Faber & Faber, 1951), for further information on these and other agencies.

1913 "to promote the well-being of mankind throughout the world." The Rockefeller Foundation's interest in public health has led it to finance several important studies, to endow between 1917 and 1950 more than thirty schools of nursing in different parts of the world, and to grant more than 700 scholarships and fellowships for advanced study to nurses of forty-seven countries. Such contributions are especially noteworthy because they were accompanied by expert advice and help for the schools concerned by nurse members of the Foundation staff who led in this new type of international service and whose influence was widely felt in the countries in which they worked. Such nurse-ambassadors had to have much more than a wide knowledge of their own professional field. Early appointees, such as Elizabeth Crowell and Mary Beard, were not only pathfinders but diplomatic and public relations experts who had to represent their profession often in countries where the popular picture of the nurse was either that of a servant or a religious sister and where medical or church officials considered themselves the final authority on what nurses should do and how they should be selected and trained. The fact that these and other nurse appointees who succeeded them were well supported by the medical and public health members of the Foundation staff was a great help in overcoming such older attitudes. The substantial endowments given to schools of nursing also made it possible to set up good examples of such institutions which made a deep impression, especially at a time when few such schools had funds of their own. It should be noted that much of the interest of the Rockefeller Foundation in nursing and nursing education grew out of the epoch-making study by Josephine Goldmark which it financed, also the report of the influential Winslow committee which preceded it.

Another example of a private agency which has contributed generously and helpfully to many important projects in nursing is the W. K. Kellogg Foundation, established in 1930 by the head of the famous breakfast food company of Battle Creek, Michigan. The original trust fund was dedicated to the health, education, and welfare of mankind. So far the Western Hemisphere has received most of the funds. Nursing is one of the four main divisions concerned with health work, each of which has its own director and advisory committee. Under Mildred L. Tuttle, who has headed this division from the start, the nursing program has expanded rapidly, has aided in many important studies and research projects, has supplemented the funds of nurses' organizations and schools of nursing during the war emergency, and has given liberal scholarships and fellowships to nurses of several countries.

OTHER AGENCIES ACTIVE IN WORLD NURSING

Among the many other agencies which have done valuable pioneering work in introducing modern nursing in many lands, the missionary societies and the individual missionaries have an important place. The names of some of these have been mentioned in preceding chapters, and several interesting biographies and histories are included in the reading list. These publications provide a record of the work of famous missionary nurses and of medical and other colleagues who have supported their efforts. Without the courage and zeal of the missionary group and their supporters, the modern nursing movement would have been unable to gain a foothold in many parts of the world where it is now flourishing. The trend toward closer collaboration between missionaries of different religious groups is a hopeful sign. In many cases, national nurses organizations were formed by missionary nurses belonging to different denominations[9] who gave an excellent example of cooperation in this and other branches of social, educational, and health work. Among these were Sisterhoods and Brotherhoods of different faiths and countries as well as Young Mens and Young Womens Christian Associations and similar groups in Jewish, and other religions.

[9] Eugenia K. Spalding, *Professional Nursing* (Philadelphia: Lippincott, 1959), Chapter 5, includes a more comprehensive and detailed discussion and bibliography of many of these agencies and individuals.

Among the voluntary agencies that have contributed greatly to the advancement of nursing in the world an important place must be given to the other professions in the medical, public health, and hospital group. Though these belong to the same family they do not always agree on specific issues. This, however, has not prevented a great deal of helpful co-operation and support among their members. Another closely related group is that of professional educators. As indicated in Chapter 1 the two professions have a common root in the broader meaning of "nurture." Especially since 1900 when leading educators began to open the doors of higher institutions of learning to graduate and undergraduate nurses, professional educators in many fields have contributed greatly to the progress of nursing. Without such opportunities little progress would have been made in preparing nurses for their widening responsibilities and in opening their eyes to the resources available in many different branches of learning. From the general public also nurses have found many friends who have served on the boards of nursing schools and of a wide variety of service agencies and professional committees. Often they have contributed generously to the funds required for carrying on such work.

In the past half-century a major contribution has been made by foundations and trusts which have not only helped to finance nursing schools, services, survey and publications, but have provided through specially prepared staff members for expert advice on such matters. In many parts of the world, as we have seen, they have been the leaders in introducing modern systems of nursing. While this young profession has received much support and help from these and many other groups, it is scarcely necessary to observe that its own members have played the chief role in the world movement. Without the creative leadership of the Founder and the stalwarts who laid the foundations of the new system in many parts of the globe there could have been no such world-wide movement. This group includes the great body of organized graduate nurses and the students who in recent years have made a substantial contribution through their associations.

SOME EVIDENCES OF NURSING PROGRESS

Though wide variations are found in nursing patterns and relationships and in levels of development the dominant trend has been toward the recognition of nursing as a distinct and separate vocation or profession closely related to medicine and public health but not subordinate to these or other forms of health service.

The widely accepted philosophy of modern nursing, which includes its aims and purposes, its basic ideas, ideals and spirit, though based on the principles laid down by Florence Nightingale has continued to develop with new demands and advancing knowledge and experience.

The professional development of nursing implies not only higher standards of education but membership in nurses organizations that require suitable educational and other qualifications and conformity with codes of ethical conduct approved by the profession as a whole.

Fields of nursing service have multiplied greatly and now put much more emphasis on preventive and health teaching procedures as well as on the social aspects of nursing. Conditions of service have also been improved as a rule, and the groups served have greatly expanded as well as the nursing personnel with their varied titles and kinds of preparation.

The education of nurses, professional and nonprofessional, basic and advanced, now receives much more careful and extended study. Schools of nursing are recognized more and more as educational institutions and nursing education as a branch of professional work that is included in the programs of higher educational institutions.

Nursing organizations have also increased greatly in numbers, in the scope of their activities, and in their influence on public opinion as well as in their value to their members. They are found on various levels including that of student nurses.

Nursing legislation for the control of nursing practice and education, by the registration of nurses, and plans for the accreditation of schools of nursing by national and state bodies or other appropriate agencies, have done much to improve educational standards and qualifications for nursing practice.

Economic conditions in nursing, including the regulation of supply and demand, salaries, pensions, hours, conditions of work, and the like, have been much improved and are increasingly regulated by government, professional, and other agencies that share in the adjustment of such conditions.

Ethical and professional codes which have been formulated and adopted by nurses' organizations, local, national and international, have done much to regulate standards of conduct and relationships with other groups of co-workers and the public, also to improve the morale and esprit de corps of nurses.

Leadership in nursing by individuals and groups has been developed through nurses' organizations and schools and is often greatly strengthened by special preparation and experience in speaking, writing and similar group activities.

The nursing press and publicity in general, including books, journals, radio, television, pamphlets, and other means of publicity, have helped to interpret nursing to the public, to keep the profession abreast of current developments, and issues in nursing, and to supplement other educational agencies in improving nursing standards and practices.

Finally, nursing investigations, surveys, reports, and basic professional scientific, social, and other studies have increased greatly in numbers, have improved in quality, and have provided the profession with a much sounder basis on which to build plans for the future. Advanced courses in research are available for qualified nurses, several of whom have become specialists in their field.

These are only a few of the more tangible evidences of the growth and development of nursing during the last century and of the wide influence which this profession is exerting in the modern world. Members of this profession and those preparing to enter it can be proud of its record.

Though much has been accomplished in nursing it would be a great mistake to assume that all its problems have been solved or that its future is secure. Among the pencilled notes left by a great nursing leader, Adelaide Nutting, are the following: "There can be no final conception of the right education for nurses; it must be a steady evolutionary process—." "All true progress in nursing depends on the creative intelligence, character and capacity of those who make up the profession of nursing . . . who breathe into it the breath of growing healthful life. Here is where we hold the future with all its inspiring potentialities in our hands."

While the future of nursing depends in large measure on nurses, it is becoming much more evident that there are other factors involved. The most important is the world situation which deeply concerns the citizens of all countries and in a special way those who are responsible for medical, nursing and other health services.

In preparing themselves for the future, nurses cannot ignore these issues which center around the conflicts between nationalism and internationalism, between a narrow patriotism and a broad concern for the health, safety, and development of the world's people. Much has been written on these subjects by historians, philosophers, religious writers and others who have delved deeply into these greatest of modern world problems. Quoting a leading historian and teacher who has written extensively on these issues for over 50 years "a great race is now beginning, a race that will be run throughout the next generation or two, between the forces of nationalism and the forces of humanity, toward the respective goals of destruction and salvation." [10] Another well known historian[11] has dramatized the exaggerated efforts given to nationalism and while it is possible to swing too far in the direction of internationalism, this movement is doing much to strengthen the brotherhood of mankind and to develop what has been called the "international mind."

Nurses have had a significant share in this movement. Its great leaders have risen above the intolerance and inhumanity

[10] Hayes, Carlton J. H. *Essays on Nationalism.* New York: Macmillan, 1926. Ch. I, VIII.

[11] Wells, H. G. *Outlines of History.* New York: Macmillan, 1920, Vol. II. Especially Ch. XXXIX, pp. 432-438.

of extreme nationalism and while they have often been militant in fighting abuses they have been fraternal in spirit and international in their aims and outlooks. This applies also to many of their followers. The best hope for the future lies in the broadening of our knowledge about other countries and in closer cooperation and friendship between their peoples. By making fuller use of the best elements in the inheritance of each nation the whole world can advance more rapidly toward peace and progress.[12]

SELECTED BIBLIOGRAPHY

Arnold, Virginia. "We Help Bring Peace," *Nurs. Outlook,* February 1953, 76-78.

Arnstein, Margaret G. *Guide for National Studies in Nursing.* Geneva: World Health Organization, 1953. WHO Bull., Suppl. #7.

"Articles and Studies on the World Health Organization 1946-1957," *Chronicle of the World Health Organization,* December 1958, 427-438.

"Basic Nursing Curriculum," *Nurs. Times,* February 10, 1956, 121. Recommendations of WHO Study Group held in Brussels, November 1955.

Beeby, Nell V. "The World's Nursing Journals," *Int. Nurs. Rev.,* July 1958, 57-67.

Breay, Margaret, and Ethel Gordon Fenwick. *History of the International Council of Nurses.* London: ICN, 1931.

Bridges, Daisy C. "Current Activities of the International Council of Nurses," *Can. Nurse,* April 1951, 287-290.

———. "Outstanding Events in the History of the ICN," *Int. Nurs. Bull.,* Summer 1949, 10-12.

———. "The Reorganization of the Florence Nightingale International Foundation with the ICN," *Int. Nurs. Bull.,* Autumn 1952, 16-17.

———, and Ellen J. Broe. "Nursing's One World," *Am. Jo. Nurs.,* January 1961, 76-78.

Broe, Ellen. "The Educational Division of the International Council of Nurses," *Int. Nurs. Bull.,* Winter 1952, 10-13.

———. "Florence Nightingale International Foundation," *Can. Nurse,* January 1954, 33-36.

Chagas, Agnes W. "The Work of WHO in Latin America," *Am. Jo. Nurs.,* April 1943, 410.

[12] This is the objective of the young organization called the Peace Corps (U.S.A.) which has already demonstrated its success in promoting a better understanding among peoples as well as in carrying out many useful projects in different countries. Among the groups selected and prepared for such services were 42 nurses (March 1962) whose experience will be followed with great interest by their professional friends. The references in the Selected Bibliography following will give a fuller account of this organization.

Chronicle of the World Health Organization. Geneva: WHO. Published monthly.

Creelman, Lyle. "The Relationship Between the World Health Organization and Professional Nursing," *Int. Nurs. Rev.*, April 1954, 35-41.

Dennis, Lawrence E. "The Training of Peace Corps Volunteers," *Higher Ed.*, Vol. XVII, No. 8 (May-June, 1961), 6-10.

———. "The Peace Corps: A New Dimension of Public Service," *Higher Ed.*, Vol. XVII, No. 8 (May-June, 1961), 3-5.

Diniz, Fernanda Alves. "WHO's European Programme in Nursing," *Int. Nurs. Rev.*, April 1958, 17-18.

Ferreira, Manoel. "The Structure, Functions, and Aims of the World Health Organization," *Int. Nurs. Rev.*, April 1954, 27-34.

First Ten Years of the World Health Organization. Geneva: WHO, 1958.

The First Twenty-Five Years The Story of a Foundation. Battle Creek: W. K. Kellogg Foundation, n. d.

"For Better Nursing Services WHO Conference on Nursing Administration," *Int. Nurs. Rev.*, April 1960, 57-59.

Forman, Douglas N., and Edward M. Dodd. "The Nurse in Mission Work," *Am. Jo. Nurs.*, May 1951, 307-308.

Fosdick, Raymond Blaine. *The Story of the Rockefeller Foundation.* New York: Harper, 1952.

Florence Nightingale International Foundation. *An International List of Advanced Programmes in Nursing Education (1951-1952).* London: ICN, 1954.

Hakola, E. A. "European Seminar on the Nurse in the Psychiatric Team," *Int. Nurs. Rev.*, April 1958, 46-48.

How to Survey a School of Nursing. A Suggested Method, Illustrated with Samples of Five Post-Basic Schools. Prepared by the Florence Nightingale International Foundation, 1952-1953. London: ICN, 1954. Report No. II.

"ICN Platform," *Int. Nurs. Rev.*, April 1960, 4.

Information About Positions in the World Health Organization. Geneva: WHO. 227A (Medical)-9/56-2500.

"International Code of Nursing Ethics," "Adopted by the Grand Council of the Int. Coun. of Nurs., São Paulo, Brazil, July 10, 1953, *Int. Nurs. Rev.*, April 1954, 62-63.

"The International Council of Nurses," *Int. Nurs. Rev.*, October 1959, 87.

International Council of Nurses. *The Basic Education of the Professional Nurse.* London: ICN, 3rd ed., 1949. Revision of *The Educational Programme of the School of Nursing.*

———. *Developing Graduate Nurse Education.* London: ICN, 1951.

———. *Exchange of Privileges for Nurses.* London: ICN, 1955.

———. Florence Nightingale International Foundation. *Basic Nursing Education,* Frances Beck. London: ICN, 1958. Report IV.

———. *International Nursing Review.* London: ICN. Published six times a year.

———. *International Nursing Review. Jubilee Issue 1899-1959.* July 1959.

An International List of Advanced Programs in Nursing Education 1951-1952. London: ICN, 1954.

The League of Red Cross Societies and World Humanitarian Problems. Geneva: LORCS, 1956. Mimeographed.

Leahy, Kathleen. "Nursing in the World Health Organization," *Pub. Health Nurs.*, April 1952, 185-186.

McLaughlin, Kathleen. *New Life in Old Lands.* New York: Dodd, Mead, 1955.

"National Nurses Associations with ICN Membership," *Int. Nurs. Rev.*, July/ August 1961, 54-58; "National Associate Representatives," 59. "ICN Standing Committees," 60-62; "New ICN Member Associations," 63-65.

Nurses: Their Education and Their Role in Health Programs. Report of the Technical Discussions at the Ninth World Health Assembly. Reprinted from *Chronicle of the World Health Organization,* July 1956, 207-227.

Odier, Lucie. *Medical Personnel Assigned to the Care of the Wounded and Sick in the Armed Forces.* Geneva: LORCS, 1953.

Organization of the League Secretariat. Geneva: LORCS, 1956.

Report of the International Committee of the Red Cross on the Training, Duties, Status, and Tenure of Enrolment of the Medical Personnel Assigned to the Care of the Wounded and Sick of the Armed Forces. XVIII. Toronto: Int. Conf. of the Red Cross, 1952.

Report on the UN. 1. "Common Sense and the United Nations," by Arthur Larsson, pp. 17-20, 62. 2. "The Trials and Triumphs of UNESCO," by George N. Shuster, pp. 21-22, 63. 3. "The UN's Hidden 85%," by John Tebbel, pp. 23-25. *Sat. Rev.,* Feb. 24, 1962.

Schroeder, Yvonne, and the staff of FNIF and ICN. *Post-Basic Nursing Education,* London: ICN, Vol. I, Report III; Vol. II, Report III; Vol. II, Report IV. 1957.

Staaff, Astrid. "Conditions of Work and Employment of Nurses," *Int. Nurs. Rev.,* October 1959, 18-24.

Stewart, Isabel M. *The Education of Nurses.* New York: Macmillan, 1943. Ch. VII-VIII.

U. S. Dept. of Health, Education, and Welfare in Cooperation with I. S. Foreign Operations Administration. *Health Abroad.* Washington: Govt. Print. Off., 1954.

World Health Organization. *Annual Reports.* Geneva: WHO.

———. "Comparative Health Legislation," *Int. Dig. of Health Legis.,* Vol. 4, No. 4, 1953, 463-489. Also available as *Nursing: A Survey of Recent Legislation.*

———. *Midwives: A Survey of Recent Legislation.* Reprint from *Int. Dig. of Health Legis.,* 1954.

———. Publications. New York: Columbia University Press International Document Service.

———. *Publications of the World Health Organization 1947-1957. A Bibliography.* Geneva: WHO, 1958.

———. *Nursing News.* Geneva: WHO. Published monthly.

"World Health Organization Symposium," *Int. Nurs. Rev.,* April 1958, 8-29.

World Health Organization. *Technical Report Series.* Geneva: WHO, various dates.

> No. 22 (1950). *Expert Committee on Professional and Technical Education of Medical and Auxiliary Personnel. Report of First Session.*
>
> No. 24 (1950). *Expert Committee on Nursing. Report of First Session.*
>
> No. 49 (1952). *Expert Committee on Nursing. Second Report.*
>
> No. 60 (1953). *Working Conference on Nursing Education. Report.*
>
> No. 69 (1953). *Expert Committee on Professional and Technical Education of Medical and Auxiliary Personnel. Second Report.*

No. 91 (1954). *Expert Committee on Nursing. Third Report.*
No. 93 (1955). *Expert Committee on Midwifery Training. First Report.*
No. 105 (1956). *Expert Committee on Psychiatric Nursing. First Report.*
No. 109 (1956). *Expert Committee on Professional and Technical Education of Medical and Auxiliary Personnel. Third Report.*
No. 167 (1959). *Expert Committee on Nursing. Fourth Report. Public Health Nursing.*
No. 199 (1960). *Post-Basic Nursing Education Programmes for Foreign Students. Report of a Conference.*
No. 212 (1961). *The Use and Training of Auxiliary Personnel in Medicine, Nursing, Midwifery, and Sanitation. Ninth Report of the Expert Committee on Professional and Technical Education of Medical and Auxiliary Personnel.*
Zachariah, Sarama. "International Nursing Seminar, Delhi," *Int. Nurs. Rev.,* April 1960, 21-24.

General Bibliography

IN ADDITION to the selected bibliography given at the end of each chapter, the following may assist the reader in gaining insight into the significance of the history of nursing: *Bibliographies on Nursing,* Vol. II, "History," pp. 23–63 (1952); *Supplements to the Bibliographies on Nursing,* "History," pp. 15–17 (1954); *Bibliographies on Nursing,* Vol. IV, "History and Developments in Nursing," pp. 31–61 (1957) (New York: National League for Nursing); Mary M. Roberts, *American Nursing: History and Interpretation* (New York: Macmillan, 1954); and Eugenia Kennedy Spalding, *Professional Nursing* (Philadelphia: Lippincott, 6th ed., 1959). Indexes to books and periodical on history and other related subjects, atlases, encyclopedias, dictionaries, and other general reference works are also of value.

1. *General References*

a. Encyclopedias, Compilations, etc.

American Hospital Association. *Cumulative Index to Hospital Literature.* Chicago: American Hospital Association, 1945-1949; 1950-1954; 1955-1959. Index also published annually.

————. *Hospital Periodical Index.* Chicago: American Hospital Association, 1954- . Published annually. Formerly *Index to Current Hospital Literature.*

American Journal of Nursing. *Cumulative Index to the American Journal of Nursing.* New York: American Journal of Nursing Company. Part I, Vol. I-X, October 1900-September 1910; Part II, Vol. XI, October 1910-September

1920; Part III, Vol. XXI-XXX, October 1921-December 1930; Vol. 31-40, January 1931-December 1940; Vol. 41-45, January 1941-December 1945; Vol. 46-50, January 1946-December 1950; Vol. 51-55, January 1951-December 1955; Vol. 56-60, January 1956-December 1960. Index also published annually.

American Journal of Public Health Cumulative Index. Chicago: American Public Health Association, 1911-1945.

American Nurses Association. *Facts About Nursing: A Statistical Summary.* New York: American Nurses Association. Published annually.

Annals of Medical History Index. New York: Schuman, 1946. Vol. 1-10, 1917-1918; New Series, Vol. 1-10, 1929-1938; Third Series, Vol. 1-4, 1939-1942.

The Canadian Nurse. Cumulative Index. Vol. 36-40, January 1940-December 1944; Vol. 41-45, January 1945-December 1949; Vol. 46-50, January 1950-December 1954; Vol. 51-55, January 1955-December 1959.

Cumulative Index to the Annual Reports of the National League of Nursing Education. 1894-1939; 1940-1950. New York: National League for Nursing, 1940, 1951.

Current List of Medical Literature. Washington: National Library of Medicine. Published monthly.

Headline Series. New York: Foreign Policy Association. Published bi-monthly.

Nursing Outlook Cumulative Index. 1953-1957; 1958-1962. New York: Nursing Outlook, 1958-1963. Index also published annually.

Nursing Research Cumulative Index. Vol. I-IV, June 1952-February 1956, published in February 1956 number; Vol. 5-8, June 1956-Fall 1959, published in Fall 1959 number. Index published annually in Fall number.

Nursing Times Index. London: Macmillan. Published annually.

Quarterly Cumulative Index Medicus. Compiled by Austin Smith. Chicago: American Medical Association, 1927-

Statesman's Yearbook: Statistical and Historical Annual of the States of the World. Edited by S. H. Steinberg. London: Macmillan. Published annually.

The World Almanac and Book of Facts. New York: World-Telegram. Published annually.

b. General History, Anthropology, and Sociology

Barck, Oscar Theodore, Jr., and Nelson Manfred Blake. *Since 1900: A History of the United States in Our Times.* New York: Macmillan, 1952.

Bernstein, David. *The Philippine Story.* New York: Farrar, Strauss, 1947.

Bernstein, Harry. *Modern and Contemporary Latin America.* Philadelphia: Lippincott, 1952.

Brockelman, Carl. *History of the Islamic Peoples.* New York: Putnam's, 1947.

Brown, G. W. (Ed.) *Canada.* Berkeley: University of California Press, 1950.

Butts, Robert Freeman. *A Cultural History of Western Education.* New York: McGraw-Hill, 2nd ed., 1955.

Childs, Marquis. *Sweden: The Middle Way.* New Haven: Yale University Press, 1947.

Coon, Carlton S. *The Story of Man: From the First Human to Primitive Culture and Beyond.* New York: Knopf, 1955. Esp. Ch. I-IX.

Halecki, Oscar. *Borderlands of Western Civilization.* New York: Ronald, 1952.

Hayes, Carleton J. H., Marshall Whitehead Baldwin, and Charles Woolsey Cole, *History of Europe.* New York: Macmillan, 1956.

Hayes, C. J. H., P. T. Moon, and J. W. Wayland. *World History.* New York: Macmillan, 1955.

Hindus, Maurice. *The Bright Passage.* Garden City, N. Y.: Doubleday, 1947.

Hitti, Philip K. *The Near East in History.* Princeton: Van Nostrand, 1961.

Hovde, B. J. *The Scandinavian Countries 1720-1865. The Rise of the Middle Classes* Ithaca: Cornell University Press, 1948. 2 vols.

Kimble, George H. T. *Tropical Africa.* New York: Twentieth Century Fund, 1960. 2 vols. Vol. II, Ch. 16, 17.

Kroeber, Alfred J. *Anthropology.* New York: Harcourt, Brace, 1948.

La Monte, John L. *The World of the Middle Ages.* New York: Appleton-Century-Crofts, 1949.

McCune, George M. *Korea Today.* Cambridge: Harvard University Press, 1950.

McGuire, Paul. *Australia: Her Heritage, Her Future.* New York: Stokes, 1939.

Montagu, Ashley. *Man: His First Million Years.* Cleveland: World, 1957.

Paton, Alan. *South Africa Today.* New York: Public Affairs Pamphlets, 1951.

Proudfoot, Mary. *Britain and the U. S. A. in the Caribbean.* New York: Praeger, 1954.

Rostovtzeff, M. *A History of the Ancient World.* Oxford: Clarendon Press, 1926-1938. 2 vols.

[Royal Institute of International Affairs]. *The Middle East.* London & New York: RIIA, 1950.

Schurz, William Lytle. *Latin America. A Descriptive Story.* New York: Dutton, 1941. Part VII.

Strakhovsky, L. (Ed.) *A Handbook of Slavic Studies.* Cambridge: Harvard University Press, 1949.

Thorndike, Lynn. *A Short History of Civilization.* New York: Appleton-Century-Crofts, 2nd ed., 1948. Esp. Part I.

Vinacke, Harold M. *A History of the Far East in Modern Times.* New York: Appleton-Century-Crofts, 1950.

c. Science, Medicine, Hospitals and Public Health

Allard, Rev. Mother. "The Beginnings of the Hôtel-Dieu of Montreal—1642," *Hospital Progress,* September 1940, 291-294.

Bachmeyer, Arthur C., and Gerhard Hartman. *Hospital Trends and Developments 1940-1946.* Cambridge: Harvard University Press, 1948.

Carlisle, R. *An Account of Bellevue Hospital.* New York: Society of the Alumni of Bellevue Hospital. 1893.

Clendening, Logan (Ed.) *Source Book for Medical History.* New York: Hoeber, 1942.

Corcoran, A. C. *A Mirror Up To Medicine.* Philadelphia: Lippincott, 1961.

Corlett, William Thomas. *The Medicine Man of the American Indian and His Cultural Background.* Springfield, Ill.: Charles C. Thomas, 1935.

Croskey, John Welsh. *History of Blockley.* Philadelphia: Davis, 1929.

Deutsch, Albert. *The Mentally Ill in America.* New York: Columbia University Press, 2nd ed., 1946.

Faxon, Nathaniel W. (Ed.) *The Hospital in Contemporary Life.* Cambridge: Harvard University Press, 1949.

Guthrie, Douglas. *A History of Medicine.* Philadelphia: Lippincott, 1948.

Hanlon, John J. *Principles of Public Health Administration.* St. Louis: Mosby, 2nd ed., 1955. Esp. Ch. 2, 29, 30, 31.

Heaton, Claude Edwin. "Medicine in New Amsterdam," *Bull. Hist. Med.,* February 1941, 125-143.

———. "Medicine in New York During the English Colonial Period 1664-1776," *Bull. Hist. Med.,* January 1945, 9-37.

Howell, William Boyman. "L'Hôtel-Dieu de Quebec," *Ann. Med. Hist.,* September 1954, 396-409.

Hume, Edgar Erskine. "The Oldest Hospital in America," *Med. Life,* September 1957, 317-330.

Lamb, Albert R. *Presbyterian Hospital and the Columbia Presbyterian Medical Center 1868-1943.* New York: Columbia University Press, 1955.

Marshall, Helen E. *Dorothea Dix, Forgotten Samaritan.* Chapel Hill: University of North Carolina Press, 1937.

Muirhead, Arnold M., and Leona Baumgartner. "The Life and Works of John Howard: An Introduction," *Bull. Hist. Med.,* May 1939, 489-534; June 1939, 595-625.

Myers, Grace Whitney. *History of the Massachusetts General Hospital June 1872 to December 1900.* Boston: Griffiths-Stillings, 1929.

Nasitir, A. P. "Royal Hospitals in Colonial Spanish America," *Ann. Med. Hist.,* November 1942, 481-503.

O'Connor, Stella. "Charity Hospital of Louisiana at New Orleans, 1736-1941," *La. Hist. Quart.,* January 1948, 1-109.

Packard, Francis R. *Some Account of the Pennsylvania Hospital from 1751 to 1938.* Philadelphia: Engle Press, 1938.

Parsons, Frederick Gymer. *History of St. Thomas's Hospital.* London: Methuen, 1932-1936. 3 vols.

Petry, Lucile. "One Hundred Fifty Years of Service," *Am. Jo. Nurs.,* July 1948, 434-435.

Saint-Marc, Rev. Mother. "The Beginnings of the Hôtel-Dieu of Quebec—1639," *Hosp. Prog.,* September 1940, 287-290.

Shryock, Richard Harrison. *National Tuberculosis Association 1904-1954: A Study of the Voluntary Health Movement in the United States.* New York: N.T.A., 1957.

Sigerist, Henry E. *History of Medicine.* New York: Oxford University Press, 1951, 1961. Vol. I and II.

Slaughter, Frank Gill. *Immortal Magyar: Semmelweis Conqueror of Childbed Fever.* New York: Schuman, 1950.

Tilton, Eleanor M. *Amiable Autocrat.* New York: Schuman, 1947.

Trevelyan, G. M. *Illustrated English Social History.* New York: Longman's Green, 1949. 4 vols.

d. Religion, Ethics, Charity and Social Reform

Benedictine Monks of St. Augustine's Abbey, Ramsgate, Comp. *Book of Saints.* New York: Macmillan, 1947.

Cohen, A. *Everyman's Talmud.* New York: Dutton, 1949.

Dehey, Elinor Tong. *Religious Orders of Women in the United States. Catholic.* Cleveland: n. p., 1930.

Frazer, Sir James George. *The Golden Bough.* New York: Macmillan, 1959. 1 vol. abbreviated edition.

Latourette, K. A. *A History of Christianity.* New York: Harper, 1953.

Lebreton, Jules, and Jacques Seiller. *The History of the Primitive Church.* New York: Macmillan, 1949. 4 vols. Esp. Vol. I. The New Testament. The Old Testament.

Public Affairs Pamphlets. New York: 22 East 38 Street.

e. Women's Work and Status

Beard, Mary. *On Understanding Women.* New York: Longman's Green, 1931.

Camden, Carroll. *The Elizabethan Woman.* Houston: Elsevier Press, 1952. Esp. Ch. II, V.

Dunbar, Janet. *The Early Victorian Woman: Some Aspects of Her Life (1837-1857).* London: Harrap, 1953.

Hughes, Muriel Joy. *Women Healers in Medieval Life.* New York: Kings Crown Press, 1943.

Langdon-Davies, J. *A Short History of Women.* New York: Viking Press, 1927.

Mead, Kate Campbell (Hurd). *A History of Women in Medicine.* Middletown, Conn.: Haddam Press, 1938.

Putnam, Emily James. *The Lady.* New York: Putnam's, 1933.

f. Nursing

Austin, Anne L. *History of Nursing Source Book.* New York: Putnam's, 1957.

Dolan, Josephine A. *Goodnow's History of Nursing.* Philadelphia: Saunders, 10th ed., 1959.

Frank, Sister Charles Marie. *The Historical Development of Nursing.* Philadelphia: Saunders, 1953.

Gibbon, John Murray, and Mary S. Mathewson, *Three Centuries of Canadian Nursing.* Toronto: Macmillan, 1947.

Hampton, Isabel A., and others. *Nursing of the Sick 1893.* New York: McGraw-Hill, 1949.

Jamieson, Elizabeth Marion, Mary Sewall, and Lucille S. Gjertson. *Trends in Nursing History.* Philadelphia: Saunders, 5th ed., 1959.

Jensen, Deborah M. *History and Trends of Professional Nursing.* St. Louis: Mosby, 4th ed., 1959.

Nutting, M. Adelaide, and Lavinia L. Dock. *A History of Nursing.* New York: Putnam's, 1907-1912. 4 vols.

Pavey, Agnes E. *The Story of the Growth of Nursing as an Art, a Vocation, and a Profession.* London: Faber & Faber, 5th ed., 1959.

Sellew, Gladys, and Sister M. Ethelreda Ebel. *A History of Nursing and Its Current Status.* St. Louis: Mosby, 3rd ed., 1956.

Seymer, Lucy Ridgely. *A General History of Nursing.* New York: Macmillan, 4th ed., 1958.

Shryock, Richard H. *The History of Nursing. An Interpretation of the Social and Medical Factors Involved.* Philadelphia: Saunders, 1959.

Stewart, Isabel Maitland. *The Education of Nurses.* New York: Macmillan, 1943.

Woolsey, Abby Howland. *A Century of Nursing.* New York: Putnam's, 1950.

Index

Abelard, Peter, 73
Abendroth, Erna von, 309
Aberdeen, Lady Ishbel, 243
Abruzzi peasants, 32-33
Acceleration of nursing programs, 221
Accreditation of schools of nursing, 224-225, 251-252
Acland, Dr. Henry W., 166
Activity Analysis of Nursing (Johns and Pfefferkorn), 227
Adams, Mildred, 412
Adams Nervine Hospital, 199
Addis Ababa hospitals, 449
Adranvala, T. K., 383
Aegle, 28
Affiliations, 203
Afghanistan, 365, 379-380; fields of nursing, 379; Ministry of Health, 379
Africa, 150, 153, 373, 438-461, 475; Institute of Central African Studies, 452
African Conference on the Development of Nursing Education in Countries South of the Sahara (WHO), 441, 441fn., 459
African Region (WHO), 474
Afrikaners, schools of nursing for, 443
Agatha, Sister Mary, 442
Agnes Karll Verband, 309
Agnes, Roman lady, 52
Alaska, 153, 231
Alaska Nurse, 231
Alcott, Louisa May, 132
Aletrinas, 319
Alexander, Bella G., 443
Alexandria, center of Hippocratic medicine, 47, 59
Alexandria University, 458
Allen, Dr. Horace, 409
Allenby, General Edmund, 370
Alline, Anna, 202, 205
All Saints Sisterhood, 130, 139, 442
Alt, Captain Grace, 406, 407, 411
Alumnae associations, 199
Alvez-Diniz, Fernanda, 337
American Army of Occupation, 394
American Association of Industrial Nurses, 220fn., 226
American Board of Missions, 403
American Bureau for Medical Aid to China, 402
American Colonization Society, 455
American Committee for Devastated France, 330

American Hospital Association (AHA), 208, 220, 229
American Hospital of Beirut, 369
American Indians, 17, 124, 231
American Joint Distribution Committee, 355
American Journal of Nursing, 140, 143, 202, 209, 230
American Journal of Nursing Company, 230
American Korean Foundation, 411
American Medical Association (AMA), 135-136, 228-229
American Nurses Association (ANA), 209, 219, 220fn., 226, 229, 232, 233-234; campaign for state registration, 201-202; code of professional ethics, 227; Co-ordinating Council of . . . and NLN, 226; economic security program, 227-228; membership in ICN, 226
American Nursing (Roberts), 211, 213, 219fn.
American Red Cross (ARC), 197, 204, 220, 231, 335, 356; Nursing Service, 222, 339
American Society of Superintendents of Training Schools for Nurses (Superintendents' Society) (See also National League of Nursing Education), 143, 200, 201, 205, 206, 208, 209, 244
American University of Beirut, 368, 369, 370
American Virgin Islands, 233, 435
American Woman's Hospital (Greece), 339
American Women's College (Turkey), 366, 367
American Women's Zionist Organization, 370
Ana Neri School of Nursing, 420, 421, 422, 423
Ancient world, care of sick in, 12-36
Anderson, Lyda, 366
Anglican Church, 93, 138, 409
Anglican sisterhoods, 130, 138, 442
Anglo-American Commission (Jamaica), 432
Angola (Portuguese West Africa), 449-450; fields of nursing, 450; nursing education, 450
Ankara University School of Nursing, 367
Anne of Bohemia, St., 69
Anne, Queen of England, 323
Antigua Certified Nurses and Midwives Association, 435
Apartheid, 444